Map It Out

Visual Tools for Thinking, Organizing, and Communicating

Elisabeth H. Wiig • Carolyn C. Wilson

Thinking Publications
Eau Claire, Wisconsin

© 2001 by Elisabeth H. Wiig and Carolyn C. Wilson

Elisabeth H. Wiig and Carolyn C. Wilson grant limited rights to individual professionals to reproduce and distribute pages that indicate duplication is permissible. Pages can be used for instruction only and must include Elisabeth H. Wiig and Carolyn C. Wilson's copyright notice. All rights are reserved for pages without the permission-to-reprint notice. No part of these pages may be reproduced in any form, electronic or mechanical, including photocopy, recording, or any information storage and retrieval system, without permission in writing from the authors.

09   08   07   06   05   04   03   02   01   10   9   8   7   6   5   4   3   2

Library of Congress Cataloging-in-Publication Data

Wiig, Elisabeth H., date.
    Map it out : visual tools for thinking, organizing, and communicating / Elisabeth Wiig, Carolyn C. Wilson.
      p. cm.
    Includes bibliographical references (p.).
    ISBN 1-888222-58-1 (pbk.)
    1. Learning disabled children—Education. 2. Communicative disorders in children—Treatment. 3. Speech therapy for children. 4. Critical thinking—Study and teaching. 5. Cognitive maps (Psychology) I. Wilson, Carolyn C., date II. Title.
LC4704 .W56 2000
302.2'071—dc21   00-060739

Printed in the United States of America
Cover design by Debbie Olson

THINKING PUBLICATIONS®
A Division of McKinley Companies, Inc.

424 Galloway Street • Eau Claire, WI 54703
(715) 832-2488 • FAX (715) 832-9082
Email: custserv@ThinkingPublications.com

COMMUNICATION SOLUTIONS THAT CHANGE LIVES®

To all the children
who contributed through their mapping

Contents

Preface viii

Part I: Introduction 1

Overview 3
Goals 3
Intended Users 4
Background 5
    From Mental Models to Conceptual Maps 5
    Conceptual Maps as Visual Tools 8

How to Use *Map It Out* 12
    Description of Conceptual Map Units 12
    Design and Use of Conceptual Maps 14
    Teaching the Conceptual Map Units with Cognitive Mediation 18
    Constructing Specialized Conceptual Maps 29

Assessing Baselines and Outcomes 31
    Using Completed Work Maps 31
    Using Checklists and Behavioral Ratings 32
    Soliciting Student Comments and Retrospectives 33

Part II: Conceptual Map Units 35

A Quick Guide 37

Section 1: Meaning and Content (Semantics) 39
    Unit 1: Word Meanings 41
    Unit 2: Word Associations 47
    Unit 3: Word Definitions 53
    Unit 4: Comparing and Contrasting Meanings 59
    Unit 5: Making Inferences and Asking *Wh*-Questions 65
    Unit 6: Verbal Analogies 71
    Unit 7: Personification 77

Map It Out

    Unit 8: Metaphors and Similes 83

    Unit 9: Analogical Metaphors 89

    Unit 10: Directional (Orientational) Metaphors 95

    Unit 11: Part-Whole and Whole-Part (Metonymy) Metaphors 101

    Unit 12: Conceptual (Ontological) Metaphors 107

Section 2: Text Comprehension 113

    Unit 13: Interpreting Text Titles 115

    Unit 14: Story Organizer 120

    Unit 15: Themes and Concepts Analysis 125

    Unit 16: Story Pentad 130

    Unit 17: *Who*—Story Analysis 135

    Unit 18: *Where*—Story Analysis 140

    Unit 19: *When*—Story Analysis 145

    Unit 20: *How*—Story Analysis for Causes and Effects .150

    Unit 21: *How*—Story Analysis for Relationship Changes 155

    Unit 22: *Why*—Story Analysis of Reasons and Rationales for Actions 160

    Unit 23: Dynamic Characterization 165

Section 3: Context (Pragmatics) 171

    Unit 24: Dimensions of Verbal Communication 173

    Unit 25: Dimensions of Nonverbal Communication 178

    Unit 26: Controlling Variables for Pragmatics 183

    Unit 27: Decision-Making for Pragmatics 188

    Unit 28: Communication Breakdown and Clarification 193

    Unit 29: Requests for Clarification 198

    Unit 30: Requests for Actions and Favors 203

    Unit 31: Cultural Features of Communication 208

    Unit 32: Pragmatic Characterization 213

    Unit 33: Perspective Taking 218

    Unit 34: Sharing, Borrowing, and Exchanging 223

    Unit 35: Negotiating Terms 228

    Unit 36: Establishing Better Relationships 233

    Unit 37: Developing Trust 238

    Unit 38: Causes for Conflict or Disagreement 243

Unit 39: Ongoing Conflict Resolution 248
Unit 40: Understanding Relationship Changes 253
Unit 41: Preparing for Role-Playing 258

Section 4: School Knowledge/Study Skills 263
Unit 42: Remembering Events 265
Unit 43: Remembering Messages 270
Unit 44: Remembering Directions to Locations 275
Unit 45: Remembering Teacher Instructions 280
Unit 46: Understanding Rules and Regulations 285
Unit 47: Social Hierarchies and Communication 290
Unit 48: School (Organizational) Culture 295
Unit 49: Understanding Cultural Diversity .300
Unit 50: Decision-Making Process for Options 305

Appendices 311

Appendix A: A Classroom Teaching Example 313

Appendix B: A Language Intervention Example 314
Background 314
Baselines for Intervention 314
Intervention Scope and Sequence 316
A Model for Intervention with Conceptual Mapping 316
Postintervention Assessments and Observations 317
Ongoing Behavioral Observations 318
Evidence of Critical Thinking 319
Summary of Observed Benefits 319

Appendix C: Behavioral Observations of Critical Thinking in Context 321

Appendix D: Critical Thinking Guide 323

Bibliography 325

References 327

Preface

> *When playing chess, tactics are for positioning the pieces and strategies are for winning the game. Mental models of chess games provide the link between the two. When communicating, tactics are for positioning yourself and strategies are for interacting with fluency, efficiency, flexibility, and versatility. Mental models of language and communication provide the link between the two.*
>
> —Elisabeth Wiig
> *Adults with Learning Disabilities*

It is now the new millennium and educational and social paradigms have undergone significant changes due to advances in technology, cognitive- and neurosciences, and education. As I listened to conversations and presentations at an international conference for educators in the late '90s, the professional terminology gave me pause. I heard the following words and expressions:

- Creating Knowledge
- Visual Tools
- Cognitive Styles
- Concept Formation
- Knowledge Management
- Intelligent Behaviors

- Mental Models
- Multiple Intelligences
- Learning Styles
- Alternatives
- Creativity

Map It Out focuses on developing an awareness of concepts and mental models that underlie language and communication through the use of visual tools—which we call *conceptual maps*. To understand the intent of our work, it is important for you to get an intuitive feeling of what mental models are and how they are developed. I can best describe the process of developing concepts and mental models by telling a story of true-life events that occurred during my childhood in Denmark.

When I was between 5 and 10 years old, Denmark was occupied by Germany. When the Germans invaded us, they removed wall posters, outdoor signs, and all other evidence of British influence. However, they forgot to remove a Chiquita banana poster that hung on a wall down a side street that I walked by on my way to school. Every morning I stopped in front of the Chiquita banana poster with a couple of my classmates. The group reminisced about what bananas were like: what they tasted like, how you opened them, where they came from, and how they used to be for sale at the greengrocers. Our little morning group attracted more and more kids, and our talks branched out to include memories of other tropical fruits, distant lands, and freedom from German occupation.

Preface

At some point, we must have attracted the attention of the Germans, for one morning we saw that the Chiquita banana poster had been removed and a poster of Hitler had been substituted. At first, we got angry. Then, we complained about the intrusion in our lives to our teachers. When the teachers told us that they could not help and cautioned us to be quiet about it, we became sad and even depressed. At that point, our sensitive classroom teacher brought us all together to talk about the banana poster and why we were so sad. She listened to us explain what we had talked about in front of the poster, and she grasped that the banana had become a symbol to us. She said that it had taught us a lot because we had shared our knowledge about bananas, tropical fruits, and the world at large. She told us that the Chiquita banana poster had become a symbol of freedom for us. It gave us hope that some day real bananas would be back in our stores and that Denmark would be free.

In the parlance of today, our teacher might have said that the banana poster evoked prior knowledge, that the knowledge was shared, that concepts related to fruits and transportation were formed, and that a mental model had been created in each of our minds for the world at large and for Denmark as a free country. She might even have said that such abstract concepts as freedom, liberty, and tyranny had been formed in the process. In other words, she would have commented on the outcomes of our active critical thinking. In a global sense, this personal experience has served as a metaphor and contribution in my professional writings.

The collaboration for this work began when Carolyn Wilson and I faced the fact that in spite of our "ingenuity" as educators, some of our students did not acquire concepts, conceptual understanding, or mental models. We recognized a need for using some sort of visual tools and for going beyond words and into conceptual mapping. As a result, we developed the conceptual maps presented in Part II as visual tools for thinking, organizing, and communicating in a stepwise process.

The first representations were created in a reactive process to meet the learning needs of specific students with specific problems. Later, we proactively developed Master Maps and Work Maps to meet anticipated student needs. We also selected examples of maps completed by students to provide models of the type of responses given by students at specific grade levels. All Master, Completed, and Work Maps in *Map It Out* were field-tested with students, clinicians, and teachers, and the final revisions were based on the constructive input they provided.

Our book *Visual Tools for Language and Communication* was first published in 1998. It has since been updated and revised based on our own experiences and feedback from our colleagues. *Map It Out: Visual Tools for Thinking, Organizing, and Communicating* is the result of this extensive revision and constructive editorial input from Nancy McKinley, Tina Radichel, and the editorial staff at Thinking Publications.

Map It Out

We respectfully acknowledge that this work had its beginnings in past and present work with other collaborators. We are especially grateful for what we learned from Jeannie Evans, Evelyn Freedman, Tom Hutchinson, Janet Lanza, Timothy Larson, Ochan Kusuma-Powell, Wayne Secord, Kathryn Thilman, Erik Wiig, Karl Martin Wiig, Russell Wilson, and Sherrie Wilson. We are thankful to our reviewers—Sandy Ladd, Vicky Lord Larson, Carla Ketter, and Linda Miller—whose contributions have improved the final version of this book. Nancy McKinley and Tina Radichel provided valuable input for this revision; they understood how to pull stored knowledge out of this author's brain and how to translate the conceptual presentations into user-friendly language and accessible formats. We would also like to thank our students for what we learned from them.

Elisabeth H. Wiig, Coauthor

Part I

Introduction

Introduction

Overview

Map It Out: Visual Tools for Thinking, Organizing, and Communicating provides professionals with a comprehensive set of visual tools for effective teaching and language intervention across four major areas: meaning and content (semantics), text comprehension, context (pragmatics), and school knowledge/study skills. The visual tools in this resource—called conceptual maps—integrate critical thinking skills and an awareness of the internal mental models that underlie language and communication.

The conceptual maps can be used with children from 6 years of age through adulthood. They are appropriate for use in therapy settings, resource rooms, or classrooms with individual students, small groups, or large groups. They can also be used for preteaching curriculum content (e.g., concepts, expressions, or themes); complementing lessons designed for listening, reading comprehension, storytelling, and writing; giving mini-lessons to establish communication rules, strategies, or processes; developing units centered around a particular theme (e.g., story analysis); providing individualized or classroom language intervention; or teaching children in the general-education classroom.

Map It Out is divided into two parts:

- Part I: Introduction provides the underlying theories and describes the organization and use of the materials and procedures presented in this book.

- Part II: Conceptual Map Units presents 50 different sets of instructions with three to four conceptual maps each. These materials develop critical thinking skills and competent performance by using targeted language and communication processes and tasks. This part contains four sections of conceptual map units for language intervention: Section 1: Meaning and Content (Semantics), Section 2: Text Comprehension, Section 3: Context (Pragmatics), and Section 4: School Knowledge/Study Skills.

Goals

The conceptual maps in *Map It Out* are designed to promote learning and increase students' capacities to take effective action and perform expertly. *Expert performance* is characterized by automatic, easy, intuitive, and effective responding and decision-making (Wiig, E.H., 1989). Experts follow the rules of communication; they refer to models in their minds and generalize to new, unfamiliar situations, seemingly without conscious effort. Expert performance requires a high level of functioning; therefore, it may not be an attainable goal for many students.

For most students, reaching a level of *competent performance* is a viable goal. Competent performers have difficulty taking action and making decisions as automatically or intuitively as experts. Competent performers still refer to stored models in their minds, but the generalization process to new, unfamiliar situations has to be regulated in a more conscious way (Wiig, E.H., 1989). Thus, they are in a transition to independent performance.

The primary goal of *Map It Out* is to help students reach the level of competent performance with regard to their thinking, organizing, and communicating. Specific goals for intervention are to:

- Augment existing knowledge of rules and conventions for language and communication
- Construct new knowledge of rules and conventions for language and communication
- Facilitate storage of the new knowledge in memory for later reference and use
- Form mental models for independent use in new contexts
- Develop critical thinking skills to integrate old and new knowledge for language and communication

The last specific goal assumes you—the professional using this resource—have knowledge of what constitutes critical thinking skills. If you need more information on this topic, these skills are highlighted in "Teaching the Conceptual Map Units with Cognitive Mediation" (see page 18).

Intended Users

Map It Out is designed to be used by a wide range of professionals. Speech-language pathologists might use the conceptual maps while providing intervention for language or learning disabilities. General educators might use the conceptual maps to complement existing teaching procedures in English, language arts, social studies, and other academic subjects. This resource can be used in counseling, vocational training, and social-skill development programs.

The maps can be incorporated into many intervention formats, such as preteaching, mini-lessons, or thematic units. They are especially useful with small groups of students who have language-learning needs either associated with various disorders or due to linguistic or culturally diverse backgrounds.

To use the conceptual maps effectively, professionals should have a background in teaching general education or special education classes or providing language intervention; be competent users of English—as a first or an acquired language; and be willing to analyze not only students' knowledge and use of the English language, but also their own. Speech-language pathologists should share the conceptual maps with other professionals to support collaboration, strengthen team teaching, and empower general educators in response to inclusion mandates.

Introduction

The conceptual map units in Part II can be used with students from 6 years of age through adulthood. Regardless of age, students can be expected to be at one of four levels of competence (Wiig, E.H., 1989). At the lowest level, Level 1, the student is essentially a beginner at the given task and needs basic training as a foundation for later acquisitions. The focus at this level is on developing awareness of significant meaning features for words, concepts, and expressions and of underlying plans for communicating (e.g., scripts and schema).

At Level 2, the student begins to extend his or her acquired knowledge to pragmatic uses. In other words, the focus is on applying knowledge of meaning features and underlying patterns and plans to academic and true-life contexts and uses.

At Level 3, the student has acquired knowledge and extended it to new communication contexts (e.g., talking to a close relative) and media (e.g., telephoning and writing). The focus is on guiding the student to generalize the acquired knowledge to increasingly more complex tasks (e.g., interviewing for a job) or higher levels of abstraction (e.g., figurative uses). Level 3 is equivalent to competent performance (see "Goals" pages 3–4).

At the highest level, Level 4, the student has learned to extend knowledge to complex tools (e.g., organizing and planning an event). The focus is on providing opportunities for self-directed training to foster spontaneous and independent application of the knowledge. Level 4 equates to expert performance (see "Goals" page 3).

The conceptual maps in this resource can be used to complement and augment teaching and intervention at each stage in this levels-of-competence model. For basic training (Level 1), follow the procedures suggested for using each conceptual map unit. As students progress, provide opportunities for extending the acquired knowledge to related texts and contexts (Level 2). At the higher levels of competence (Levels 3 and 4), guide students to complete the maps independently or in collaborative teams.

Background
From Mental Models to Conceptual Maps

In the Preface, Elisabeth Wiig gives a true-life instance of how a group of children in German-occupied Denmark developed mental models from daily discussions of a Chiquita banana poster. Their mental models probably shared common features but took different forms. Some children may have formed images in their minds. Some may have developed concept hierarchies, verbal scripts, or multidimensional diagrams. Some children may have even formed mental models for higher level concepts, such as freedom and tyranny. Still, all of them could talk about bananas even though there were no real bananas to be had.

Map It Out

As human beings, we naturally seek to make order out of the seeming chaos of the external world. We do this by forming *mental models*—structured, internal representations of what we experience or observe. They are abstractions of real-life, teaching, and vicarious experiences in the form of simplified, organized, and dynamic images or maps. They are constructed over time and are constantly modified as a result of new experiences. In other words, mental models are living and growing representations of reality in the mind's eye. Mental models have been defined as internalized, reduced dimension representations of events, encounters, relationships, or problem situations (Wiig, K.M., 1994a). Senge (1990) states, "Mental models are deeply ingrained assumptions, generalizations, or even pictures or images that influence how we understand the world and how we take action" (p. 8). He elaborates on this definition by stating, "Working with mental models starts by turning the mirror inward; learning to unearth our internal pictures of the world, to bring them to the surface and hold them rigorously to scrutiny" (p. 9).

The existence of mental models is generally accepted, although researchers have called the inner representations and the stages of their development by different names (e.g., Bruner, 1973, 1983; Elkind and Flavell, 1969; and Vygotsky, 1986). Gardner (1991) delineates early stages in the development of mental models. Table 1 presents an overview.

Table 1

An Overview of Stages in the Early Development of Mental Models

Stage	Age (in years)	Development
I. Event or Role Structuring	1½–2	Symbolic play acquired; agent, action, and object roles in language recognized
II. Topological Mapping	3	Spatial and temporal relations comprehended and produced
III. Digital Mapping	4	Emergence of ability to number and understand numerical relationships
IV. Notational or Second-Order Symbolization	5–7	Schemes established to remember information; second-order symbols (i.e., symbols for symbol systems) developed
V. Embeddedness	8	Emergence of ability to form higher order, abstract mental systems

Source: Gardner (1991)

The developmental progression outlined by Gardner (1991) supports the position that mental models are abstracted and internalized in a process that is active, relatively slow, hierarchically organized, and dependent on repeated exposures. Theories and investigations of learning and instruction assure us that educators can provide instruction to support the abstraction and internalization of mental models (Bruner, 1973; Costa, 1991; Dansereau and Cross, 1990; De Bono, 1992; Elkind and Flavell, 1969; Feuerstein, 1980; Hyerle, 1996).

Conceptual maps, however, are outside our minds. They may or may not be designed to represent the mental models that reside inside our minds. Conceptual maps are a type of visual tool. Visual tools are used for structuring known information and constructing new knowledge. Visual tools encompass physical representations of events, encounters, relationships, or problem situations (Wiig, K.M., 1994a). Commonly used visual tools in our society include maps, diagrams for statistical data presentation, and the two- or three-dimensional drawings or blueprints used to guide the construction of a house.

There are some features that are especially important in a comparison of mental models and conceptual maps. One is that nobody can ever tap all the knowledge and mental models that reside in an individual's mind. Outsiders can only see the tip of the iceberg; the majority is hidden. Since mental models are tacit, others can only get at the parts of a model that the owner can consciously think about. This means that to probe what mental models people form for a given task, one needs to elicit information from several competent performers, expert performers, or both. This also means that it is difficult to arrive at and design a conceptual map that will fit how every person thinks. Some people will construct concrete or analogical mental models of reality. Others will construct more abstract and often metaphoric mental models. Some may even construct multidimensional visual images in their mental models. The characteristics of mental models and conceptual maps are compared in Table 2 on page 8.

A second important characteristic is that cultural and linguistic factors will influence the construction and use of mental models. In classrooms where students represent a wide cultural and linguistic diversity, there may be several different types of mental models students bring to the classroom. One of the authors had the opportunity to travel to Africa and work with teachers of children from the local African communities. The teachers there believed that their students did not bring mental models to the classroom. After working with the author, however, the teachers learned that their students did bring mental models to the classroom and that those models were primarily visual. Their models were representations for tasks, such as weaving cloth and baskets, painting imaginary and metaphoric representations of animals, and hunting or herding cattle to protect them from wild animals. The task of the classroom teachers became to expand the children's innate abilities and to construct mental models for verbal, symbolic, and academic interactions.

Table 2

A Comparison of Mental Models and Conceptual Maps

Mental Models	Conceptual Maps
• Representations in the mind • Formed in an innate process • Tacit and often not consciously accessible • Simple or complex in representation • Can take the form of visual images • Internalized over the long term • May be a direct analog to real life or metaphoric in representation • Used in a generalization process • Interpretation depends on all prior knowledge (e.g., cultural, linguistic); this introduces diversity	• Representations in physical reality • Designed as visual-graphic representations • Explicit and accessible to self and others • Simple or simplified in structure • Often take the form of diagrams or charts • Formalized in a translation process • May represent concepts, relationships, processes, or sequences • Used in a teaching-learning process • Interpretation and use is initially guided; potential diversities are modified through feedback and teaching

Source: Wiig and Wiig (1996)

A third important point is that just as mental models are dynamic and change with experience, so, too, must conceptual maps be flexible. The maps used for teaching must never become static in the way professionals use them. Instead, professionals must be willing to adapt or modify maps, allowing students to determine where to begin the process of analyzing, categorizing, and forming relationships to complete a conceptual map. For example, the African students had mental models for tasks of daily living and for survival. The challenge for the teachers was to help students see the relationship between those mental models and the mental models needed within academic situations. (This is not unlike the challenges faced by teachers outside of Africa!)

Conceptual Maps as Visual Tools

Conceptual maps are visual representations of ideas that reside in the mind. At the same time, conceptual maps are part of a larger set of visual tools. Visual tools can be used to promote understanding, critical thinking, and strategy development. Visual tools can take many forms. As an example, the most commonly used visual tools for teaching geography are maps, atlases, and globes. These visual tools present an abstraction of physical reality that allows a student to form a mental model of something that is too vast to be explored by physical means. Visual tools can also represent abstractions of mental models or problem-solving processes.

Significant attention has been given to using visual tools in business and education (Glasgow, Narayanan, and Chandrasekaran, 1995; Hyerle, 1996; Senge, 1990; Wiig, K.M., 1994a, 1994b, 1995). With advances in computer technology, organizations have the means to create visual tools. According to Hyerle (1996), visual tools for teaching and learning can be grouped into three categories, based on the interaction between format and function.

1. *Webs* record associations and relations that result from brainstorming. In classrooms, webs are often used to elicit a variety of associations in response to a word, theme, or topic. As an example, the educator may write the word *spring* in an oval on a chalkboard. Students are then asked to say what comes to their minds when they think about spring. The educator records the students' responses, often by categorizing them according to underlying dimensions (e.g., activities, weather, or plant life).

2. *Organizers* provide a structure for eliciting responses, thinking, and problem solving. They often take the form of a table, sometimes with three, four, or five columns. Each column is labeled to indicate the type of information to be entered in it. As an example, a simple organizer for storytelling might have three columns labeled "Beginning," "Middle," and "End." Organizers can also use a block or rubric format, sometimes with four blocks (two-by-two) and sometimes with sixteen blocks (four-by-four). This design is often used when there are different levels associated with a given type of information. As an example, consider a two-by-two block design for charting aspects of early child development. The left set of blocks is labeled "Nutrition" and the right set "Motor Milestones." The two upper blocks are labeled "Infant" and the lower blocks "Toddler."

3. *Process maps* establish relationships between content, ideas, themes, and issues. Process maps can take many different forms; however, they all organize a progressive sequence or process of evolution. As an example, educators in vocational workshops often translate a set of verbal instructions into a stepwise progression with boxes and connectors to indicate the flow of actions (i.e., a flow diagram). Sophisticated process maps can also be used to develop an understanding of how meanings change with each transmission. For example, play Telephone Message and discuss how the message gets altered with each transmission.

Wiig and Wiig (1996), however, categorize visual tools in a somewhat different way. They begin with the assumption that visual tools for thinking, organizing, and communicating must capture and represent aspects of a competent language user's underlying, internalized mental models. These internalized mental models can be translated into one or more types of visual representations—as the authors have done in this book through the use of conceptual maps.

Map It Out

The conceptual maps in *Map It Out* come in seven different formats to serve different functions. Different conceptual map types can be combined and sequenced to form larger teaching units. The categorization system is somewhat more detailed than the one presented above by Hyerle (1996). Wiig and Wiig's (1996) taxonomy closely relates the form and function of the visual tool:

1. *Concept maps* (not to be confused with the general category of conceptual maps) focus on analyzing the meaning features of words, concepts, or expressions. These maps elicit an analysis of four to six dimensions of meaning for a given verbal stimulus. They provide metastructures for developing knowledge of significant dimensions and features. Concept maps can be used for analyzing and constructing meaning for concrete and abstract words, concepts, expressions, and themes and to start the process of creating a broader meaning base. They have a centered oval with four to six surrounding boxes for responses. An example of a concept map is in Unit 1: Word Meanings (see page 43).

2. *Associative maps* are also called *webs* or *semantic nets* and the process of completing them is often referred to as *mind mapping* (Buzan, 1991; Wykoff, 1991). These maps record free associations in response to a given stimulus. They provide a metastructure for eliciting associated responses for words, concepts, or expressions. Associative maps can be used to give insight into the amount of prior knowledge students have about a given verbal stimulus. They have a centered oval with many surrounding boxes for responses. An example of an associative map is in Unit 2: Word Associations (see page 49).

3. *Comparison and contrast maps* vary in design complexity, depending on the number of related words, concepts, or themes the comparisons involve. They provide metastructures for knowledge of shared and nonshared dimensions and features. Comparison and contrast maps are used to identify and record similarities and differences in dimensions and features between two critical components (i.e., words, concepts, expressions, or themes). Each map has two ovals, one box for shared features, and two boxes for different features. An example of a comparison and contrast map is in Unit 4: Comparing and Contrasting Meanings (see page 61).

4. *Underlying-structure maps* represent components of the underlying structure of fixed expressions, such as verbal analogies and metaphors, dialogue, narratives, or other forms of discourse. They show the organization of the unique components of a given task, expected product, or interaction. They provide metastructures for knowledge of the underlying organization. An underlying structure map can help students visualize and internalize the organization as a script or schema. They have a structure identified

with two or more boxes for recording the segments of it. An example of an underlying structure map is in Unit 11: Part-Whole and Whole-Part (Metonymy) Metaphors (see page 103).

5. *Theme maps* analyze oral and written discourse in a format similar to the concept map category. These maps are designed to elicit analysis of categories (e.g., components, dimensions, or aspects) of a single theme or of multiple themes in a text. They provide metastructures for building knowledge about critical details and logical relations and for arriving at multiple interpretations of text. They have a centered oval for the theme with four to six surrounding boxes for responses. They may also include an option to map out secondary themes. An example of a theme map is in Unit 15: Themes and Concepts Analysis (see page 127).

6. *Process and sequence maps* represent segments or components of an evolving process. These maps may show a series of steps for completing, for example, a written paper, lab report, or vocational study assignment. These maps build awareness of and assist in constructing knowledge about steps or stages in an overall procedure. They provide metastructures for procedural knowledge for implementing an action, process, or sequence. They have the process in an oval followed by a sequence of boxes for responses. An example of a process and sequence map is in Unit 27: Decision-Making for Pragmatics (see page 190).

7. *Dynamic relationship maps* represent changing or evolving interactions or relationships. They provide metastructures for knowledge of dynamic and changing interrelations. The purpose is to assist students in seeing relationships, identifying and analyzing sources of change over time, and constructing knowledge about the whole of an interaction or a relationship. A dynamic relationship map usually identifies the early relationship and the conditions before, during, and after the turning point (i.e., the critical action or event that caused the relationship to change). The turning point is identified in the oval, and related boxes are provided for recording outcomes. An example of a dynamic relationship map is in Unit 40: Understanding Relationship Changes (see page 255).

For many students—especially those who have language disabilities, learning disabilities, or both—conceptual maps provide a means of understanding complex relationships that can escape them when described only in words. Using conceptual maps as visual tools in teaching or intervention minimizes the burden on the students' auditory processing and memory abilities because the maps structure thinking and make the critical thinking process a conscious one. The conceptual maps can be referred to while students are engaged in thinking, organizing, and communicating. This allows students with visual memory abilities to store the conceptual maps of their mental models, provided that the maps are not too complex.

How to Use *Map It Out*
Description of Conceptual Map Units

There are 50 conceptual map units in Part II. The units are designed to be used in combination with existing language intervention approaches, procedures, and materials. The conceptual map units are grouped in sections according to four linguistic categories: Meaning and Content (Semantics), Text Comprehension, Context (Pragmatics), and School Knowledge/Study Skills. Within a section, the conceptual map units are grouped and sequenced by presenting tools for developing awareness of underlying dimensions, parameters, and dynamics first, basic tools next, and more advanced conceptual maps and communication functions last. You can select an entire section or just a few related units to teach within a circumscribed category. As an alternative, individual units can be used to teach with a more specific focus, such as for a targeted grade level. Each unit is labeled with a suggested educational level (not to be confused with the levels of competence described on page 5): elementary (grades 1–3), upper elementary (grades 4–6), or secondary (grades 7–12). A number of maps span multiple levels (e.g., upper elementary and secondary). The levels do not appear on the maps so they can be used with older students who may need lower-range maps.

The format of the conceptual map units is intended to support collaborative discussion and planning for language intervention and team teaching in classrooms and is similar across sections. Each unit starts with an introduction that states the suggested educational level(s) and objectives, describes how the conceptual maps can be used in intervention, gives example dialogue for presenting the Work Map to students, and provides suggestions for extended activities. It is important to note that some of the objectives are covered in the extended activities only. The introduction is followed by the conceptual maps: first a Master Map, second one or two Completed Maps, and third a Work Map.

Master Maps

The first map in each unit is called a Master Map. It is a tool for introducing the underlying dimensions, features, processes, or relationships associated with a given concept, expression, or theme.

The Master Maps were designed by a team of speech-language and learning disabilities professionals who examined their individual mental models for a given concept, expression, or theme. After sharing their mental models, the team members worked to develop and design a generic conceptual map that captured the important features of their collective mental models. The team members also used professional resources, such as texts that dealt with normal progressions in language acquisition and presented models for language content and use, to guide the final representations.

The Master Map shows and labels the critical component (i.e., the concept, expression, or theme) and the major dimensions of meaning for the critical component. It also indicates the overall process or application the professional can use as a teaching tool (see pages 14–18 for an expanded discussion of the Master Map). Before using a unit with students, review the Master Map for the organization and labeling of dimensions, features, or relationships and look at the entries in the response boxes. If it would be beneficial, show students the Master Map, and discuss its organization and expected types of entries. In that way, the Master Map serves as an introduction to the later mapping activities.

Use the fact that the Master Maps were developed by a team to illustrate to students that in conceptual mapping, there is no right or wrong—there are only best attempts at capturing the knowledge and models that reside in their minds. This fact should also make it easier for you to consider how to modify existing maps for instruction or intervention (e.g., enlarging them, dividing them into two or more maps with related sections of the original, or combining or sequencing the maps).

Completed Maps

The Completed Maps show representative responses given by individual students or groups of students at various grade levels during mediated conceptual mapping in inclusive classrooms or settings for language intervention. These maps provide an example of how students responded to mapping activities that used a constructive, mediated learning process. See pages 18–29 for a full discussion of teaching with cognitive mediation. The Completed Maps are not to be viewed as final answers; they should be shown to students as illustrative examples only, and the content should be discussed and modified as necessary. The map content is printed in a font that resembles printing to show students that they are examples given by their peers.

The Completed Maps should be used as models for demonstrating the tasks involved. They should be shared and discussed with students before giving group or individual mapping assignments. The Completed Maps can be made into overheads or enlarged to poster size so that students can share them. Guide the students by asking questions, such as:

- *What do you think is important in or about this example of a Completed Map?*
- *What do you think could be added to make the map responses more complete?*
- *Is everything written in an appropriate box or circle?*

Work Maps

The Work Maps are tools for analysis, synthesis, evaluation, and elicitation of responses during mapping tasks. Make copies of Work Maps as needed to complete mapping tasks and activities.

Map It Out

Also use copies of the Work Map to complete extended activities. When working with younger students, it may be helpful to make enlarged copies of the Work Maps. The teaching and learning process should be interactive, multidirectional, iterative (i.e., repetitive), and recursive (i.e., determine steps in a process by an initial event); that is, it should provide "hooks" to access the students' thoughts and ideas for constructing knowledge. Always introduce the Completed Map(s) and walk through their elements before completing a Work Map. The Work Maps, once completed by students, can be used as baseline measures. They can also be used to chart the knowledge acquired by students and to document progress. The use of completed Work Maps for assessment will be discussed in greater detail in "Assessing Baselines and Outcomes" (see page 31).

Design and Use of Conceptual Maps

The overall design of the conceptual maps in *Map It Out* is illustrated in Figure 1. Each component of the map is described in the sections that follow.

Figure 1

Basic Conceptual Map Components

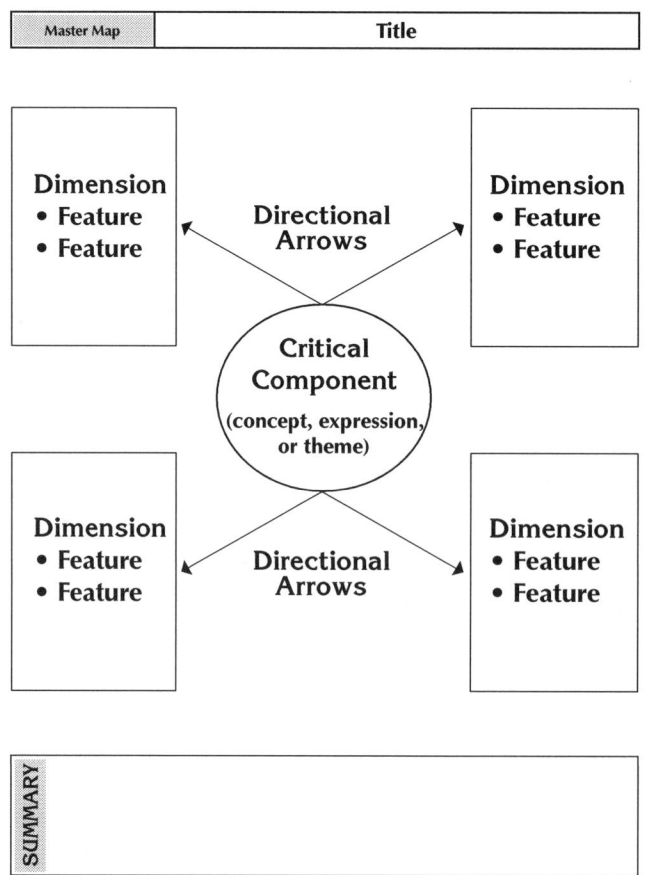

Title

The title on each conceptual map relates to the objectives listed on the introduction page of each unit (see "Description of Conceptual Map Units" page 12).

Critical Component(s)

Critical concepts, expressions, or themes (i.e., the critical components) appear or are entered by the professional in one or more ovals either at the center or top of conceptual maps. If there is more than one critical component, the primary one appears or is entered in the larger oval. This larger oval will also have a darker border. Occasionally there will be two ovals with a dark border. In these cases, both ovals are primary. Secondary components appear or are entered in smaller ovals. Shaded ovals provide further organization to assist the student in the mapping activity. The shading indicates that no written entry is necessary.

When the oval for a critical concept or theme is placed in the center of the map, it indicates that the mapping activity requires analysis and identification of essential dimensions and features. The boxes that surround a centered oval indicate the number of dimensions and features to be identified and provide spaces for recording the features associated with each dimension. You will find examples of this design on the Master Map in Unit 25: Dimensions of Nonverbal Communication (see page 180).

When the oval for the critical concepts is placed at the top of the map, it indicates that the mapping activity requires analysis to identify levels, components, or steps in a process or to compare and contrast items or events. The boxes for the dimensions and features of these levels, components, or steps are arranged with or without arrows. When the response boxes include arrows between them, it means that the order is hierarchical and that one step builds on the previous one and leads to the next (see the Master Map in Unit 39: Ongoing Conflict Resolution, page 250). When the arrows do not exist between boxes, it means that the order in the process is not important (see the Master Map in Unit 7: Personification, page 79).

In some mapping units, it is easy to make students aware of what the critical components are. For example, on the Completed Map in Unit 33: Perspective Taking (see page 221), the concept is a person and it is provided in the center oval. In other units, it is not as easy to spot what the critical components are, so you may need to help students identify and understand them. This is often the case when there are several critical components. You will find an example of this on the Master Map in Unit 42: Remembering Events (see page 267).

Map It Out

Dimensions and Features

The critical component (i.e., concept, expression, or theme) should be broken into dimensions and their features. Thus, the oval(s) for the critical component(s) on a map are associated with the surrounding boxes (i.e., squares or rectangles). Students use these boxes on the Work Maps to write individual features. (For younger students, it helps to make lines in the boxes to write on.)

On the Master Map in Unit 1: Word Meanings (see page 43), the critical component (in this case, a word) is broken down into its dimensions and features. You can teach the process of identifying dimensions and features of the critical component by saying, for example:

Each word can be broken down into separate dimensions of meaning. Consider the word apple. *When I use that word in a sentence, story, or recipe, it calls up many meanings in your minds. The many meanings can be grouped into dimensions. In the case of the word* apple, *the dimensions can refer to the actions associated with it, the functions it can serve in your life, its physical attributes, or other things that come to mind.*

In addition to the boxes, quote bubbles are occasionally used when dimensions or features refer to spoken language or dialogue. On the Master Map in Unit 30: Requests for Actions and Favors (see page 205), the dimensions include different forms of spoken requests, which are expressed in the quote bubbles.

Directional Arrows

The ovals for critical components and the boxes for identifying and analyzing the associated dimensions and features are usually connected by directional arrows. If an arrow points from a critical component oval to a box for an associated dimension, it means that the concept, expression, or theme should be broken down into its significant dimensions and features. If an arrow points toward a critical component oval, it means that the dimensions and features influence the critical component or that it depends on what the dimensions or features are. In other words, an arrow pointing away from an oval indicates an analysis or breaking into dimensions and features, and an arrow pointing toward an oval indicates a synthesis by integrating the dimensions and features into a whole. In addition, some arrows may point in both directions when the relationship is reciprocal (i.e., the two sides or ideas mutually influence each other). Some directional arrows may connect two ovals or two boxes. In that case, similar rules (i.e., pointing away means breaking into parts, pointing toward means synthesis, and pointing both ways means a reciprocal relationship) apply.

The directional arrows are significant in the mapping process. You can teach the significance of the arrows by explaining the process indicated by each arrow on a map as you use it. You can also teach the principles associated with the different directions of the arrows. To explain the purpose of the arrows that point away from a critical component oval, you may say, for example:

When the arrows point away from an oval, it means that the word or concept in the oval must be broken down into its major components and characteristics. So the arrow tells you to analyze the concept, expression, or theme and break it down into the dimensions and features associated with it.

To explain the purpose of arrows that point toward a critical component oval, you might say, for example:

When the arrows point toward an oval, it means that the components and characteristics can vary depending on the situation or relationship. So the central word is influenced by the components and their characteristics. The arrows tell you to identify and pull together the dimensions and features associated with the concept, expression, or theme to construct its meaning.

To explain the purpose of arrows that point both ways, you might say, for example:

When the arrows point in both directions, it means that each part is related to another in some way. The arrows remind you to think about how each idea, person, or strategy influences and is influenced by another.

In general, students in upper-elementary and secondary grades will understand and remember the principles. Students in elementary grades may need to be reminded of the purposes of the arrows for every mapping activity.

Summary

A space for writing definitions, notes, outcomes, or summaries is given in a rectangle at the bottom of each conceptual map. Students often must be taught how to write a definition or a summary. Explain that the elements for a definition or summary can be pulled from what is written in the boxes.

You can use examples from Completed Maps as illustrations for teaching. For instance, the Completed Map in Unit 16: Story Pentad (see page 133) can be presented as you say, for example:

Map It Out

> *Look at the summary the students wrote. Let's take the sentences in the summary apart and find where the words and ideas came from and where they are written in the boxes.*

After this analysis, ask the students to synthesize the information given to come up with a different summary. Cover the summary on the map and say to the student, for example:

> *Look at the information the students gave in the response boxes. Now pull out concepts and ideas you think could be used to write a summary.*

Guide students in the process of synthesis, write the summary, and compare your students' summary with the Completed Map summary for that unit.

Teaching the Conceptual Map Units with Cognitive Mediation

Cognitive mediation is an active and interactive process in which the professional guides students in thinking, organizing, and communicating. It provides dynamic guidance for learners on how to think critically. Without cognitive mediation to foster a critical thinking process, the conceptual maps in Part II are no more useful than regular worksheets for rote learning and practice. The verbal script provided by cognitive mediation brings life to teaching with conceptual maps and transforms the teaching process into conceptual mapping. The conceptual maps provide structure and organization for thinking, organizing, and communicating and act as visual tools for guiding and recording the results of a critical thinking process.

The use of cognitive mediation is supported by recent discoveries in brain research that suggest these discoveries have implications for general education (Caine and Caine, 1991, 1997). They emphasize that teaching for memorization of meaningless facts leads to a downshifting in which learners fail to think creatively or use higher level cognitive processes. Instead, Caine and Caine view learners as active participants. They recognize that concepts are easier to remember than details, that information must be shared in meaningful experiences, and that the end goal is for the learners to construct adaptive mental models. The authors of this book share these views, as reflected in their use of conceptual maps and cognitive mediation during language intervention.

Simply giving students information or answers, without involving them in a problem-solving process, is not enough to support the development of critical thinking. This is because imparted information may not be processed and integrated. Conceptual mapping with cognitive mediation fosters critical thinking and allows learners to construct their own knowledge. They come to own the new knowledge, which in turn empowers them.

In cognitive mediation, the role of the professional is to serve as mediator first and facilitator second while students gain competence in thinking critically. Mediators and facilitators share many characteristics. They both listen actively and without bias, show no judgment of students' contributions, guide the process step by step, keep participants in line and the process flowing, and make sure every contributor is heard. There are, however, essential differences that should be noted. As mediators, professionals need to be knowledgeable about the subject matter and give positive, constructive content contributions. As facilitators, professionals need little or no knowledge about the subject and cannot give content-related contributions, only process-related directives. Mediation is most needed at Levels 1 and 2 of the competence model; facilitation is best used at Levels 3 and 4 (see discussion on page 5).

It should be clear from the distinctions between mediators and facilitators that cognitive mediation is essential in the early stages of acquiring and constructing knowledge in a critical thinking process. The role of facilitator should be limited to contexts in which students already possess the knowledge needed to work with conceptual maps.

Six Principles of Cognitive Mediation

It is impossible to provide an exhaustive list of the behaviors that characterize a good mediator. However, the authors have found the following principles to be especially helpful in supporting a learner-driven mediation process (Wiig, E.H. and Kusuma-Powell, in press).

Principle 1. Guide the student to see, understand, and accept the usefulness of the new knowledge in his or her own life. This stage in the mediation process is intended to develop what has been called *idealistic knowledge*. This type of knowledge can motivate a student, empower him or her, and assist in transferring and generalizing a critical thinking process. An example of developing idealistic knowledge is found in the mapping activities in Unit 37: Developing Trust (see page 238) where students address the concept and features of trusting another person using examples from their own lives. You might start by telling students one or two concrete examples of a relationship with trust and then one without trust (e.g., between educators and students or between students and peers). For example, you might say:

When a teacher or boss trusts you to get an assignment done on time, he or she gives you an assignment and lets you work independently until the job is done. If the teacher or boss doesn't trust you, he or she may stand over your shoulder every moment or ask you about the project everyday.

You may want to give several additional examples that apply directly to your students' lives.

Principle 2: Make thinking explicit by thinking aloud, drawing, diagramming, or webbing. During the mapping activities, it is important to make the thinking process explicit. This can be done by talking about your thinking process (i.e., thinking aloud) while demonstrating how to complete a Work Map. It can also be done by allowing students to express themselves in nonverbal ways (e.g., drawing, gesturing, and diagramming) and in less than standard-form language (e.g., telegraphically). Then put students' thinking into words in a question, paraphrase, or elaboration. Webbing, an established teaching technique in classrooms, can also be used. In that case, write the critical component (i.e., concept, expression, or theme [e.g., spring]) at the center of a page, poster, or chalkboard, and ask students to come up with associations or thoughts. Categorize the contributions by drawing an arrow from the critical component (e.g., spring) to each category mentioned by students (e.g., weather, play, and clothing).

Principle 3: Facilitate responses by identifying a "hook," providing a concrete anchor, and eliciting the student's prior knowledge or experiences. Find a "hook" that will motivate the students. As an example, when using Unit 37: Developing Trust (see page 238) with a teenage student, the hook may be to talk about the trust that often exists between best friends. In that case, the purpose of the activity may be to analyze how an existing trust relationship can be maintained, rather than developed.

Providing a concrete anchor for a mapping activity is similar to yet different from providing a hook. A concrete anchor can be thought of as using a current example from students' lives to provide the basis for later mapping activities. A commonly required area of study in the secondary curriculum may be titled "Ancient Civilization," "Ancient Societies," or "Early Cultures and Civilizations." Whatever the title, most students cannot jump back and imagine what life must have been like in ancient times. They may benefit from exploring concrete examples of different cultural expressions (e.g., arts, music, food, and clothing) as a lead-in or an anchor. They may benefit from a cultural field trip (e.g., walking down a street with multicultural stores and restaurants), videos and films, hearing people from different cultures talk to the group, or asking students from different cultures to talk about their backgrounds. Once the concepts of cultural differences and cultural diversity are understood, a comparison of the concepts of culture and civilization could be guided. With this knowledge as a base, students should be ready to learn about ancient cultures and civilizations, compare them, and contrast the ancient forms with the modern-day representations.

To elicit prior knowledge, use general, open-ended questions or requests, such as:

What do you already know about _____? or *Tell me what you know about _____.*

Follow up by using guided questioning to focus the student's attention on features or specifics that were not mentioned. Examples would be to ask:

Do you know anything else about _____? or *Think a little more about _____ and tell me what else comes to your mind.*

The guided questions can also be made more specific to probe for details by asking, for example:

You told me about _____ (e.g., the parts of a telephone). *Can you tell me something about _____* (e.g., how telephones work)?

Principle 4: Guide the student through the process of completing conceptual maps in active, multidirectional, iterative, and recursive ways. When talking about a Completed Map or demonstrating the use of a Work Map for a unit, be careful not to fall into a rote pattern. It is very easy to work in a linear fashion, moving from left to right or from top to bottom in a rigid way. During conceptual mapping, rote or rigid patterns must be avoided because they limit students' active, creative, and critical involvement. The process of describing a Completed Map and demonstrating or guiding how to complete a Work Map must be flexible. This means that a given Work Map can be completed from any direction and in any pattern. Students should also be encouraged to go back to previous responses in an iterative or recursive fashion. The design of the conceptual maps for a given unit will help encourage structured thinking and provide a framework for organized critical thinking without limiting a creative workflow.

Principle 5: Do not comment on or judge the student's responses or suggestions; the final judgments must occur through peer or self-evaluation. Students should respond to and evaluate their performance in all conceptual mapping activities. The professional's role is to guide thinking and mediate learning. By giving them lead roles and encouraging peer- and self-evaluation of their responses and products, students are empowered. Giving students the lead does not mean that you cannot provide a response or an evaluation. It does mean, however, that such tasks must be kept to a minimum and should occur only when students ask for help.

Principle 6: Continuously question the student using guided questioning techniques and reframe and refine the student's contributions. The questioning process is intended to encourage students to contribute as much as they know to the mapping activity. In guided questioning, start with a general question that is likely to be answered by students. After the first question, focus questions more and more to elicit additional knowledge and information from students. All questions should be open-ended and preferably allow students to give more than one answer. Return to Unit 37: Developing Trust (see page 238) for some illustrative examples. You may begin by asking, for example:

How many people do you know that you feel you can trust? Name some of them.

Then you may want to narrow the questioning and ask, for example:

What are some of the behaviors that made you trust each of these people?

Map It Out

If a student gives an answer that is unclear, seems incomplete, or is off the topic, you should rephrase the initial question, reframe the student's answer, or add refinement to the answer. This can be done by saying, for example:

I asked you how people you trust behave toward you. You answered that they are kind to you. Besides being kind, what do the people you trust do that makes you trust them? While you think about my question, I will give an example of how people I trust behave.

Strategies for Teaching with Cognitive Mediation

Using cognitive mediation while teaching conceptual mapping provides a number of strategies that are effective for students. For example, asking open-ended questions guides the student in thinking about what he or she is saying. Additionally, using a framework for sequencing questions allows the professional to increase the complexity of questions from easiest to hardest. Another strategy involves the process of critical thinking as a goal-oriented approach to problem solving and evaluation of ideas. Finally, using metaphors provides a strategy that offers a creative way for students to engage in the cognitive mediation process at their own level.

Asking Open-Ended Questions

As highlighted in Principle 6 (see page 21), questioning is a major component of cognitive mediation and it is important to evaluate every question before asking it (Costa, 1991). The best questions are open-ended and can be answered with more than one answer. In other words, they can elicit multiple responses to promote divergent thinking. Fortunately, this type of questioning becomes automatic after a few sessions. Open-ended questions usually contain one of the *wh-* words alone (i.e., *who, what, when, where, why,* and *how*) or embedded in phrases (e.g., "In what ways...?" or "What types of...?"). When a question uses a *wh-* word, the tendency is to use a verb that leads to a single answer (e.g., "Who is the main character?"). Because one of the goals of cognitive mediation is to encourage multiple responses and divergent thinking, open-ended questions should be used so that students can give several answers, whenever possible. This requires only a small change in how open-ended questions are asked. Table 3 uses *Little Red Riding Hood* to illustrate how single-answer questions can be changed to elicit multiple answers.

Sequencing Questions

It is helpful to use a framework for sequencing questions in an order from least to most difficult. Costa (1991) reframed and simplified Bloom's (1956) structure for questioning, calling his new framework "The Three-Story House." This metaphor is useful as a guide for questioning students during cognitive mediation. Questions at the three stories are called *input* (level 1), *process* (level 2), and *output* (level 3) questions. Figure 2 on page 24 illustrates Costa's framework applied to a discussion of Mother Teresa.

Table 3

A Comparison of Single- and Multiple-Answer Questions for *Little Red Riding Hood*

Single-Answer Questions	Multiple-Answer Questions
Q. *Where did Little Red Riding Hood go?* A. Her grandmother's house.	Q. *What are some of the places Little Red Riding Hood went on her outing?* A. The woods and her grandmother's house.
Q. *How did Little Red Riding Hood feel when she saw the wolf?* A. Scared.	Q. *How did Little Red Riding Hood feel at different times in the story?* A. Happy to visit her grandmother; scared when she saw the wolf; shocked when she saw the wolf in Grandma's clothes.
Q. *Who shot the wolf?* A. The hunters.	Q. *In what ways was the problem with the wolf solved?* A. Little Red Riding Hood was brave when she saw the wolf in bed; the hunters happened to appear; the hunters shot the wolf.

1. *Input questions* are questions at the first and lowest level. They ask for specific information that was given as part of a story, a text, or a lesson. Input questions essentially ask for facts and details that are important or are used to elaborate on the content. Questions about the input (i.e., the content of the story, text, or lesson) should be asked first in the sequence of questioning.

2. *Process questions* are questions at the second level. They ask for answers that require the students to process the given information. Process questions use verbs such as analyze, compare, and explain. Questions that require cognitive processing should be asked second in the sequence of questions or intermixed with questions at the output level.

3. *Output questions* are questions at the third and highest level. They are framed to elicit inferences, predictions, evaluations, and applications. They use wordings like the following:

    What might…? Evaluate…, What effects…? Predict…, Imagine if…, and *How does this apply…?*

Output questions require the students to apply critical and creative thinking processes.

Map It Out

Figure 2

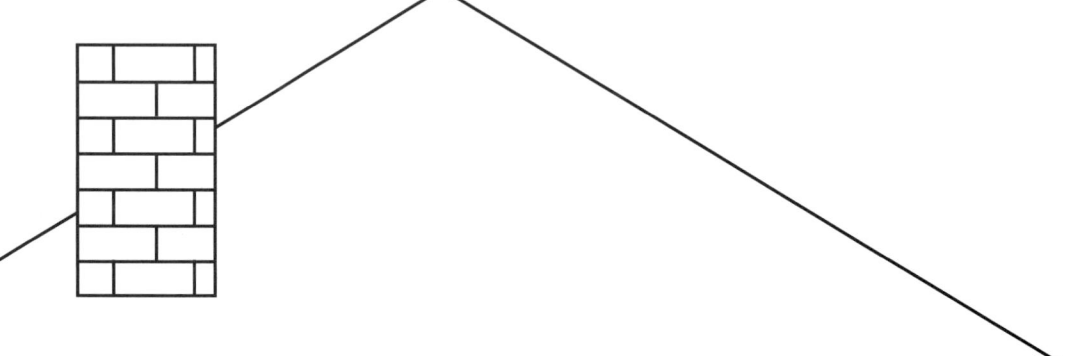

The Three-Story House Framework (Costa 1991) Applied to Mother Teresa

3. Output Questions
- *How might future generations remember and honor Mother Teresa?*
- *Evaluate the impact of Mother Teresa's work in Indian society and in the world.*
- *How do think Mother Teresa would have continued her work if she had lived 10 more years?*
- *Imagine what the lives of the people of India would have been like if Mother Teresa had not been there.*

2. Process Questions
- *Compare Mother Teresa's work to the work of Mahatma Gandhi.*
- *What were some of the reasons for Mother Teresa's choice of work?*
- *What were Mother Teresa's philosophies that supported her work?*
- *Analyze and describe the stages in Mother Teresa's personal development.*
- *Explain why Mother Teresa will be remembered.*

1. Input Questions
- *What roles did Mother Teresa play in Indian society?*
- *What causes did Mother Teresa support?*
- *What were some of Mother Teresa's personal qualities?*
- *What were some characteristics of Mother Teresa's background?*

Fostering Critical Thinking

Critical thinking is a process, not a product. It is an approach to thinking and problem solving that involves evaluation, as well as other cognitive processes. It involves abilities such as formulating inferences, calculating likelihood, setting priorities, and making decisions. Halpern

(1989) uses the term *critical thinking* to describe a thinking process that incorporates goals, has purpose, and employs reason. Empirical evidence shows that critical thinking can be taught (Finke, Ward, and Smith, 1992; Gilhooly, 1988; Halpern, 1989). If the thinking process is analyzed, the components of critical thinking might be considered as illustrated in Figure 3 on page 26. The fact that critical thinking is a process with identifiable components makes it easier to teach the skills involved.

The literature provides specific suggestions for teaching and promoting critical and creative thinking (Finke, Ward, and Smith, 1992). These can be grouped as either avoidance or support strategies; some of the suggestions are general in nature while others are more specific. Teaching behaviors to avoid include (1) having preconceived expectations for conceptual or creative responses, which impose demands for conventional and convergent responding, satisfying the professional rather than the students; (2) making authoritative comments or evaluating student responses instead of maximizing the opportunities for discovery and self-evaluation; and (3) using results from an assessment of individual differences in cognitive styles and creativity as a static profile for the student. The diversity in cognitive styles and creativity among students should be welcomed and opportunities should be given for students to demonstrate their specific strengths and talents.

Conversely, supportive teaching strategies allow you to generate commitment and active involvement from the students, fostering independence, student empowerment, and a sense of ownership. You must provide (1) appropriate, gentle constraints for beginning critical thinking and creative responding; (2) a structure that will allow the reinforcement of multiple responses and divergent thinking to support mental flexibility, diversity, and multiple conceptual or artistic perspectives; (3) an opportunity for internal sources of motivation (e.g., through a talent or an interest) for becoming a critical thinker or creative artist; and (4) an anchor for students' critical thinking efforts in the prevailing academic, social, and cultural environment, whether in a specific subject area (e.g., English) or in an artistic domain (e.g., music). The end goal for teaching with conceptual mapping is to promote understanding and internalization of the critical thinking processes and to facilitate transfer and generalization to abstract, global applications. (An example of using conceptual maps in the classroom is provided in Appendix A.)

Map It Out

Figure 3

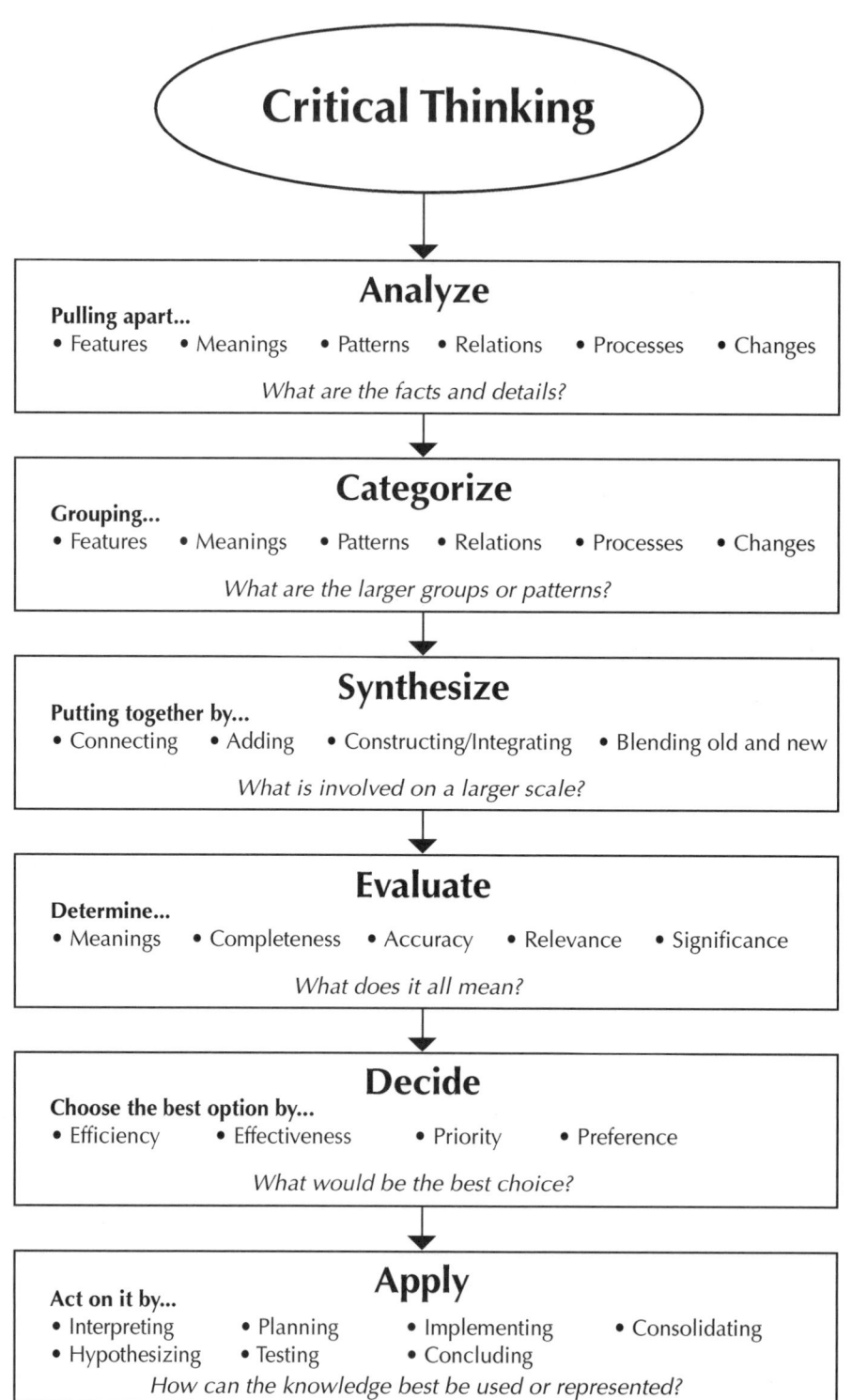

Some Components of Critical Thinking

There are 10 essential principles for teaching critical thinking:

1. Assess and accept individual differences in cognitive styles and creativity.
2. Avoid demands or preconceived expectations for conceptual or creative responses.
3. Provide appropriate constraints during beginning efforts at critical thinking by using, among others, conceptual maps and cognitive mediation.
4. Foster divergent thinking, encourage mental flexibility, and support multiple conceptual perspectives.
5. Minimize authoritative evaluation and maximize discovery and self-evaluation.
6. Identify, activate, and encourage internal sources of motivation.
7. Generate commitment, involvement, independence, ownership, and empowerment.
8. Promote insight in different knowledge domains (e.g., social studies and sciences) and of the critical thinking processes involved.
9. Anchor critical thinking efforts in the prevailing academic, social, and cultural environments.
10. Promote understanding and internalization of the critical thinking processes and facilitate abstract and global applications.

Using Metaphors

While developing *Map It Out*, students' behaviors and responses were observed while they discussed the Completed Maps and performed the mapping tasks given to them. A pattern emerged in student behaviors that revealed what students thought and what behaviors needed to be modified. These patterns are captured in what is termed the *Garden of Knowledge* metaphor. This metaphor provides a way for educators and students to analyze what the student does without being judgmental. Students may require time and repetition to use the Garden of Knowledge metaphor effectively. When they do, however, this strategy can be an extremely valuable tool for language intervention (Lakoff and Johnson, 1980). The following are characteristic Garden of Knowledge behaviors, listed and described in order from least to most favorable:

- *Closing the gate*—Indicates an unwillingness to be taught or let any new knowledge into the garden
- *Fencing the garden*—Tends to say, "I know my territory," or "I know what I know;" or tends to put a fence around what is already known to make it inaccessible

Map It Out

- *A garden of perennials*—Indicates a preference for or tendency to stay with what is already known and to avoid the bother of constructing new knowledge (i.e., replanting)

- *A garden of annuals*—Signals a preference for or tendency to forget what was learned from other conceptual mapping experiences; always wants the excitement of newness

- *Blaming the weather*—Shows a tendency to blame the conceptual map for difficulties in completing a task

- *No more space*—Indicates an unwillingness to consider new ideas or ways of thinking

- *No fancy plants here*—Signals that the conceptual map or concepts in it are too difficult and that preteaching with simpler conceptual maps or concepts may be needed

- *Don't mess with my garden*—Indicates that new concepts, ideas, relations, structures, or representations create confusion or messiness among already existing or familiar ones

- *Wow! What a garden!*—Expresses excitement about what has been organized and discussed

- *Let's get rid of that weed*—Suggests that something does not fit or belong with the map focus (i.e., metaknowledge)

- *Let that rabbit go*—Indicates that an idea will take her or him totally off course (i.e., metaknowledge)

- *What kind of garden next year?*—Suggests that the conceptual map format can be used for a different concept, expression, theme, or context (i.e., metaknowledge)

Introduce the Garden of Knowledge metaphor to students during conceptual mapping. As an example, you might say the following:

Inside ourselves, everyone has a lot of valuable knowledge. Everyone also has some knowledge that is incomplete and needs to be expanded. Think about the knowledge you have as if your mind is a garden. Then think about all the knowledge you have as being made up of plants and flowers that are arranged, planted, and sheltered in different ways. Let's talk a little about what a garden is like and how your knowledge can be compared to plants in a garden.

Then use the garden metaphor in a guided discussion. Afterward, introduce the idea of evaluating one's own knowledge by saying, for example:

Sometimes, what you think is accurate knowledge may be inaccurate. In your garden, incorrect knowledge is like a weed that sometimes needs to be removed. Other times, you may feel that you already know enough and don't want to know any more. In your garden, this feeling is like closing the gate. As we work with conceptual mapping, we will talk about how what you do or how you react is like tending a garden.

An example of using the Garden of Knowledge metaphor in intervention with an individual student is presented in Appendix B.

Constructing Specialized Conceptual Maps

Overview

In the past, visual tools were created primarily by architects, artists, designers, engineers, and scientists. Today, anyone can design visual tools by using computer software programs. The visual tools (i.e., conceptual maps) in this book were originally laid out using the professional version of software called Inspiration (1997). With the increasing number of computers in schools and homes and with the development of software like Inspiration and Microsoft PowerPoint (1998), creating, modifying, and using conceptual maps is becoming accessible and relatively easy for educators and students alike.

No single resource can provide an exhaustive or all-encompassing selection of conceptual maps for language intervention. For this reason, you may want to develop your own conceptual maps to suit your students' particular needs. The process of constructing new conceptual maps begins with "mining your own minds." It requires that you uncover the mental models for language and communication that are hidden in your mind. While you can construct specialized maps on your own, a team process (whether professionals only, students only, or both groups together) in which the elicitation of models is guided and mediated by a leader results in more complete and generic maps.

Design Process

The team process for eliciting mental models and representing them in conceptual maps can be broken down into steps. A summary of these steps is provided in Table 4 on page 30. The first step in the process of eliciting a new conceptual map is to identify, define, and label the task or sequence of activities for which the conceptual map is being developed. It is helpful to begin with a label that captures the purposes of the map and that can later be used as a title. The team will need to give a short description of the purposes and goals they see for the task. The objective statements for each conceptual map unit in this book can be used as models for this activity.

The second step is to specify the underlying cognitive processes demanded by the task. This means that the team must identify if the task requires analysis, synthesis, analogical reasoning, or other reasoning strategies. Identifying the cognitive processes involved will lead

Map It Out

Table 4

Steps, Activities, and Outcomes in Constructing Conceptual Maps

Steps	Activities	Outcomes
1. Identify	• Identify, define, and label the concept, problem, or issue.	• Label or short description
2. Specify (Sequence is interchangeable.)	• Specify the underlying cognitive processes. • Select a map format for representing the processes. • Identify and specify four to six major underlying dimensions. • Delineate the content of each major dimension.	• Specification according to a taxonomy for cognition • Preliminary map design • Identification of major underlying dimensions • Specification of map content
3. Synthesize	• Integrate the identified dimensions, features, or processes.	• Assessment of the new knowledge or meaning
4. Evaluate	• Apply to an example and evaluate to identify needed elaboration.	• Modification, elaboration, and refinement
5. Apply	• Use the developed Master Map in teaching or intervention.	• Judgment of efficacy as a teaching tool

From *Visual Tools for Critical Thinking in Classrooms: Conceptual Mapping and Cognitive Mediation* by E.H. Wiig and O. Kusuma-Powell, in press, Arlington, TX: Schema Press. © 2001 by KRI. Adapted with permission.

directly to selecting an appropriate map format. The team should then try to identify four to six underlying dimensions or parameters of the concept, expression, or theme. Then they can delineate the content or features of each major dimension or parameter. Refer to "Conceptual Maps as Visual Tools" (see pages 8–11) for an overview of how conceptual map formats can be classified and for suggestions to help identify one or more appropriate formats for representing a generic model.

Third, the team leader guides the participants in synthesizing multiple design ideas and opinions through a compare-and-contrast process to make a final decision. If the members of a design team come up with two or more different solutions for designing a conceptual map, each suggested design can be enlarged and posted on a board. The leader may ask some or all of the following types of questions and record the answers to guide the decisions for a consolidated, generic map design:

- *How are the formats you suggested alike?*
- *How are the formats you suggested different?*
- *What are the most essential features of each map?*
- *Do you think those features should be included in a generic map model?*
- *How can the essential features be incorporated into a consolidated map?*
- *What conceptual map formats do you think would best capture the features we have identified?*

The fourth step requires the team to evaluate the knowledge that can be elicited and constructed by using the conceptual map. In a way, this step is the first test of whether the map representation can do what it is intended to do. This step requires the team to evaluate if the conceptual map is complete in terms of the processes and the content. If the map is incomplete, the team will need to elaborate or modify the map content.

The fifth step in the design process is to use the first draft of the generic conceptual map in teaching or intervention and evaluate its performance. Then the team can assess whether the conceptual map will do for the students what it did for them. It is important to listen to all students' comments. If they say that something is missing, elicit what it might be. If they want the design modified, listen to the suggestions and evaluate if the suggestions can or should be incorporated into the map.

Assessing Baselines and Outcomes
Using Completed Work Maps

One method for assessment is to ask students to complete a Work Map independently. This assignment can be given before and after teaching or intervention with conceptual mapping. Before instruction begins, ask students to complete a Work Map for a rather simple task that constitutes the basis for the instruction to follow. For example, students could map the meaning features associated with a grade-level appropriate word (e.g., flower and plant names), theme (e.g., plant life during the seasons of the year), or broader topic (e.g., plant life cycles). The baseline Work Maps can be collected and saved. After teaching or intervention for the theme or topic has been completed, ask each student to complete another Work Map for the same or a related word, theme, or topic that has been taught. A simple comparison of the Work Maps that were completed before and after instruction should show improvements in both the quantity and quality of the features and summaries recorded. The two completed Work Maps can be kept and used as authentic work samples for showing a student's progress.

As cited in *Visual Tools for Critical Thinking in Classrooms* by E.H. Wiig and Kusuma-Powell (in press), a Grade 6 teacher in an inclusive English as a Second Language classroom described the differences between the baseline mapping results and the responses given after teaching with conceptual mapping.

> *The initial exposure of students to the concept of mapping is crucial, if the process is to succeed. This seems particularly true for younger students. Hindsight offers preferred alternatives. In this case, I would have chosen to introduce the mapping activity at the start of the human senses unit as an assessment tool to determine the extent of student prior knowledge on the subject. The comparison to the Work Map at the end of the unit would have provided me with valuable information on the breadth and depth of student learning. I did, however, see remarkable differences between the first student maps on the human senses and the third map on hypothesis. Progress was evident not only in the level of conceptual analysis, but also in the way students approached the activity—with more confidence and authority. My goal is to continue using cognitive mapping and eliciting student responses on the process and have them meta-cogitate on their own thinking patterns and on the value(s) of the process.*

Using Checklists and Behavioral Ratings

Behavioral observations and ratings can provide a second authentic source of information for assessing critical thinking in action. A checklist—*Behavioral Observations of Critical Thinking in Context*—is provided in Appendix C and can be used by professionals to guide their observations of student responses during conceptual mapping and problem solving. The checklist contains five groups of critical thinking components: (1) Analysis, (2) Synthesis, (3) Prediction, (4) Evaluation, and (5) Application. The items are stated in positive terms (e.g., "The student recognizes…") to emphasize identifying strengths and providing teaching support for ameliorating weaknesses.

The checklist items should be rated on a four-point scale. Because the behaviors are stated as positive occurrences, the best rating is Always, indicating that the positive behavior described occurs consistently over time. The second rating is Often, indicating that the positive behavior occurs frequently, but not consistently. The third rating is Sometimes, indicating that the positive behavior occurs only some of the time and infrequently. The least favorable rating is Rarely, indicating that the behavior occurs very infrequently or never. This rating scale is commonly used and has been applied in the Clinical Evaluation of Language Fundamentals–3: Observational Rating Scales (CELF–3 ORS) (Semel, Wiig, E.H., and Secord, 1996).

The observations and ratings of critical thinking behaviors can be judged against variable performance criteria. For a criterion-referenced interpretation, a student's performance level is expressed as the percentage obtained when the ratings in the Always and Often categories are added and a percentage of the total is calculated. For example, if a student's observer rated 20 out of the 27 criteria as Always or Often, the percentage would be 74 percent. This resulting percentage of top ratings can then be judged against variable performance criteria. The percentage of top ratings obtained by a student determines the interpretation of the quality and level of the student's performance. The levels used for interpreting the percentages of top ratings are as follows:

- Level 4: Top ratings between 80 and 100 percent indicate that the student is an independent performer. In other words, the student has acquired a level of competence that makes it possible to use critical thinking spontaneously and to generalize it to other tasks.

- Level 3: Top ratings between 50 and 79 percent indicate that the student is competent but needs classroom or other intervention to become an independent performer. At this level, a transition is in progress and needs to be supported through cognitive mediation and facilitation.

- Level 2: Top ratings between 30 and 49 percent indicate that the student needs team intervention by a speech-language pathologist, learning disabilities specialist, or other professional to improve critical thinking and classroom performance. The student shows considerable weakness and can only apply a critical thinking process when supported by cognitive mediation.

- Level 1: Top ratings between 0 and 29 percent indicate that the student is a beginner and needs intensive team-based intervention to meet his or her educational needs. The student shows a severe weakness in using critical thinking for problem solving, and basic training is required to facilitate progress to the next level of performance.

Students should also be given a method of observing and evaluating their own critical thinking during conceptual mapping and other academic activities. Students who have been taught with a conceptual mapping approach soon learn to discriminate and label stages when they are involved in analysis, synthesis, prediction, evaluation, and application. They have acquired a level of metacognition and metaknowledge that allows them to step back and analyze a task and then evaluate what they need to consider in the process of critical thinking to solve a problem or complete a project. The *Critical Thinking Guide* provided in Appendix D can be used as a template for self-questioning and evaluation as well as for completing steps during cognitive mediation. The *Critical Thinking Guide* can also be given to students in upper-elementary and secondary grades as a template for completing classroom or homework assignments.

Map It Out

Soliciting Student Comments and Retrospectives

Spontaneous or elicited comments from students immediately after completing a conceptual mapping activity or reflections after a period of time can reveal much about the impact of using conceptual mapping for teaching and intervention. During field-testing of the approach in inclusive classrooms in the International School of Tanganyiaka (Africa), teachers asked students for their comments or reflections both before using conceptual maps and after. The teachers recorded and summarized representative student comments. Most comments indicated that the students learned and acquired metaknowledge of their thinking styles; a few comments were not as positive. The following examples of student comments from a Grade 8 science class were collected by E.H. Wiig and Kusuma-Powell (in press); the comments illustrate what a professional can evaluate by asking for spontaneous comments:

Organization and Categorization

- *It helped me organize my ideas.*
- *If I had a test on it, I think the map would help me.*
- *It helped me pull apart and recategorize information from the booklet.*

Clarify Procedures and Focus Thinking

- *The boxes gave detailed instructions, which were easy to follow.*
- *The boxes show you what to do.*
- *By reading the questions in the boxes, we knew what we had to do.*
- *The questions focused our thinking.*
- *I had to think carefully about every box and search for the details in each of them.*

Extend Understanding

- *The different categories helped me learn more than I already knew.*
- *It gave me a better look at adaptations.*

Part to Whole

- *The questions in the boxes made it easy. We only had to think and look closely at the adaptation.*
- *My biggest problem was understanding how the structure and function were related. Doing the map helped me understand.*
- *I had a problem understanding what the benefit and problems would be, but after doing the relationship of the structure and function, I could see very clearly that there would be many problems* [it could be used for] *and benefits.*

Filing student comments using a portfolio system allows for qualitative comparisons to be made over time. As the conceptual maps within *Map It Out* become integrated with the curriculum, students will have many additional opportunities for improving their thinking, organizing, and communicating skills.

Part II

Conceptual Map Units

Conceptual Map Units

A Quick Guide

This quick guide is provided to orient you—the professional who has previous experience using conceptual maps—to the unique features of *Map It Out*. You should also review a few of the conceptual map units to get a sense of their design, implementation, and applications. After doing so, you should feel confident enough to experiment with the conceptual maps; these maps will complement the methods and tools you currently use for teaching, language intervention, or both. In addition, the Bibliography lists more readings and resources to help you get started.

Professional Activities	Student Activities
Prepare Review the lead-in information, the Master Map, and the Completed Map before using them in a session or class.	None
Introduce Guided Mapping Task Introduce, distribute, and discuss the content of the Work Map with students. You may want to use the Master Map as a model when introducing and discussing the Work Map.	**Question and Discuss** Students listen to explanations of concepts, dimensions, or themes. They ask questions and discuss important or unfamiliar aspects.
Illustrate Introduce and lead a discussion of the Completed Map with students.	**Discuss** Students discuss the completed concepts, dimensions, or themes.
Apply Guide students as they complete the Work Map for a unit. Follow up with discussion and independent work (i.e., extended activities).	**Complete Guided Mapping Task** Students complete the Work Map as guided by the professional.
Introduce Independent Mapping Task(s) Introduce additional Work Map tasks (found in the extended activities) as needed to respond to curriculum objectives and reach educational goals.	**Complete Independent Mapping Task(s)** Students complete additional Work Maps independently or in small groups.
Test (Educational Outcomes) Use related Work Map tasks (found in the extended activities) and Appendices C and D for evaluating baselines and progress.	**Complete Test** Students complete a Work Map for a related but unfamiliar task. Students complete the *Critical Thinking Guide* in Appendix D.

Section 1
Meaning and Content
(Semantics)

Unit 1: Word Meanings 41

Unit 2: Word Associations 47

Unit 3: Word Definitions 53

Unit 4: Comparing and Contrasting Meanings 59

Unit 5: Making Inferences and Asking *Wh-*Questions 65

Unit 6: Verbal Analogies 71

Unit 7: Personification 77

Unit 8: Metaphors and Similes..83

Unit 9: Analogical Metaphors 89

Unit 10: Directional (Orientational) Metaphors.............................95

Unit 11: Part-Whole and Whole-Part (Metonymy) Metaphors 101

Unit 12: Conceptual (Ontological) Metaphors 107

Unit 1: Word Meanings

> ### Educational Levels
>
> Elementary through secondary
>
> ### Objectives
>
> (1) Understand meaning features for words, concepts, and expressions by recording word type, category name, actions, uses, features, characteristics, and other aspects as appropriate; and (2) prepare for defining words, comparing and contrasting word meanings, and forming concepts

Completed Maps

For the first map, students in Grade 1 were asked to analyze the word *carrot*. The teacher first wrote the word meanings the students knew in the surrounding boxes. Then the teacher elicited the name of the grammatical class the word *carrot* belonged to. Next the teacher reviewed the students' responses (i.e., their prior knowledge) and elicited additional meanings in a multidirectional, recursive process to facilitate in-depth understanding.

Show the Completed Map to students and say, for example:

> *This map shows how a class took apart the meanings for the word* carrot.
> *Let's talk about what the students said and what the teacher wrote.*

You may want to follow up by asking, for example:

> *What do you think is special about carrots? In what ways are carrots different from other vegetables?*

The second map shows how students in Grade 6 analyzed the concept of fairness. The analysis was triggered by students squabbling over another teacher's apparent unfairness. The teacher elicited and recorded prior knowledge and then expanded and modified meanings to create a more appropriate and complete understanding.

Map It Out

Work Map

Select a word. Show the Work Map to students and say, for example:

This map is empty. Let's talk about this word. Then we'll consider which category and grammatical class it belongs to. Then we'll analyze the word.

Emphasize that a word has many meaning features, is used in a certain way in sentences (e.g., as a noun or a verb), and is one of many examples of a word category (i.e., semantic class).

Extended Activities

1. Ask students to suggest one or more words related to the lesson content to analyze.

2. Ask students to use the word(s) they analyzed in two or more different sentences.

3. Ask students to write a short paragraph about the object or concept that was analyzed.

4. Select two grade-level-appropriate words and help students analyze each word separately for its meaning features. Then compare the two words to identify similarities and differences.

5. Make a game of identifying a word from its meaning. Show a Completed Map with the word (i.e., the main concept) missing. Ask students to tell the word that is missing on the map.

6. Play a word analysis game in which Completed Maps for two or more words are cut up to separate the response boxes. Ask the students to put together the boxes that belong to each word to form a complete map.

Meaning and Content (Semantics)

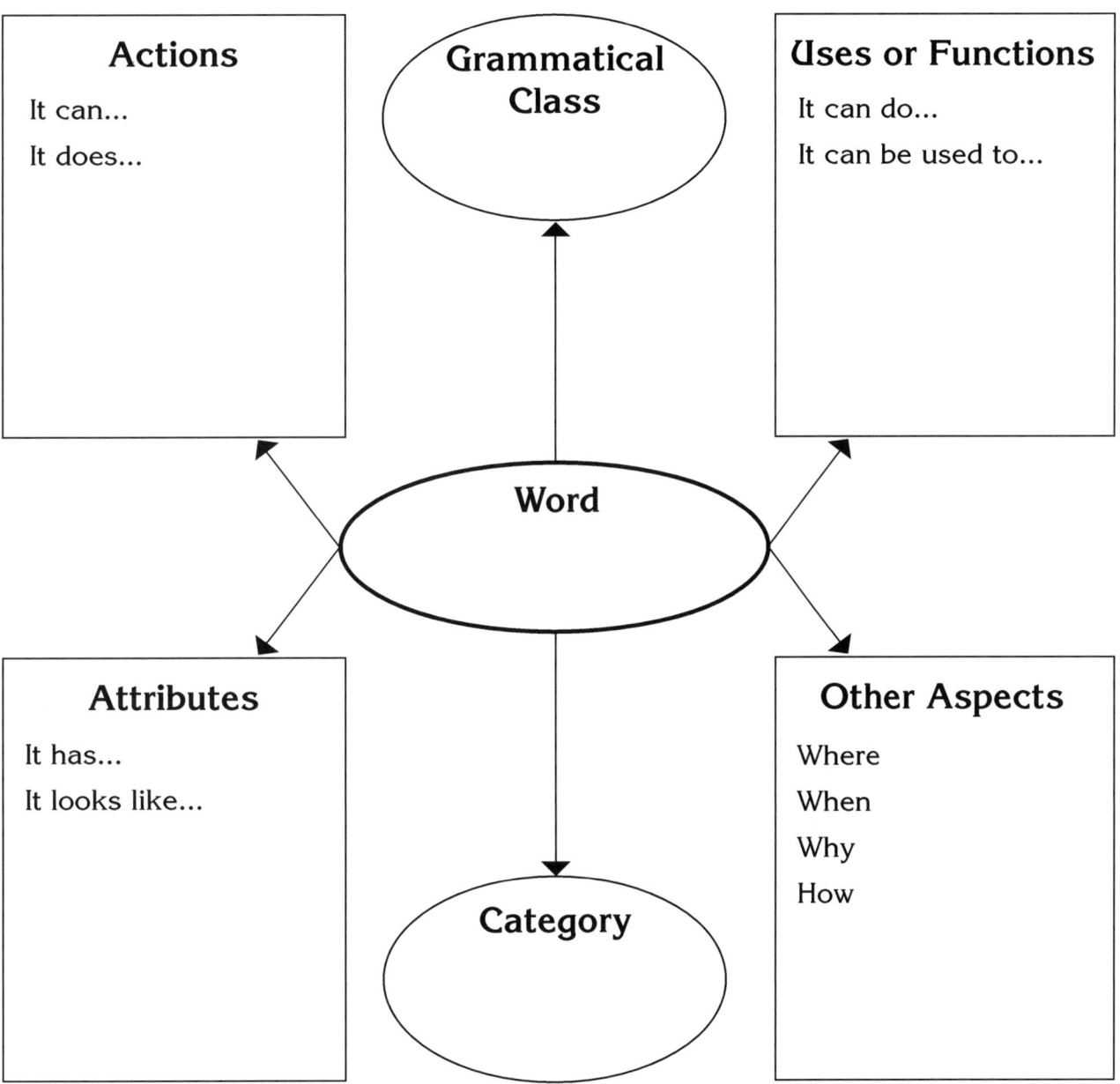

© 2001 by E.H. Wiig and C.C. Wilson
Duplication permitted for educational use only.

43

Map It Out

| Completed Map | Word Meanings |

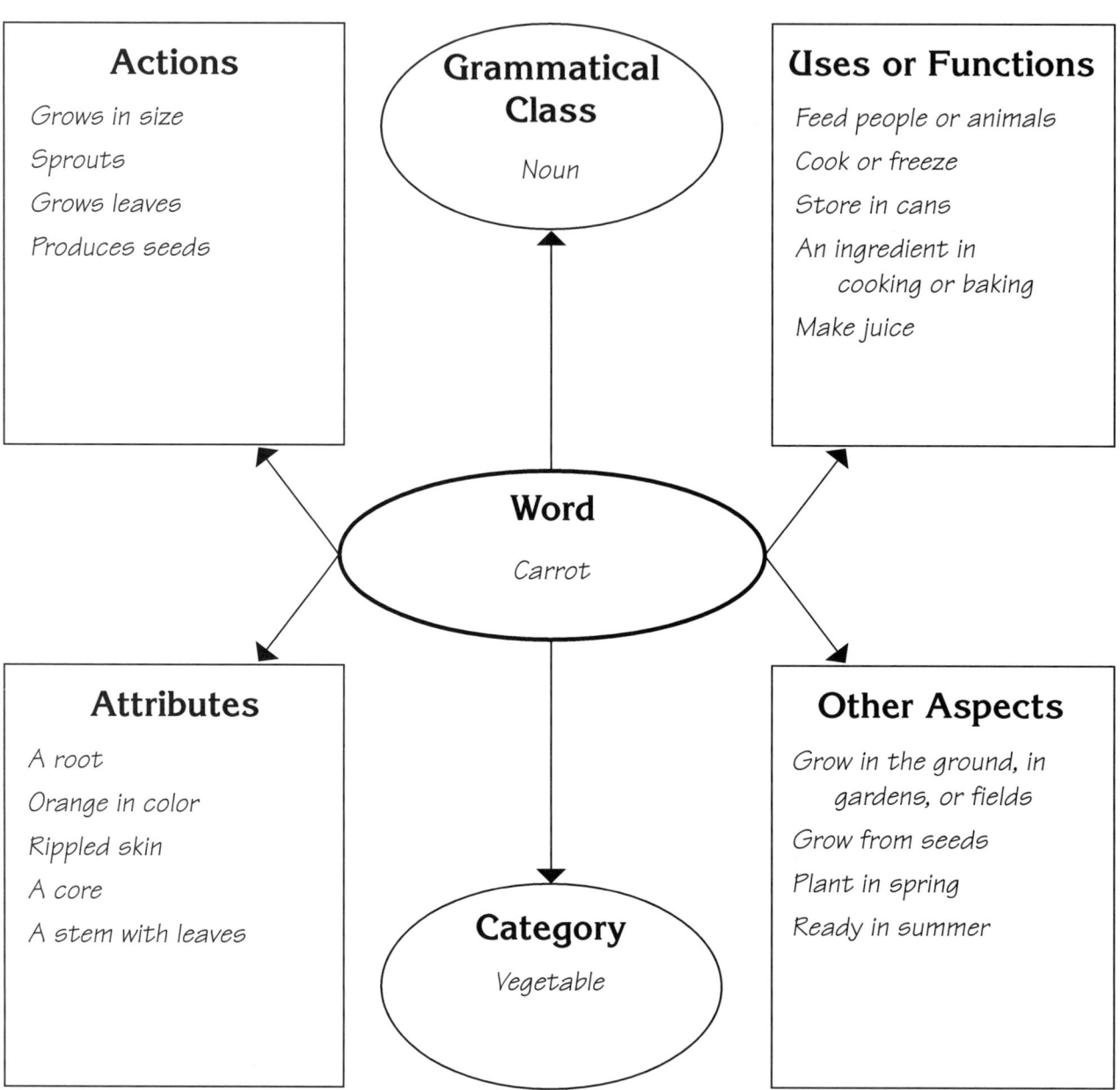

Grammatical Class
Noun

Actions
Grows in size
Sprouts
Grows leaves
Produces seeds

Uses or Functions
Feed people or animals
Cook or freeze
Store in cans
An ingredient in cooking or baking
Make juice

Word
Carrot

Attributes
A root
Orange in color
Rippled skin
A core
A stem with leaves

Other Aspects
Grow in the ground, in gardens, or fields
Grow from seeds
Plant in spring
Ready in summer

Category
Vegetable

SUMMARY
I eat raw carrots for snacks and cooked carrots for dinner.

44

© 2001 by E.H. Wiig and C.C. Wilson
Duplication permitted for educational use only.

Meaning and Content (Semantics)

| **Completed Map** | **Word Meanings** |

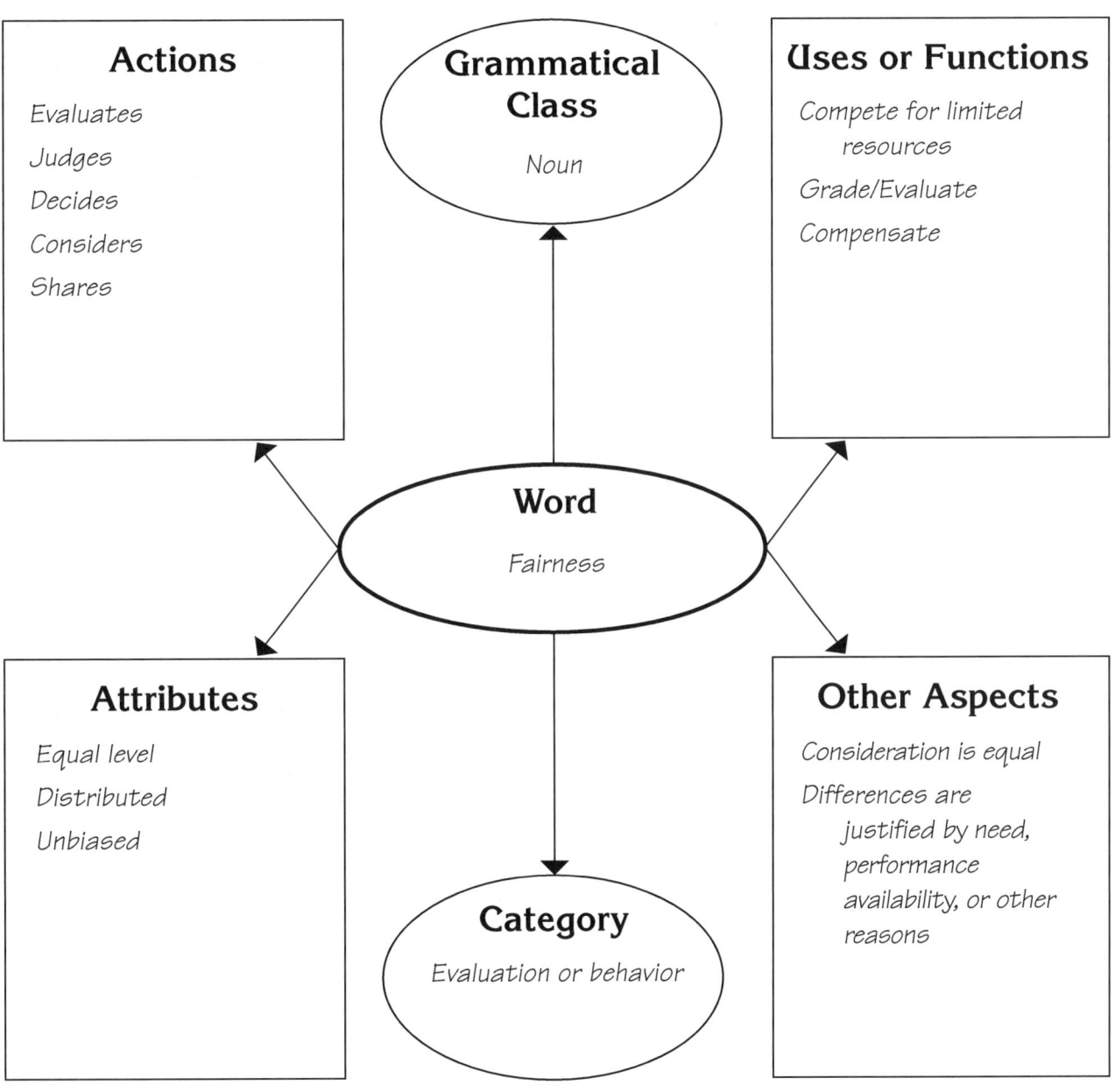

Actions
Evaluates
Judges
Decides
Considers
Shares

Grammatical Class
Noun

Uses or Functions
Compete for limited resources
Grade/Evaluate
Compensate

Word
Fairness

Attributes
Equal level
Distributed
Unbiased

Category
Evaluation or behavior

Other Aspects
Consideration is equal
Differences are justified by need, performance availability, or other reasons

SUMMARY
Sharing punishment for a group act
Receiving the support that is needed and appropriate for someone
Getting equal time in class

© 2001 by E.H. Wiig and C.C. Wilson
Duplication permitted for educational use only.

Map It Out

| Work Map | Word Meanings |

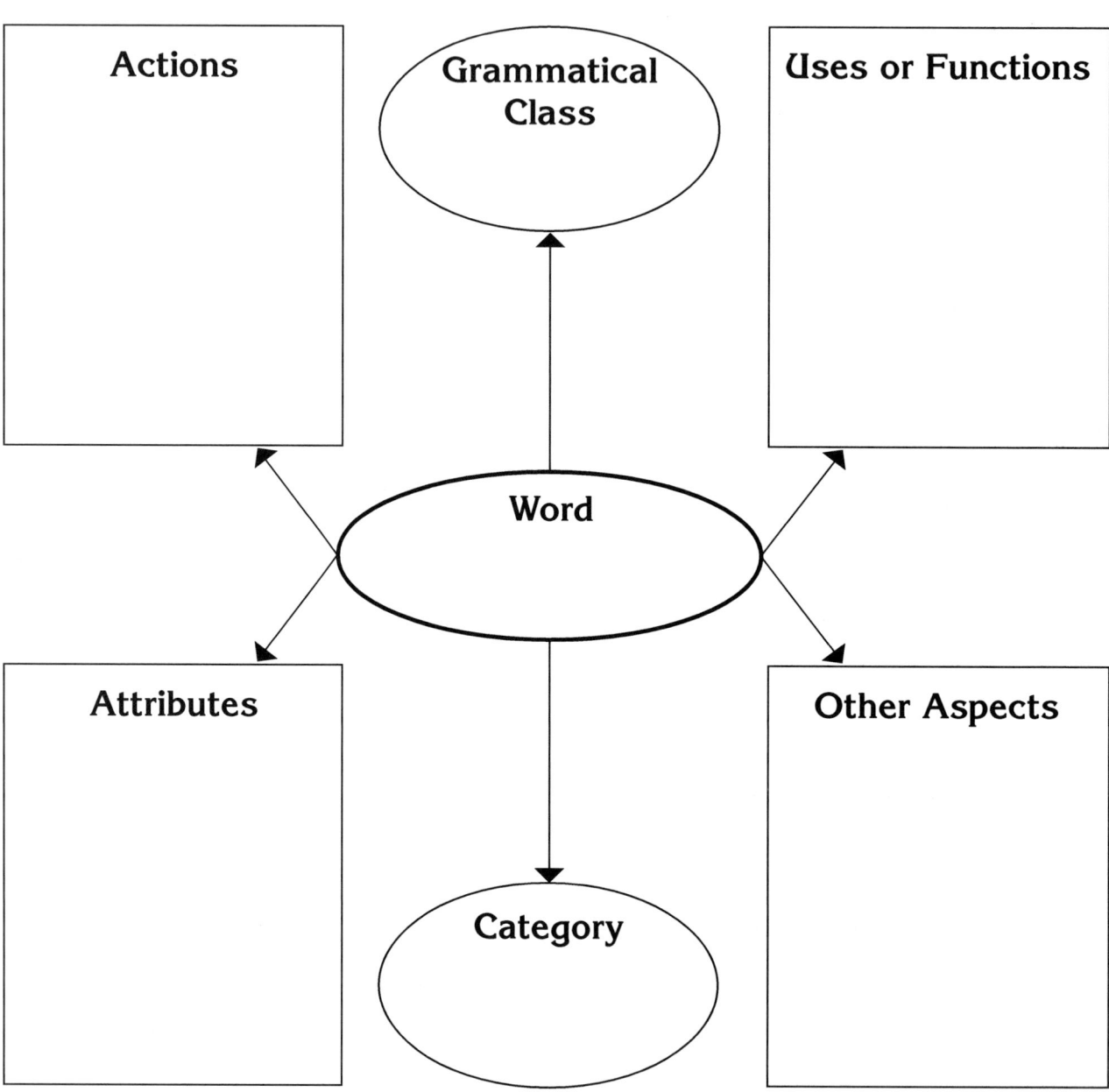

SUMMARY

46

© 2001 by E.H. Wiig and C.C. Wilson
Duplication permitted for educational use only.

Meaning and Content (Semantics)

Unit 2: Word Associations

> **Educational Levels**
>
> Elementary through secondary
>
> **Objectives**
>
> (1) Understand that word associations are triggered in the mind by a given word or concept; (2) identify and explain differences and similarities among word associations; (3) form categories for word associations; (4) broaden the meaning base for words and concepts; and (5) prepare for comparing and contrasting concepts and defining words

Completed Maps

For the first map, a student in Grade 4 generated word associations for the word *lemon* during a 1–2 minute brainstorming session. The student said the words, and the teacher wrote them down in the order they were said. The teacher then guided an analysis of how the associations were related in the student's mind.

Show the Completed Map to students and say, for example:

> *This map shows an example of the word associations a student gave for a word. Let's start by looking at the word* lemon *and the word associations for it.*

After reviewing the map, you may want to ask:

> *How does each word association relate to the word in the center? For example,* lemon *and* grapefruit *are connected by color and word category.*

For the second map, students in Grade 7 were engaged in a session on human relationships. They did not appear to understand the concept of trust. Each student completed a map for the word *trust*. Students then shared their associations, talked about similarities and differences, and developed a composite map.

Map It Out

Work Map

Select a word. Show the Work Map to students and say, for example:

This map is empty. Tell me what words come to your mind when you think about this word. I'll record your responses. Afterward we can talk about how the words are related.

Extended Activities

1. Have each student independently complete a map for a highly familiar word. Then compare two or three of the student maps to see which associations are the same and which are different.

2. Give students a Completed Map for a given word. Then ask them to color-code the different word categories (e.g., animals or parts) represented by the associated words.

3. Play a word association game. Ask students for a word to write in the center of a map. Then go from student to student and ask for a word associated with the one in the center. After the game, discuss why many of the word responses were repeated. Then ask students to find unique responses on the map and explain how that association came to someone's mind.

4. Play an "association hopscotch" game. In this game, someone chooses a word and writes it in the center of the map. Then each student gives a word that is associated with the last word given. Record the responses on the map. After the map is complete, students can discuss how the chain of word associations progressed and why the words came to mind.

Meaning and Content (Semantics)

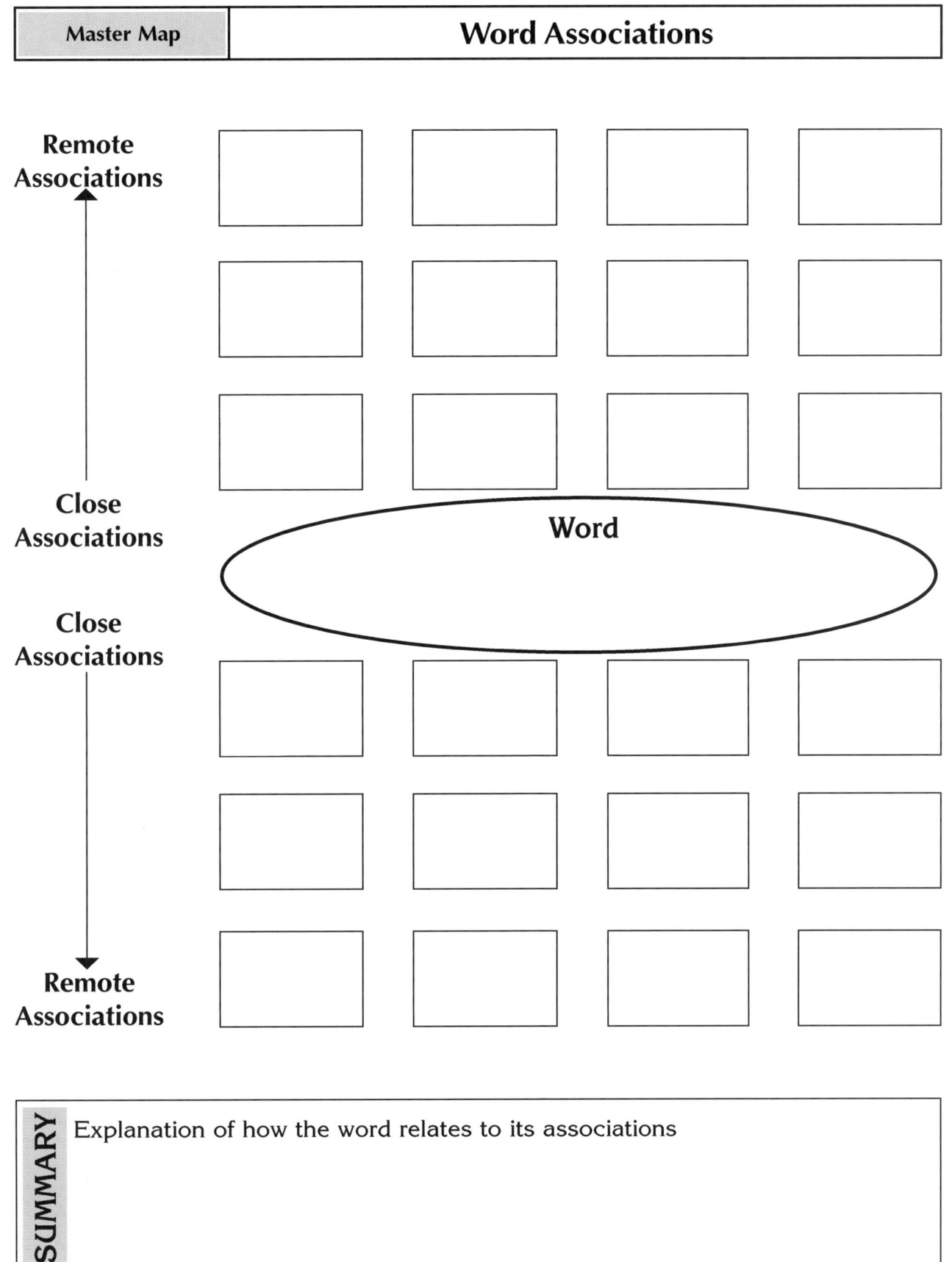

Map It Out

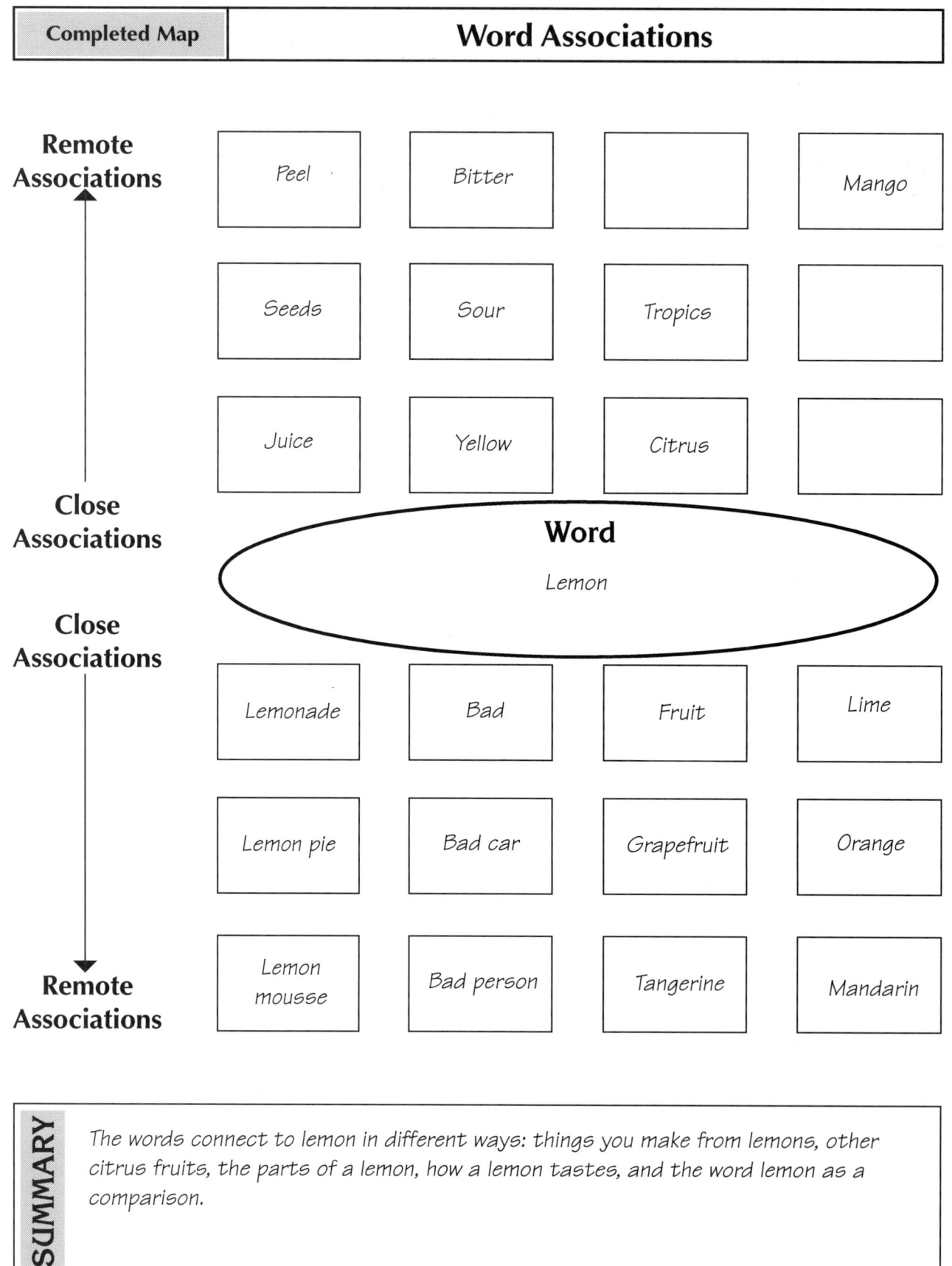

Meaning and Content (Semantics)

Completed Map	**Word Associations**

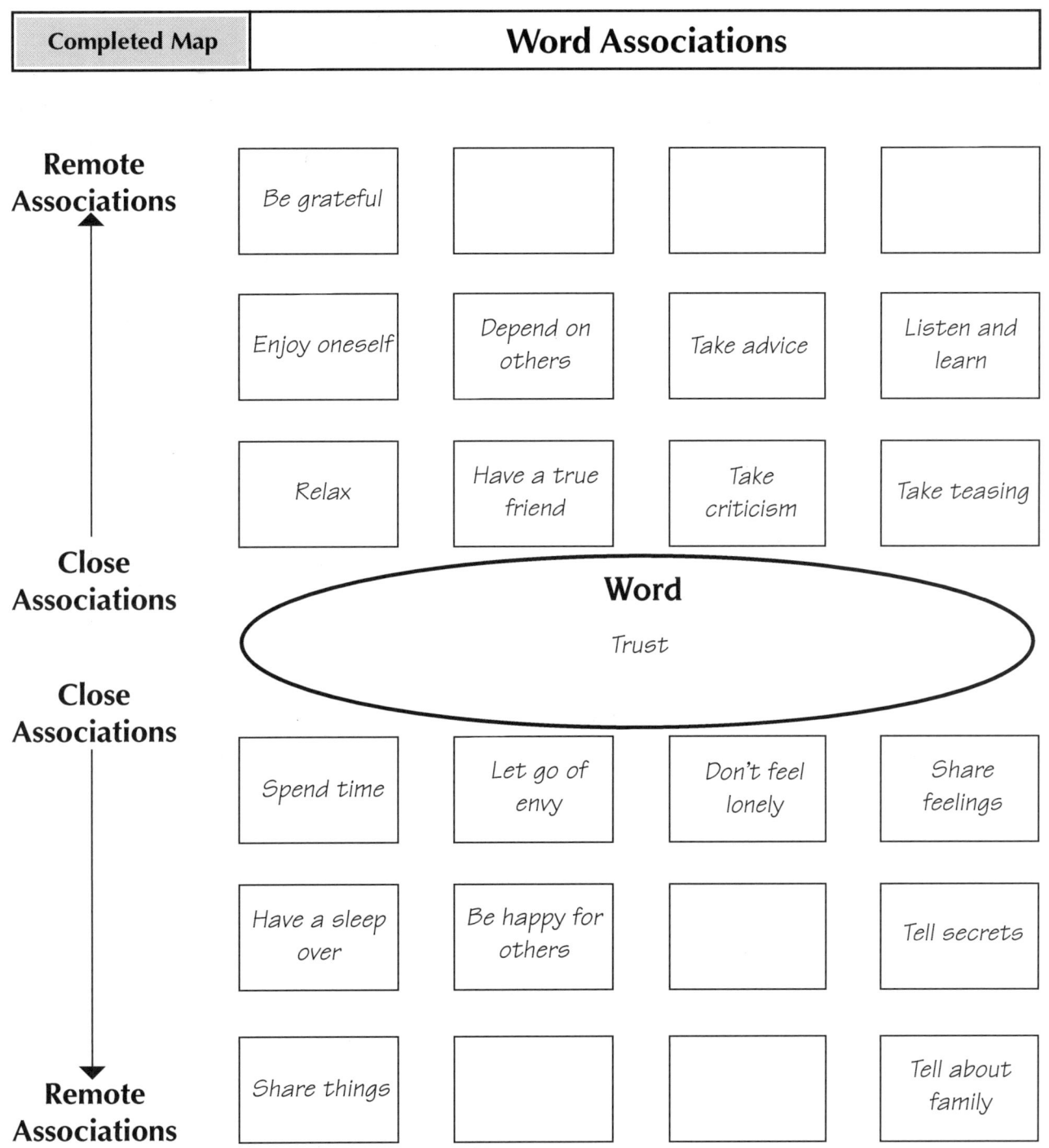

SUMMARY

Trusting someone can be hard, but lots of good things happen when you do: feeling good inside, being able to express many kinds of things, and being able to respond to criticism or negative comments more easily.

© 2001 by E.H. Wiig and C.C. Wilson
Duplication permitted for educational use only.

Map It Out

| Work Map | **Word Associations** |

Remote Associations ↑

Close Associations

Close Associations

Remote Associations ↓

Word

SUMMARY

Meaning and Content (Semantics)

Unit 3: Word Definitions

> **Educational Levels**
>
> Elementary through secondary
>
> **Objectives**
>
> (1) Recognize parts of word definitions; (2) synthesize meaning features into a whole; (3) define words in a dictionary-like fashion by referring to word class (i.e., presupposition) and concrete and abstract features; and (4) compare and contrast definitions for similarities and differences

Completed Maps

The first map shows the responses students in Grade 2 gave for the word *apple*. Students identified the class the word belongs to. Then the teacher guided them in identifying important features.

Show the Completed Map to students and say, for example:

> *This map shows an example of how some students defined the word* apple. *Let's look at the group of things they said an apple belonged to. Then we'll look at some of the important concrete and abstract features that go with the word* apple.

After reviewing the map, you may want to ask:

> *What is special about fruits that set them apart from other kinds of food? What is special about an apple that sets it apart from other fruits?*

Emphasize that definitions of words include a category name and descriptive features.

For the second map, students in Grade 10 discussed the meaning of the word *treaty* as it related to one of their lessons in history class. Students identified the larger category it belonged in. Then they wrote down concrete and abstract features of treaties.

Map It Out

Work Map

Show the Work Map to students and say, for example:

> *This map is empty. Let's select a word and list its category name. Then we'll consider the concrete and abstract features of the word.*

Extended Activities

1. Ask students to analyze a word and give a definition. Then ask them to compare their definition with one found in a dictionary resource. Discuss how they are alike and different.

2. Ask students to define a new word and write two or more different sentences with the word they defined.

3. Give students a dictionary definition for one or more words. Let them analyze each definition and identify abstract and concrete features.

4. Make a game of completing word definitions. Write the target word's class (i.e., presupposition) and let each student complete the definition with two or more features. Then compare the different words the students come up with.

Meaning and Content (Semantics)

| Master Map | **Word Definitions** |

Presupposition
Class or semantic category a word belongs to

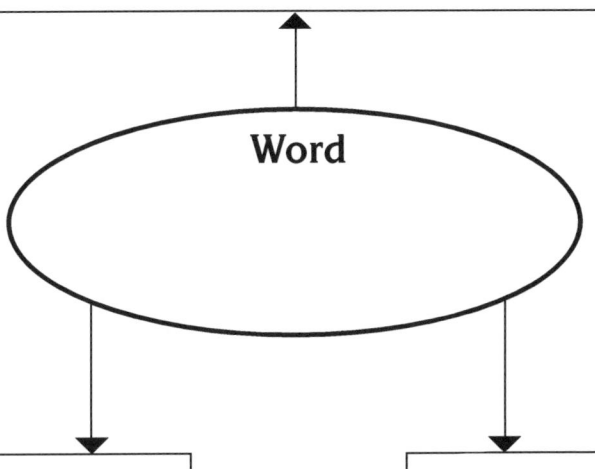

Concrete Features
Colors
Shapes
Sizes
Textures
Parts

Abstract Features
Actions
Functions
Uses
Values

SUMMARY Definition of the word and examples

© 2001 by E.H. Wiig and C.C. Wilson
Duplication permitted for educational use only.

Map It Out

| Completed Map | Word Definitions |

Presupposition

Fruit

Word

Apple

Concrete Features

Round
Red, yellow, or green
Seeds
Skin
Core
Meat

Abstract Features

Eat
Cook
Bake
Make pies
Bob

SUMMARY

Definition—An apple is a meaty fruit that can be eaten raw, cooked, or baked and can be red, yellow, or green.

Examples—Washington, golden delicious, red delicious

Meaning and Content (Semantics)

Completed Map	**Word Definitions**

Presupposition

Formal, legal, and written document

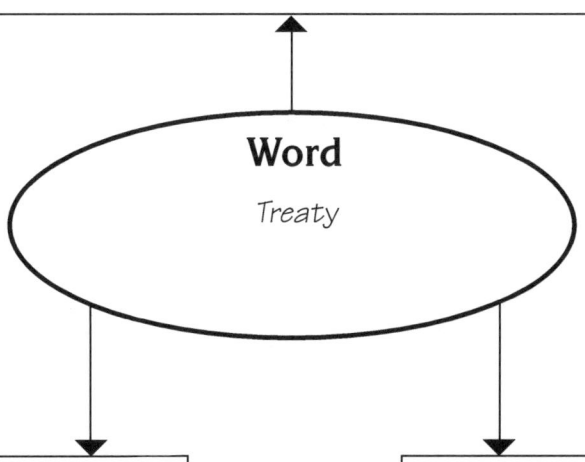

Word

Treaty

Concrete Features

Written
Document
Contractual
Negotiated by countries, groups, governments
States the compromise
Sets limits and conditions

Abstract Features

Guides relationships
Limits aggressive actions
Makes guarantees
Ends hostilities (war)
Reflects consensus

SUMMARY

Definition—A treaty is a written document that sets conditions and guides relations between two opposing parties and is arrived at through negotiation.

Examples—Nuclear weapons ban, peace treaty, cease-fire agreement

Map It Out

| Work Map | Word Definitions |

Presupposition

Word

Concrete Features

Abstract Features

SUMMARY

© 2001 by E.H. Wiig and C.C. Wilson
Duplication permitted for educational use only.

Meaning and Content (Semantics)

Unit 4: Comparing and Contrasting Meanings

Educational Levels

Elementary through secondary

Objectives

(1) Understand shared (i.e., similar) and nonshared (i.e., different) meanings of related words; (2) compare and contrast related words or concepts in speech or text; and (3) construct definitions that differentiate related words (i.e., words in the same category) or similar words (e.g., synonyms)

Completed Maps

For the first map, students in Grade 4 compared how snakes and salamanders were similar and how they were different. They independently completed maps, shared their responses, and added any similarities or differences they had missed. Then the teacher guided a discussion of the features.

Show the Completed Map to students and say, for example:

This map shows an example of comparisons between two words and their meanings. Let's look at the words and talk about how they are similar in meaning and how they are different.

The second map was completed by students in Grade 10 who were involved in a history lesson on treaties. The students did not completely understand the similarities and differences between two actions involved in negotiating a treaty. The teacher guided the completion of the map and posted it for easy reference.

Map It Out

Work Map

Show the Work Map to students and say, for example:

> *This map is empty. Let's select two words that have related or similar meanings. We'll talk about the meanings the words share—that is how they are similar. Then we'll talk about the meanings that are different.*

Note that students may find it easier to start with meaning differences and then identify similarities.

Extended Activities

1. Give the students antonym word pairs (i.e., pairs of word opposites) from lessons or texts to compare and contrast.

2. Ask students to select a pair of related words or word classes from lessons or texts. Then have them compare and contrast the words' meanings and write two different sentences—one with each word—that show the similarities or differences, but not both, between the two words.

3. Ask students to write word definitions for words they have compared. Then ask them to compare their definitions to those in a dictionary resource.

4. Ask students to look up and copy the dictionary definitions for two related words or word classes. Then ask them to discuss how the dictionary definitions point out the similarities and differences in meanings between the words.

5. Make a game of guessing words. Give students a Completed Map without the words that are being compared. Ask students to come up with the words and discuss how they figured them out.

Meaning and Content (Semantics)

| Master Map | **Comparing and Contrasting Meanings** |

Similar

Shared descriptions (what actions, functions, or attributes?)

Shared spaces (where?)

Shared times (when?)

Shared causes (how?)

Shared values/Importance (why?)

Shared equivalences (what is it like?)

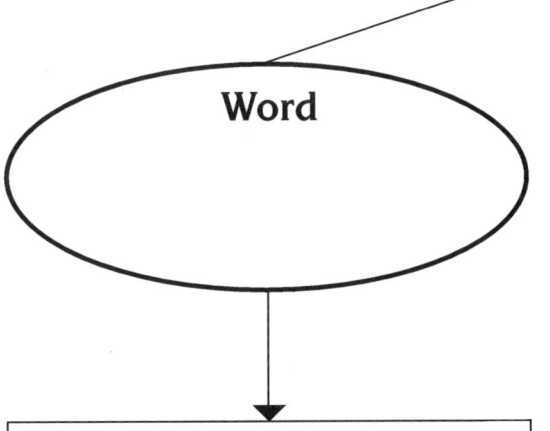

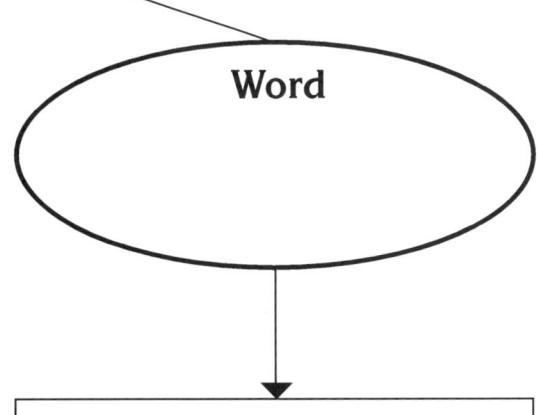

Different

Descriptions (what actions, functions, or attributes?)

Spaces (where?)

Times (when?)

Causes (how?)

Values/Importance (why?)

Equivalences (what is it like?)

Different

Descriptions (what actions, functions, or attributes?)

Spaces (where?)

Times (when?)

Causes (how?)

Values/Importance (why?)

Equivalences (what is it like?)

SUMMARY — Summary of similarities and differences

© 2001 by E.H. Wiig and C.C. Wilson
Duplication permitted for educational use only.

Map It Out

| Completed Map | **Comparing and Contrasting Meanings** |

Similar
Reptiles
Cold-blooded
Hibernate in cold weather or winter
Live in dry places

Word: Snakes

Word: Salamanders

Different (Snakes)
Wind their way
Eat small animals
Have no legs
Have scales
Can be poisonous and dangerous

Different (Salamanders)
Run and climb
Eat insects
Have four legs
Have long tails
Can lose their tails if scared
Are not dangerous

SUMMARY: Snakes and salamanders are cold-blooded reptiles that live in dry places and hibernate. They are different in how they move, what they eat, what they look like, and their dangerousness.

Meaning and Content (Semantics)

| Completed Map | **Comparing and Contrasting Meanings** |

Similar

Verbal interactions

Word
Discuss

Word
Negotiate

Different

State opinions, views, attitudes, beliefs, and preferences on a topic in a supportive situation

No outcome needed—the conversation itself is most important

Different

Give and take opinions and points of agreement/disagreement in a hostile situation

Outcome is intended—both sides must find a way to compromise

SUMMARY

Having a discussion and participating in a negotiation are both verbal interactions. But discussions are held to simply share opinions, and negotiations are held to make a compromise when two groups don't agree.

© 2001 by E.H. Wiig and C.C. Wilson
Duplication permitted for educational use only.

Map It Out

| Work Map | **Comparing and Contrasting Meanings** |

Similar

Word

Word

Different

Different

SUMMARY

Meaning and Content (Semantics)

Unit 5: Making Inferences and Asking *Wh*-Questions

> ### Educational Levels
> Upper elementary through secondary
>
> ### Objectives
> (1) Understand what information, given or implied, is needed for drawing inferences and asking *wh*-questions (i.e., who, what, where, when, why, and how); and (2) make several inferences about statements, expressions, song or text titles, summary statements, slogans, or ads (i.e., develop divergent thinking)

Completed Maps

For the first map, students in Grade 5 could not make inferences from a lead-in statement in a short story. The teacher guided the students in identifying and recording possible inferences based on their past experiences or other prior knowledge. The class generated inferences and came up with *wh*-questions to ask and answer as they read the short story. The teacher helped students find cues in the text that narrowed the options for inferences. Then the teacher helped students ask and answer *wh*-questions while they were reading.

Show the Completed Map to students and say, for example:

> *Let's look at the inferences and discuss how each could help make a perfect day. Then we'll choose some and put them together to describe what the day could have been like.*

For the second map, a student in Grade 10 could not explain to his counselor why he had problems completing school assignments. The counselor guided a process of helping the student ask *wh*-questions that resulted in identifying and recording tasks to be done, actions to be taken, when actions and tasks needed to be completed, and sources of interference. The student and counselor then discussed each item and came up with ways the student could improve his study habits and modify his free-time activities.

Map It Out

Work Map

Select a statement, assertion, or expression. Show the Work Map to students and say, for example:

> *This map is empty. Let's look at this expression and talk about what it makes us think about. We'll organize each thought based on which category it belongs to. Then we'll make guesses about what the expression means.*

Extended Activities

1. Ask students to analyze a few comments or statements from a famous speech or text and come up with inferences. Then ask students to make up some *wh-*questions they could ask the speaker or author to get more information. Read the entire speech or text, and discuss how their inferences fit the content.

2. Select some familiar song titles, and ask students to write multiple inferences about the content of the songs.

3. Ask one student to come up with a general statement or expression that relates to his or her life. Ask the other students to come up with inferences. Then have students ask *wh-*questions of the student who made the statement.

4. Select one or more ads with general statements from newspapers, magazines, or TV. Ask students to come up with multiple inferences about the product in the ad. Discuss how to verify which inferences make sense based on experiences with products.

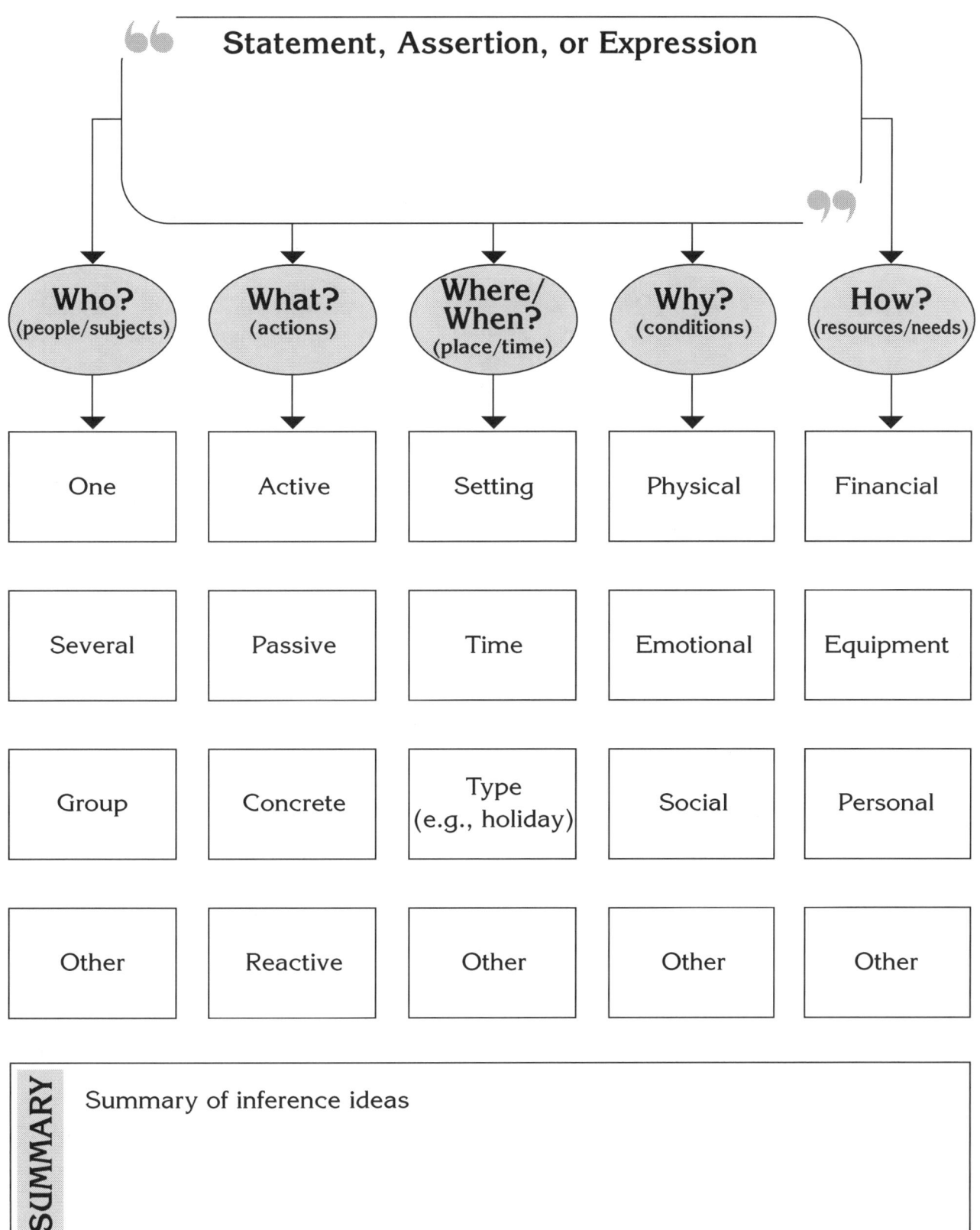

Map It Out

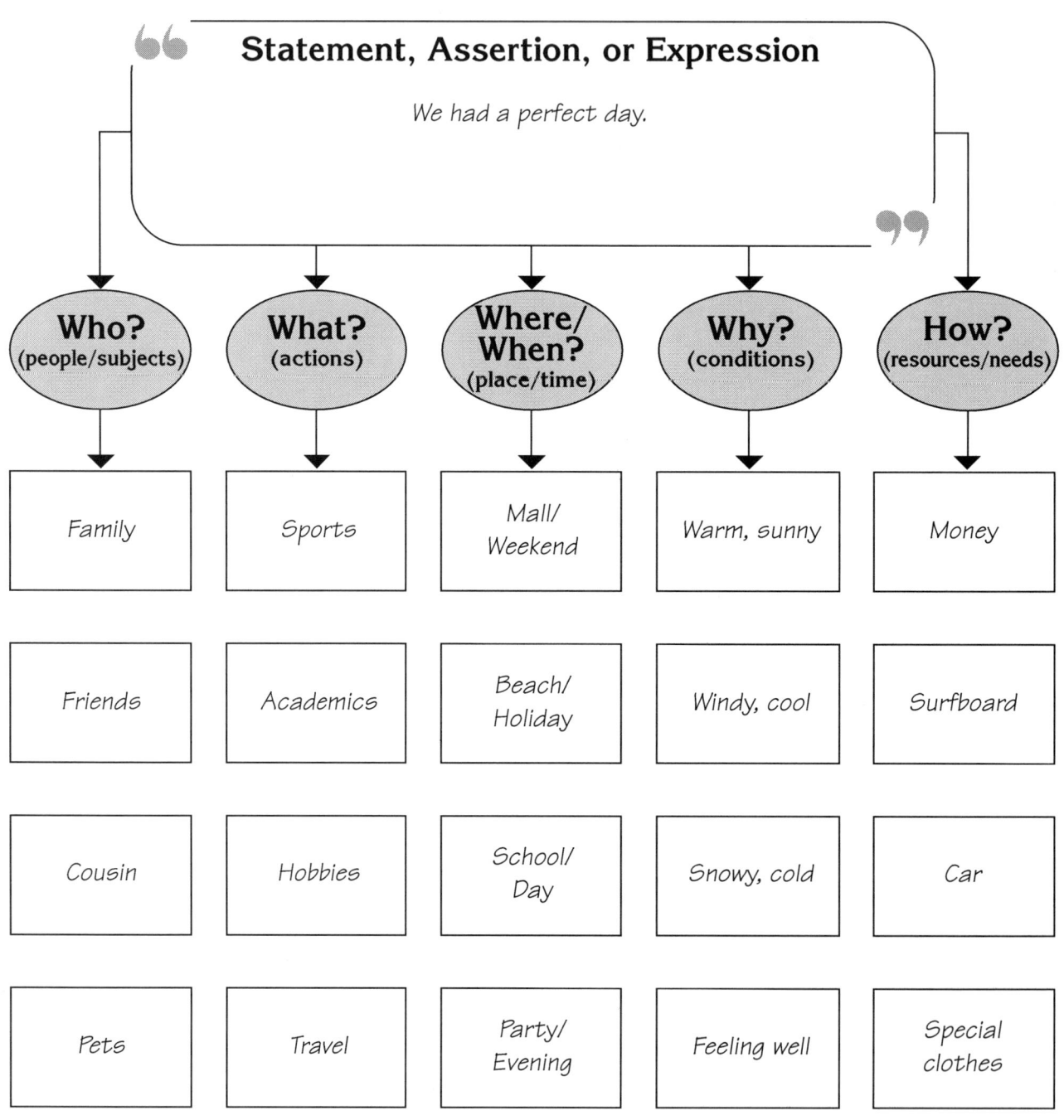

Meaning and Content (Semantics)

| Completed Map | **Making Inferences and Asking *Wh*-Questions** |

Statement, Assertion, or Expression

I can't keep up with all the assignments!

Who? (people/subjects)	What? (actions)	Where/When? (place/time)	Why? (conditions)	How? (resources/needs)
Math test	Study for math	Math class/ Tomorrow	Band practice	Make more time for homework
History essay	Research topic	History class/ Next week	Family time	Learn to research
Science project	Go to library	Science class/ Three weeks	Sick last week	Organize/Have better habits
Team project	Write paper	Team meeting place/ End of term	Girlfriend	Reduce other activities

SUMMARY: I have trouble completing my assignments because there is a lot to do and there are lots of different due dates. I also have many other activities I am involved in. I think I need some help with study skills and habits. Maybe if I get more organized I'll be able to keep up.

© 2001 by E.H. Wiig and C.C. Wilson
Duplication permitted for educational use only.

Map It Out

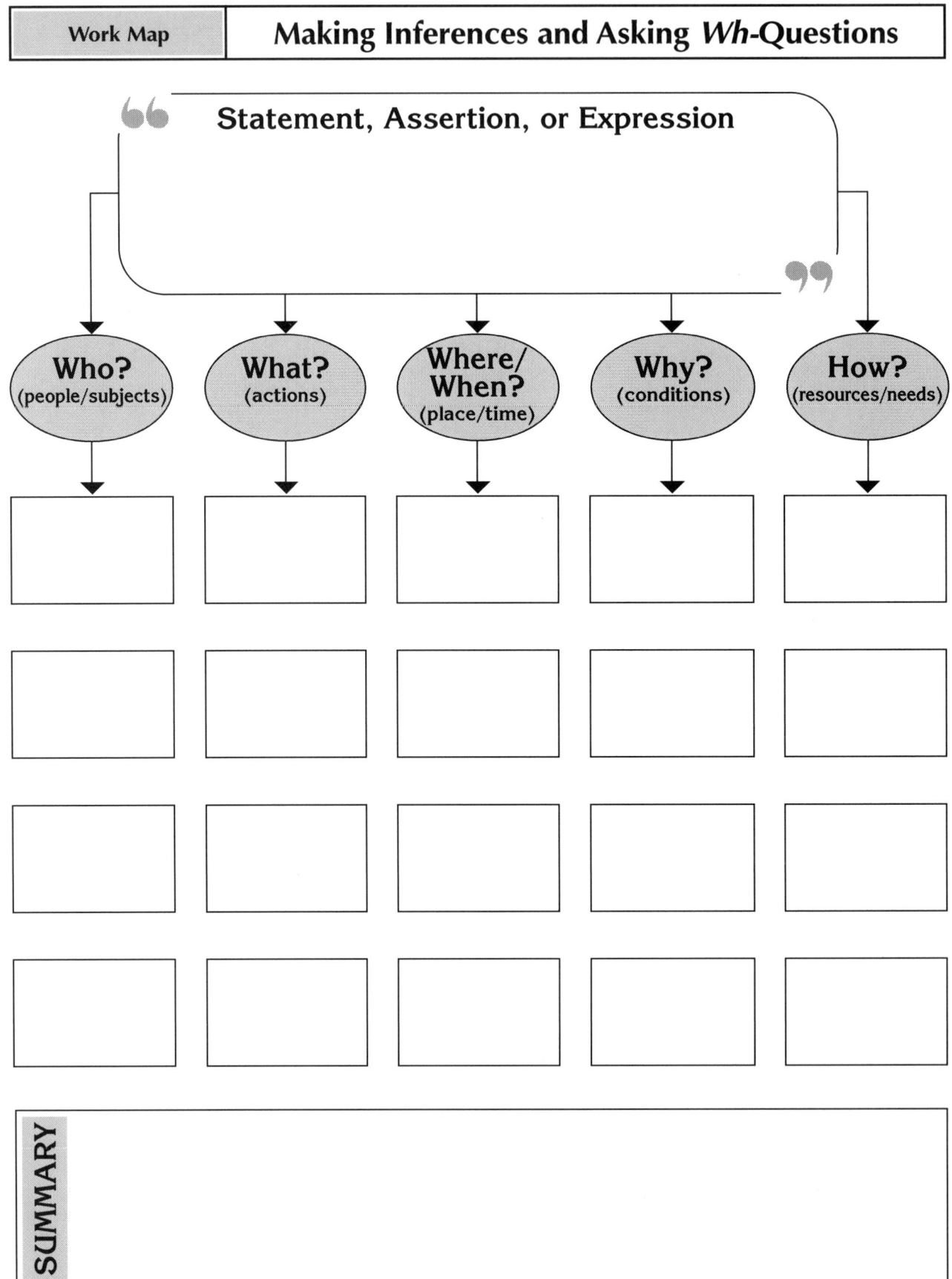

Unit 6: Verbal Analogies

> **Educational Levels**
>
> Elementary through secondary
>
> **Objectives**
>
> (1) Understand the formats used for verbal analogies; (2) identify shared underlying dimensions; and (3) extend underlying meaning relationships to complete a verbal analogy

Completed Maps

The first map was completed by students in Grade 5. They had learned about mammals, defined the word, and compared mammals to other subclasses of animals. The teacher then played a verbal analogy game with the class to practice the new knowledge in a testlike format. Students identified the underlying relationship from the list of "Underlying Meaning Relationships" and transferred it to the map to complete the analogy.

Show the Completed Map to students and say, for example:

> *This map shows an example of a comparison of meanings called a verbal analogy. Look at the word* fur *and the word* mammals *and find the meaning relationship between them. Then we'll look at the word* feathers, *discuss what word would show the same relationship, and complete the comparison.*

The second map was created by students in Grade 8. The class was interpreting poetry with metaphoric expressions specifically related to particular attitudes and feelings. The teacher guided the students through completing a figurative verbal analogy. The teacher then introduced students to the underlying structure of directional metaphors (see Unit 10: Directional [Orientational] Metaphors, page 95).

Map It Out

Work Map

Pick a relationship topic. Show the Work Map to students and say, for example:

This map is empty. Let's think of a relationship topic. Then we'll come up with two words and find the relationship between the words. Then we'll complete the analogy with two more words that have the same relationship.

Extended Activities

1. Start by writing a sentence that contains an analogy listed in the "Underlying Meaning Relationships" list. Ask students to take the sentence apart and find the critical word parts.

2. Ask students to build a verbal analogy by choosing an underlying meaning relationship (e.g., part-to-whole) and a relationship topic (e.g., types of fruit). Then ask them to find four words to complete an analogy.

3. Give students a map with only two words in the ovals. The order and placement of the words can be changed to make it more difficult. Challenge students to make as many different analogies as possible for each word set.

4. Ask students to make up a verbal analogy for each relationship in the "Underlying Meaning Relationships" list that is appropriate for their grade and age. The first half (i.e., the left column) of the list is generally easier than the last.

Meaning and Content (Semantics)

| Master Map | Verbal Analogies |

Relationship Topic

Word A1 is/are to Word A2 as Word B1 is/are to Answer

Underlying Meaning Relationships (circle)

- Action/Reaction
- Opposite
- Synonym
- Part-to-Part
- Part-to-Whole
- Whole-to-Part
- Quality/Value
- Quantity/Number
- Sequence/Order
- Space/Location
- Temporal/Time
- Figurative
- Affective/Feelings
- Other

Analogy Relationship

Example

SUMMARY: Written or paraphrased analogy

© 2001 by E.H. Wiig and C.C. Wilson
Duplication permitted for educational use only.

Map It Out

Completed Map	**Verbal Analogies**

Relationship Topic

Animal kingdom

Word A1: Fur is/are to **Word A2**: Mammals as **Word B1**: Feathers is/are to **Answer**: Birds

Underlying Meaning Relationships (circle)

- Action/Reaction
- Opposite
- Synonym
- Part-to-Part
- (Part-to-Whole)
- Whole-to-Part
- Quality/Value
- Quantity/Number
- Sequence/Order
- Space/Location
- Temporal/Time
- Figurative
- Affective/Feelings
- Other

Analogy Relationship

Part-to-Whole

Example

Covering for the body

SUMMARY: Mammals have fur, and birds have feathers.

74

Meaning and Content (Semantics)

| Completed Map | Verbal Analogies |

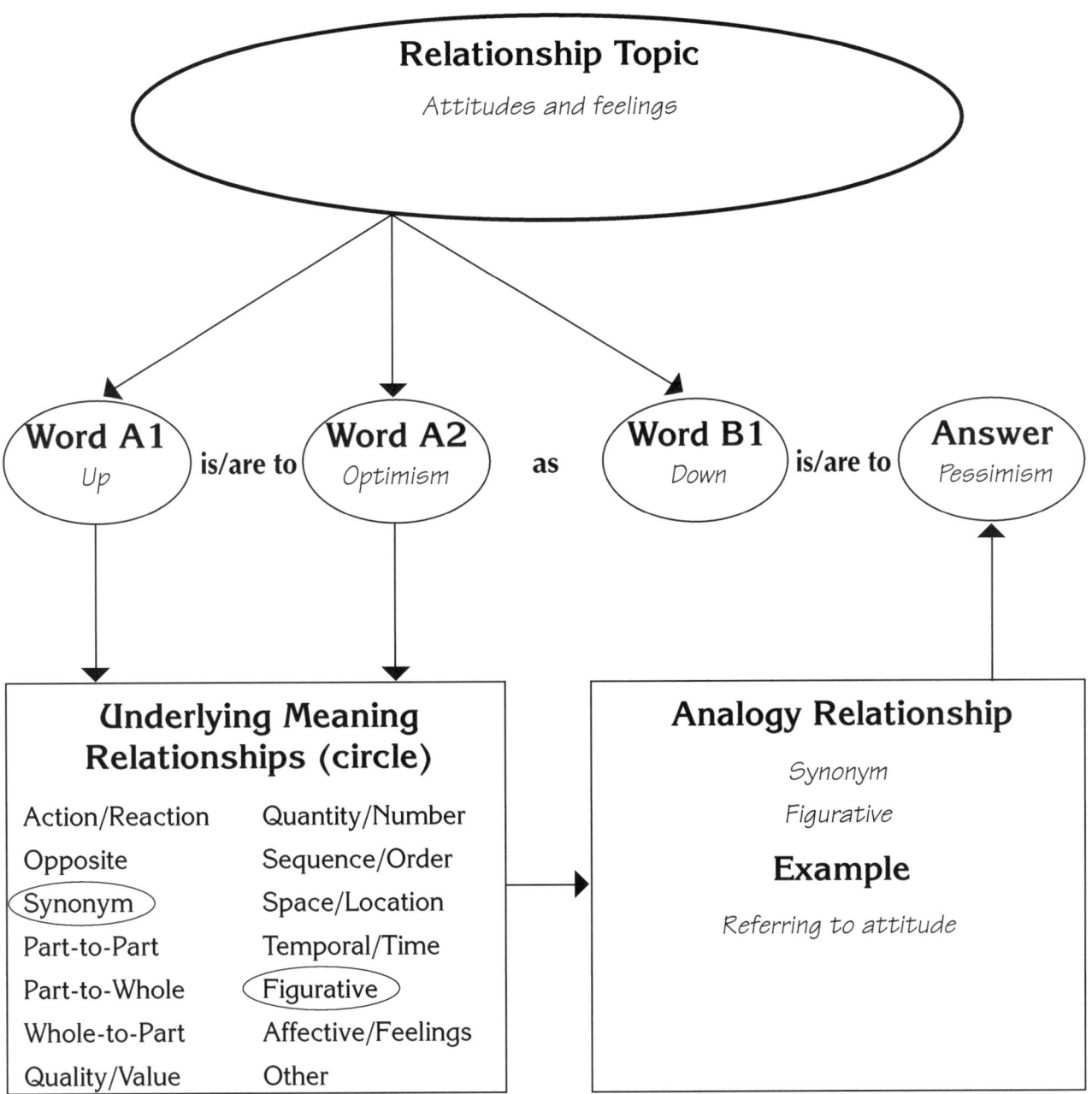

Relationship Topic
Attitudes and feelings

Word A1 *Up* is/are to **Word A2** *Optimism* as **Word B1** *Down* is/are to **Answer** *Pessimism*

Underlying Meaning Relationships (circle)

- Action/Reaction
- Opposite
- (Synonym)
- Part-to-Part
- Part-to-Whole
- Whole-to-Part
- Quality/Value
- Quantity/Number
- Sequence/Order
- Space/Location
- Temporal/Time
- (Figurative)
- Affective/Feelings
- Other

Analogy Relationship

Synonym

Figurative

Example

Referring to attitude

SUMMARY: *Optimistic people are often called "up" (positive and happy) while pessimistic people are called "down" (negative and unhappy).*

© 2001 by E.H. Wiig and C.C. Wilson
Duplication permitted for educational use only.

Map It Out

| Work Map | **Verbal Analogies** |

Relationship Topic

Word A1 is/are to Word A2 as Word B1 is/are to Answer

Underlying Meaning Relationships (circle)

Action/Reaction	Quantity/Number
Opposite	Sequence/Order
Synonym	Space/Location
Part-to-Part	Temporal/Time
Part-to-Whole	Figurative
Whole-to-Part	Affective/Feelings
Quality/Value	Other

Analogy Relationship

Example

SUMMARY

76

© 2001 by E.H. Wiig and C.C. Wilson
Duplication permitted for educational use only.

Meaning and Content (Semantics)

Unit 7: Personification

> **Educational Levels**
>
> Elementary through secondary
>
> **Objectives**
>
> (1) Recognize personification in stories, poems, and plays; and (2) use personification to create images for story and poetry writing

Completed Maps

The first map shows how a student in Grade 2 analyzed the extension of human characteristics and features in *The Giving Tree* by Shel Silverstein.

Show the Completed Map to students and say, for example:

> *This map shows examples of personification a student found in* The Giving Tree. *Let's look at each example and talk about the thoughts or images it brings to our minds.*

The second map shows how students in Grade 9 prepared to write a short story or a poem. The teacher guided the students in creating examples of personification they might use in their writing to describe a perfect storm.

Work Map

Select a story, poem, or play that uses personification. Show the Work Map to students and say, for example:

> *This map is empty. Let's find some examples of personification in this piece of writing. We'll categorize each personification. Then we'll discuss the personifications you find and how you reacted to them.*

Map It Out

Extended Activities

1. Ask students to create examples of personification. Write the name of an object (e.g., clouds), and ask students to use human features to make up examples of personification.

2. Play a personification game. Select an object in the immediate setting (e.g., a table), and ask students to give it human characteristics and express each characteristic in a sentence.

3. The personification game can also be extended into writing. Ask students to write a short poem or story about a distant object (e.g., the moon) and use personification.

4. Give students the name of a familiar object (e.g., a TV) or entity (e.g., clouds). Ask them to use personification to describe it (e.g., "My TV has its eyes on the world").

Meaning and Content (Semantics)

Master Map	Personification

Object or Entity

- **Actions or Behaviors**
  - Object and verb expression
  - Object and verb expression
  - Object and verb expression
  - Object and verb expression

- **Characteristics or Emotions**
  - Object and modifier expression
  - Object and modifier expression
  - Object and modifier expression
  - Object and modifier expression

- **Physical Features**
  - Object and modifier expression
  - Object and modifier expression
  - Object and modifier expression
  - Object and modifier expression

SUMMARY: Description of the object and its personification

© 2001 by E.H. Wiig and C.C. Wilson
Duplication permitted for educational use only.

Map It Out

| Completed Map | Personification |

Object or Entity
The Giving Tree

Actions or Behaviors
- The tree gives.
- The tree talks.
- The tree feels.

Characteristics or Emotions
- The tree was happy.
- The tree was sad.

Physical Features
- The tree stretched to the sky.

SUMMARY: The tree in this story was much like a person, maybe a parent. It gave everything it had to the boy it loved. It also felt sad when the boy did not visit and was happy when he did visit.

Meaning and Content (Semantics)

Completed Map	**Personification**

Object or Entity
A perfect storm

Actions or Behaviors

- The clouds were boiling.
- The clouds were seething.
- The sky threw a tantrum.
- The winds yelled and screamed.

Characteristics or Emotions

- The sky was angry.
- The sky caused fear.
- The winds were violent and threatening.

Physical Features

- The clouds towered over.
- The seas were majestic.
- The green and white waves warned.
- The waves came like big fists.

SUMMARY

The weather in our stories will have human characteristics. The clouds, wind, sky, and water could be like angry people with many emotions and physically violent actions. A scary place to be!

© 2001 by E.H. Wiig and C.C. Wilson
Duplication permitted for educational use only.

Map It Out

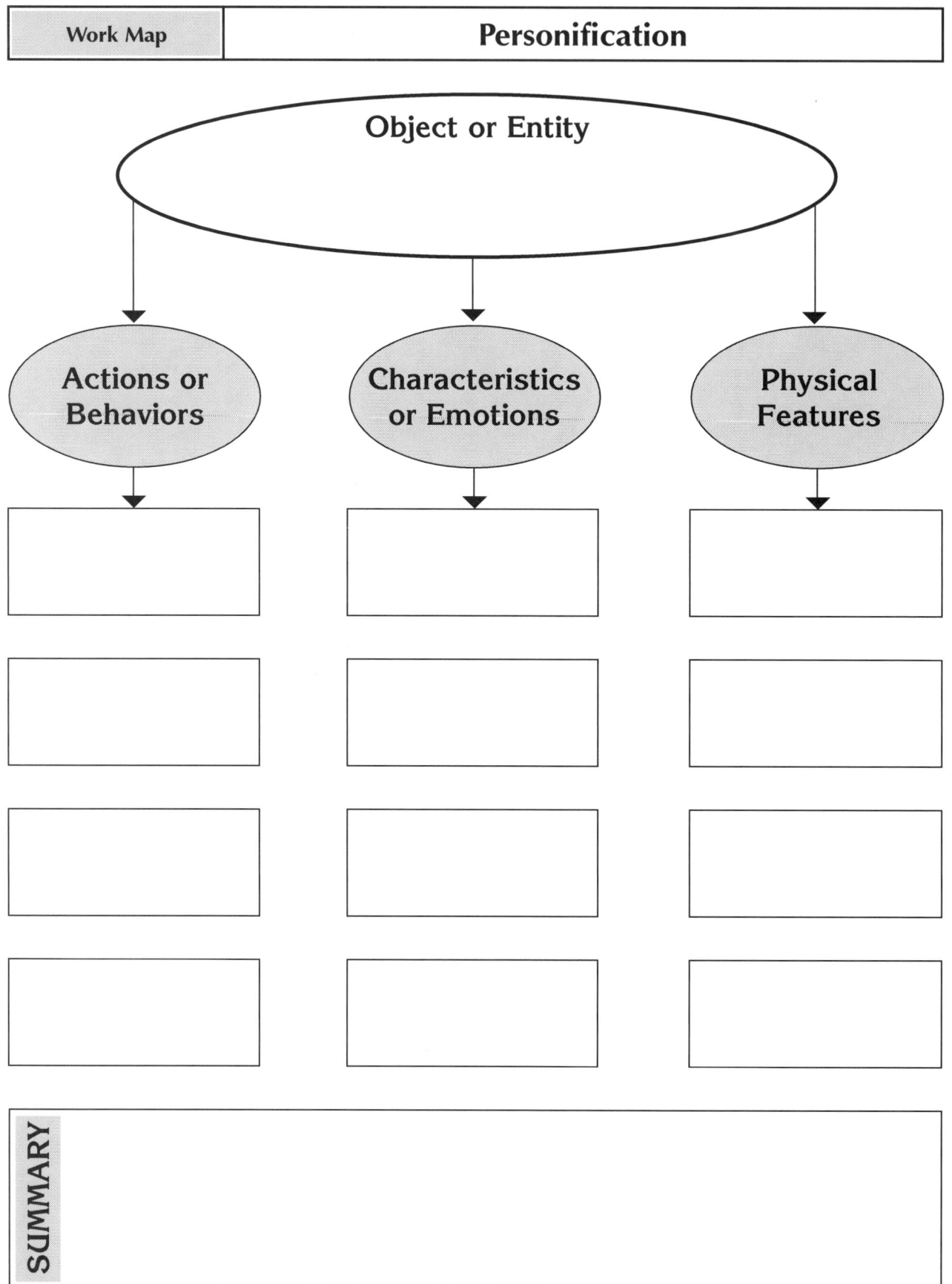

Meaning and Content (Semantics)

Unit 8: Metaphors and Similes

Educational Levels
Elementary through secondary

Objectives
(1) Understand the format of metaphors and similes; (2) analyze and extend comparisons using the structure of metaphors and similes; and (3) construct metaphors and similes to express comparisons and create mental images

Completed Maps

The first map shows how students in Grade 2 learned the structure of metaphors and similes and created expressions about one person in their class, Sue.

Show the Completed Map to students and say, for example:

> *This map shows comparisons of how a person and several objects are alike. Let's look at the characteristics of the person and objects. Then we'll look at the metaphors and similes the students wrote.*

Remind students that objects can include living and nonliving objects.

The second map shows examples of metaphors and similes made by students in Grade 7. The class had completed a discussion of emotions. The map activity was completed as a follow-up to this discussion.

Work Map

Show the Work Map to students and say, for example:

> *This map is empty. Let's choose a person and one or more objects. Then we'll identify some of the person's characteristics and the object's characteristics. We'll make a metaphor first. Then we will use the same words to make a simile.*

Map It Out

Extended Activities

1. Discuss the characteristics of some animals, objects, or entities that are often used for comparisons in metaphors and similes. Then discuss how the characteristics of the chosen animal, object, or entity are transferred to a person as a comparison in a metaphor or simile.

2. Ask students to analyze metaphors and similes used in a story, text, or play. Have them explain what characteristics each metaphor or simile stresses.

3. Ask students to view TV commercials and find examples of metaphors and similes in the ads.

4. Have each student describe himself or herself using two or more metaphors and similes (e.g., "I sing like a crow"). After each characterization, ask the other students to discuss the meanings and effects (e.g., sarcasm).

5. Ask students to make up one or more metaphors or similes to advertise familiar objects (e.g., about a book they have read, "It reads like a dream").

Meaning and Content (Semantics)

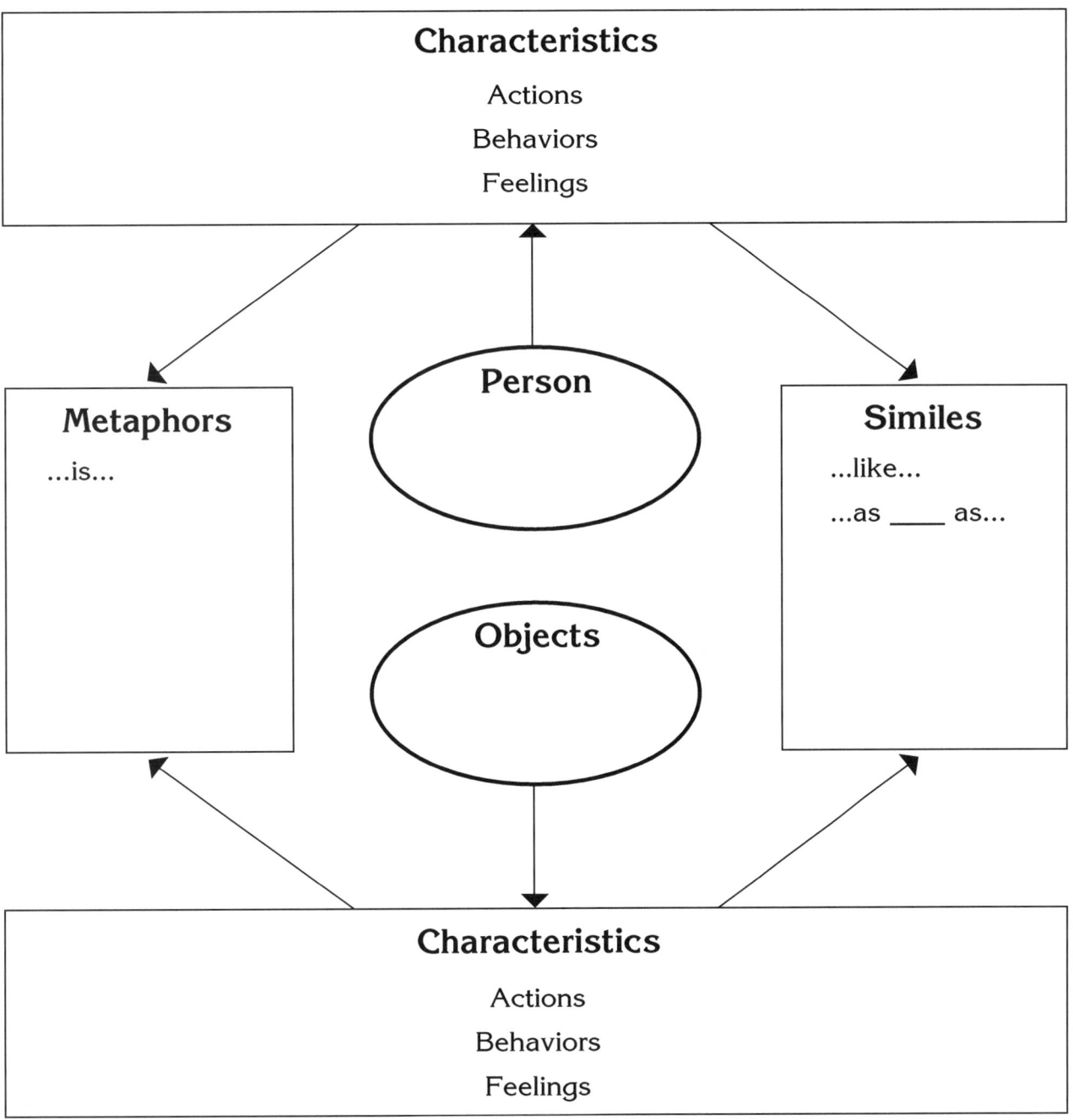

85

Map It Out

| Completed Map | **Metaphors and Similes** |

Characteristics

Eats, sings, hears

Metaphors

Sue is a sparrow at lunchtime.

Sue is a songbird.

Person

Sue

Similes

Sue sings as pretty as a songbird.

Sue hears like an owl.

Objects

Songbird
Sparrow
Owl

Characteristics

Songbird—has a beautiful voice

Sparrow—eats very little

Owl—has sharp ears/hearing

SUMMARY

We compared Sue to three animals. She sings as pretty as a songbird. She eats like a sparrow. She can hear like an owl.

Meaning and Content (Semantics)

| Completed Map | **Metaphors and Similes** |

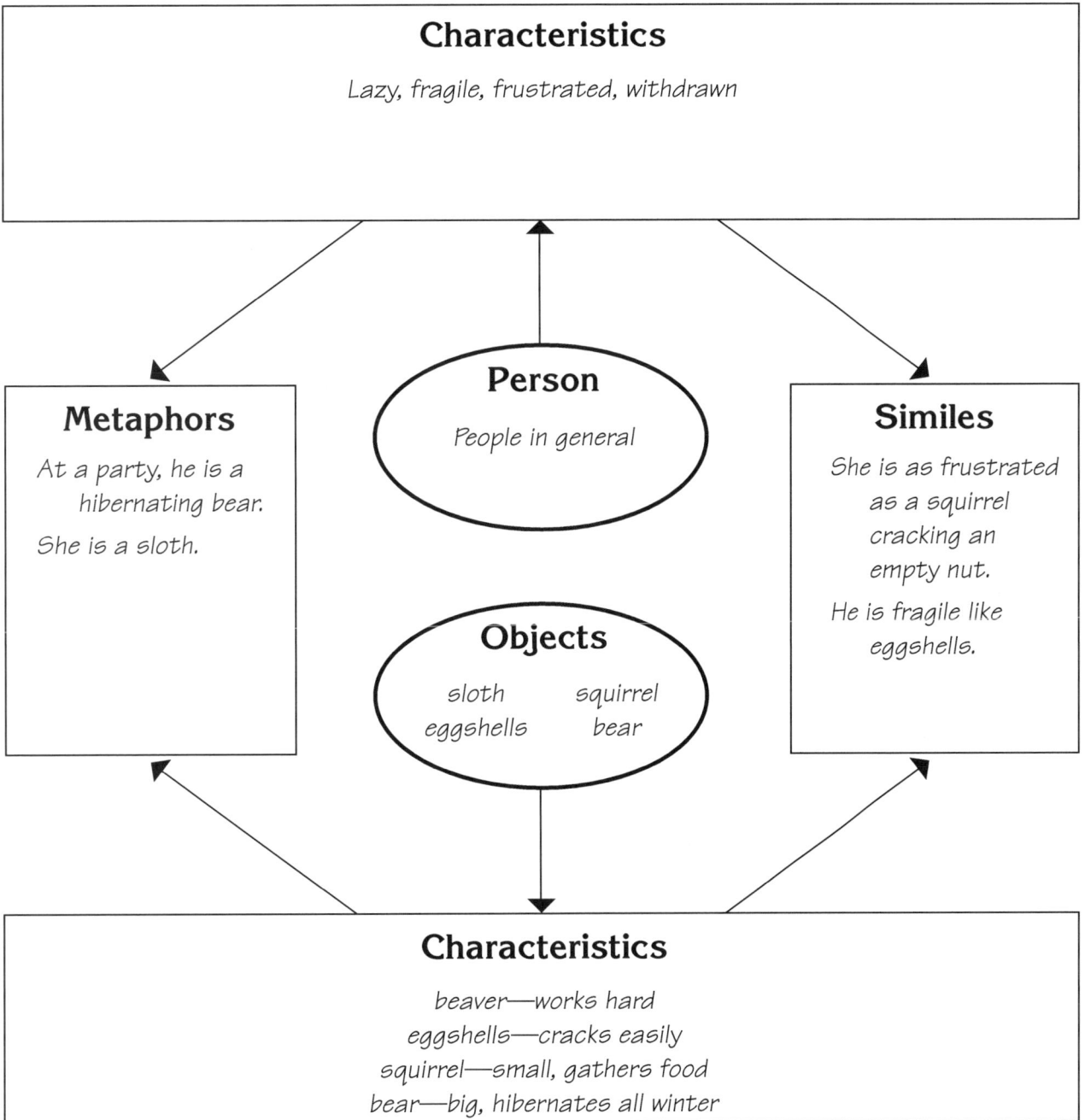

Characteristics
Lazy, fragile, frustrated, withdrawn

Person
People in general

Metaphors
At a party, he is a hibernating bear.

She is a sloth.

Similes
She is as frustrated as a squirrel cracking an empty nut.

He is fragile like eggshells.

Objects
sloth   squirrel
eggshells   bear

Characteristics
beaver—works hard
eggshells—cracks easily
squirrel—small, gathers food
bear—big, hibernates all winter

SUMMARY

We compared people in general to four objects. She is a sloth today. His ego is fragile like eggshells. The woman is as frustrated as a squirrel cracking an empty nut. He is withdrawn like a bear in hibernation.

© 2001 by E.H. Wiig and C.C. Wilson
Duplication permitted for educational use only.

Map It Out

| Work Map | **Metaphors and Similes** |

Characteristics

Metaphors   Person   **Similes**

Objects

Characteristics

SUMMARY

Meaning and Content (Semantics)

Unit 9: Analogical Metaphors

> **Educational Levels**
>
> Elementary through secondary
>
> **Objectives**
>
> (1) Understand, analyze, and extend comparisons in analogies; and (2) use the structure of analogical metaphors to express comparisons in a simplified form

Completed Maps

The first map was completed by students in Grade 3. The teacher showed the class examples of analogical metaphors and discussed their parts with the students. Then the teacher asked the students to team up and figure out their meanings.

Show the Completed Map to students and say, for example:

This map contains some examples of metaphors that compare famous people or entities to everyday behaviors. Let's come up with the meaning for each expression. Afterward we will share the meanings and talk more about metaphors.

The second map shows how students in Grade 6 explained the meanings of analogical metaphors that the teacher heard and collected from students around the school.

Work Map

Select an expression. Show the Work Map to students and say, for example:

This map is empty. Let's look at this expression. Then we'll compare the behaviors or qualities to the famous people or entities in the expression.

Discuss with the students that analogical metaphors can be positive or negative depending on the situation and tone of voice. Remind students that negative comparisons are often used in sarcastic remarks.

Map It Out

Extended Activities

1. Ask students to analyze the analogical metaphors in a text. Have them explain what characteristics each metaphor stresses.

2. Discuss the characteristics of some famous people who are often referred to in classes (e.g., literature or history). Then discuss what characteristics each person has that could be used for a comparison in an analogical metaphor.

3. Ask students to make up positive analogical metaphors that use the names of famous contemporaries in sports, music, or politics.

4. Ask students to use the names of famous contemporaries to make a sarcastic or negative remark about someone in the news. Make sure that the sarcasm is not aimed at other students.

5. Ask students to make up one or more analogical metaphors to advertise familiar objects (e.g., about a new school computer, "It's like having an Einstein in class").

Meaning and Content (Semantics)

| Master Map | Analogical Metaphors |

Behaviors or Qualities

Actions
Achievements
Chores/Tasks/Work
Past experiences

Expressions

Metaphors that use names of well-known people, objects, or events to allude to a person's behaviors or qualities in a positive or negative way

Well-Known People or Entities

People	Time periods
Places	Films/Plays
Objects	Songs
Events	Art

SUMMARY: Explanations of the metaphors in the expressions

© 2001 by E.H. Wiig and C.C. Wilson
Duplication permitted for educational use only.

Map It Out

| Completed Map | **Analogical Metaphors** |

Behaviors or Qualities

Lover, romantic
Calculated thinking
Lack of genius
Unsuccessful

Expressions

"He is a Romeo.
Get out of computer mode.
Way to go, Einstein.
Foiled again, Wily Coyote."

Well-Known People or Entities

Romeo
Computer
Einstein
Wily Coyote

SUMMARY

A "Romeo" is romantic; he is focused on love.
"Get out of computer mode" means slow down and stop thinking so hard!
"Way to go, Einstein" is sarcastic when someone does something stupid.
"Foiled again, Wily Coyote" means the person should not have expected to succeed since Wily never does.

Meaning and Content (Semantics)

| Completed Map | **Analogical Metaphors** |

Behaviors or Qualities

Poor condition

Poet, writer

Very old

Humorous

Expressions

" My dad says his car is a lemon.
My English teacher is a Shakespeare.
Our neighbor is a fossil.
My uncle is a regular Jay Leno. "

Well-Known People or Entities

Lemon

Shakespeare

Fossil

Jay Leno

SUMMARY

If a "car is a lemon," it's in poor shape.

The "English teacher is a Shakespeare" because he or she likes to read plays, poetry, and other literature.

"Our neighbor is a fossil" means that he or she is very, very old!

"A regular Jay Leno" means the uncle is funny or thinks he is funny.

© 2001 by E.H. Wiig and C.C. Wilson
Duplication permitted for educational use only.

Map It Out

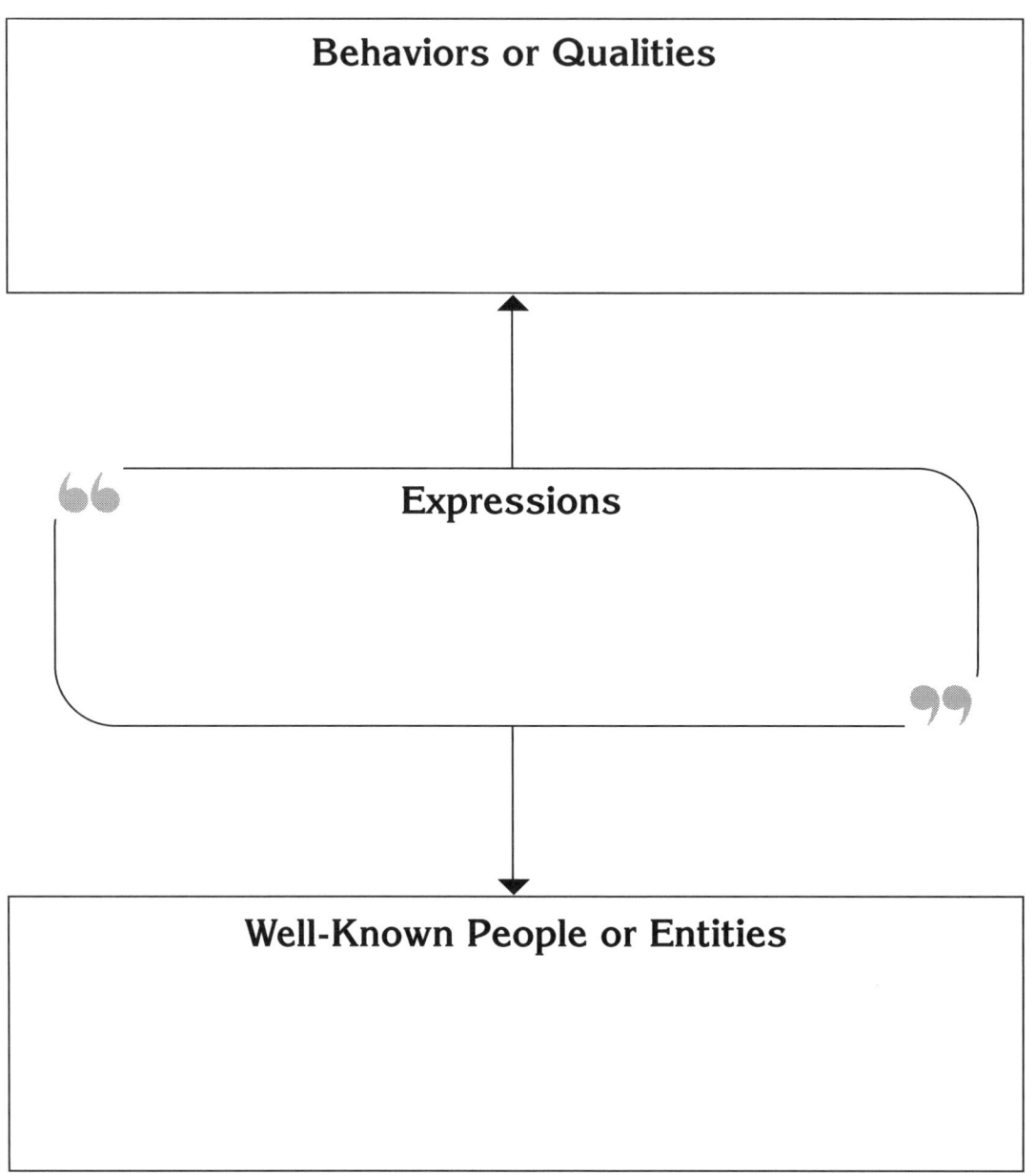

Unit 10: Directional (Orientational) Metaphors

> **Educational Levels**
>
> Upper elementary through secondary
>
> **Objectives**
>
> (1) Analyze and interpret underlying positive or negative meanings in directional (orientational) metaphors in stories, texts, plays, poetry, and other educational materials; and (2) use directional words to create novel expressions and imagery

Completed Maps

The first map shows how students in Grade 7 analyzed metaphors in Martin Luther King, Jr.'s famous speech *I Have a Dream*. To begin, the students found and wrote down a passage from the speech that had metaphors. Then they identified metaphors with directional words and analyzed whether they indicated positive or negative feelings or actions. They were reminded that positive and negative directional elements could be implied or inferred.

Show the Completed Map to students and say, for example:

> *This map shows some of the metaphors from a very famous speech. Let's look at the passage. Then we'll talk about how words that refer to a direction in space can be used to tell about important positive and negative feelings and actions. Then we'll look at the directional words Martin Luther King, Jr. used to make positive and negative expressions about America.*

The second map shows how students in Grade 4 identified and interpreted some directional metaphors in the song "Somewhere Over the Rainbow" from the film *The Wizard of Oz*. The teacher obtained copies of the lyrics from the Internet. The students first worked in small teams to identify directional metaphors. Then the teacher guided the class in interpreting them.

Map It Out

Work Map

Select a speech or poem that uses directional metaphors. Show the Work Map to students and say, for example:

> *This map is empty. Let's find an expression in this text that uses a word for a direction in space. Then we'll look for positive and negative references in the expression related to feelings or actions.*

Extended Activities

1. Identify and discuss directional words that can be used in a metaphor to describe people's actions or achievements. Discuss that the words can be either positive (e.g., up or ahead) or negative (e.g., down or behind) in meaning.

2. Ask students to select a topic and come up with directional metaphors to describe its positives and negatives.

3. Ask students to identify directional metaphors in a play (e.g., *A Midsummer Night's Dream* by William Shakespeare) or story (e.g., *The Outsiders* by S.E. Hinton). Then ask them to interpret each metaphor and tell if it was meant to be positive or negative.

4. Play a directional-metaphor game that focuses on understanding the positive or negative impact of words. Give everyday examples of people and events. Then ask students to select a directional word for each example and make up a directional metaphor about it.

Meaning and Content (Semantics)

| Master Map | **Directional (Orientational) Metaphors** |

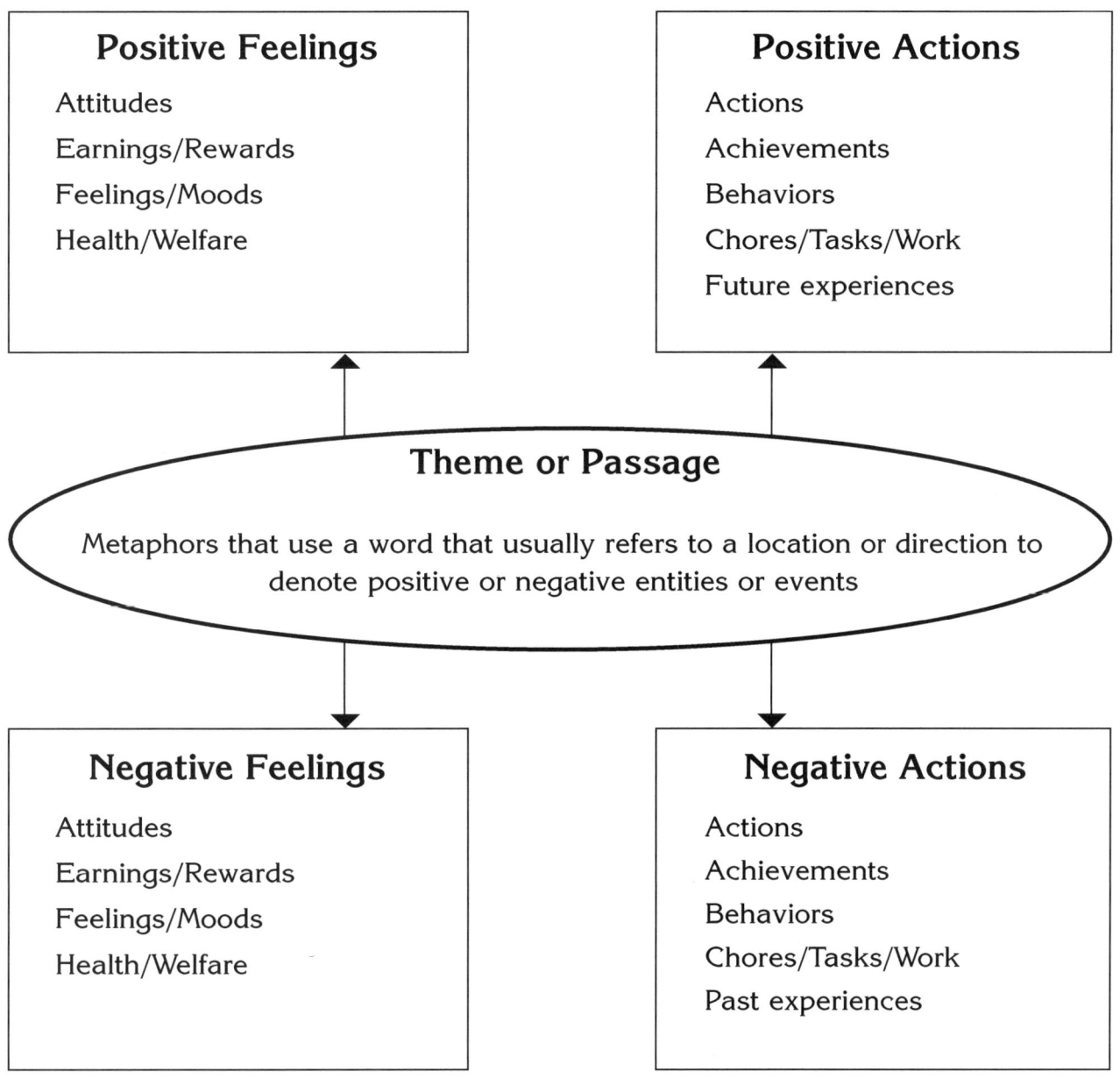

Positive Feelings
- Attitudes
- Earnings/Rewards
- Feelings/Moods
- Health/Welfare

Positive Actions
- Actions
- Achievements
- Behaviors
- Chores/Tasks/Work
- Future experiences

Theme or Passage

Metaphors that use a word that usually refers to a location or direction to denote positive or negative entities or events

Negative Feelings
- Attitudes
- Earnings/Rewards
- Feelings/Moods
- Health/Welfare

Negative Actions
- Actions
- Achievements
- Behaviors
- Chores/Tasks/Work
- Past experiences

SUMMARY: Interpretations of the metaphors in the theme or passage

© 2001 by E.H. Wiig and C.C. Wilson
Duplication permitted for educational use only.

Map It Out

| Completed Map | **Directional (Orientational) Metaphors** |

Positive Feelings

Sunlit path—hope and happiness

Positive Actions

To rise from—leave the gruesome past and embrace a better future

Rise to majestic heights—remain nonviolent in demonstrations for racial equality

Soul force—use a strong spirit, not violence

Theme or Passage

...to rise from the dark and desolate valley of segregation to the sunlit path of racial justice.

Again and again we must rise to the majestic heights of meeting physical force with soul force.

Negative Feelings

Dark and desolate valley—sadness and despair

Negative Actions

Physical force—implies use of violence

SUMMARY

Martin Luther King, Jr.'s classic speech uses many positive metaphors to inspire people to persist and create harmony. He uses both positive feeling and positive action metaphors to help people feel stronger and continue to do more work.

Meaning and Content (Semantics)

| Completed Map | **Directional (Orientational) Metaphors** |

Positive Feelings
...wake up where the clouds are far behind me—bad feelings are gone, happiness is coming

Positive Actions
Birds fly over the rainbow—Dorothy wishes to follow the birds toward happiness and away from sadness

...melt like lemon drops/Away above the chimney tops—problems went away

Theme or Passage
...wake up where the clouds are far behind me
Where troubles melt like lemon drops
Away above the chimney tops
Birds fly over the rainbow

Negative Feelings

Negative Actions
Where troubles melt like lemon drops—bad feelings and sorrows built up at one point

SUMMARY

Dorothy sings a song about getting happier. She knows that everything doesn't always go well but that things will get better. She uses words like behind, above, and over to express her feelings.

© 2001 by E.H. Wiig and C.C. Wilson
Duplication permitted for educational use only.

Map It Out

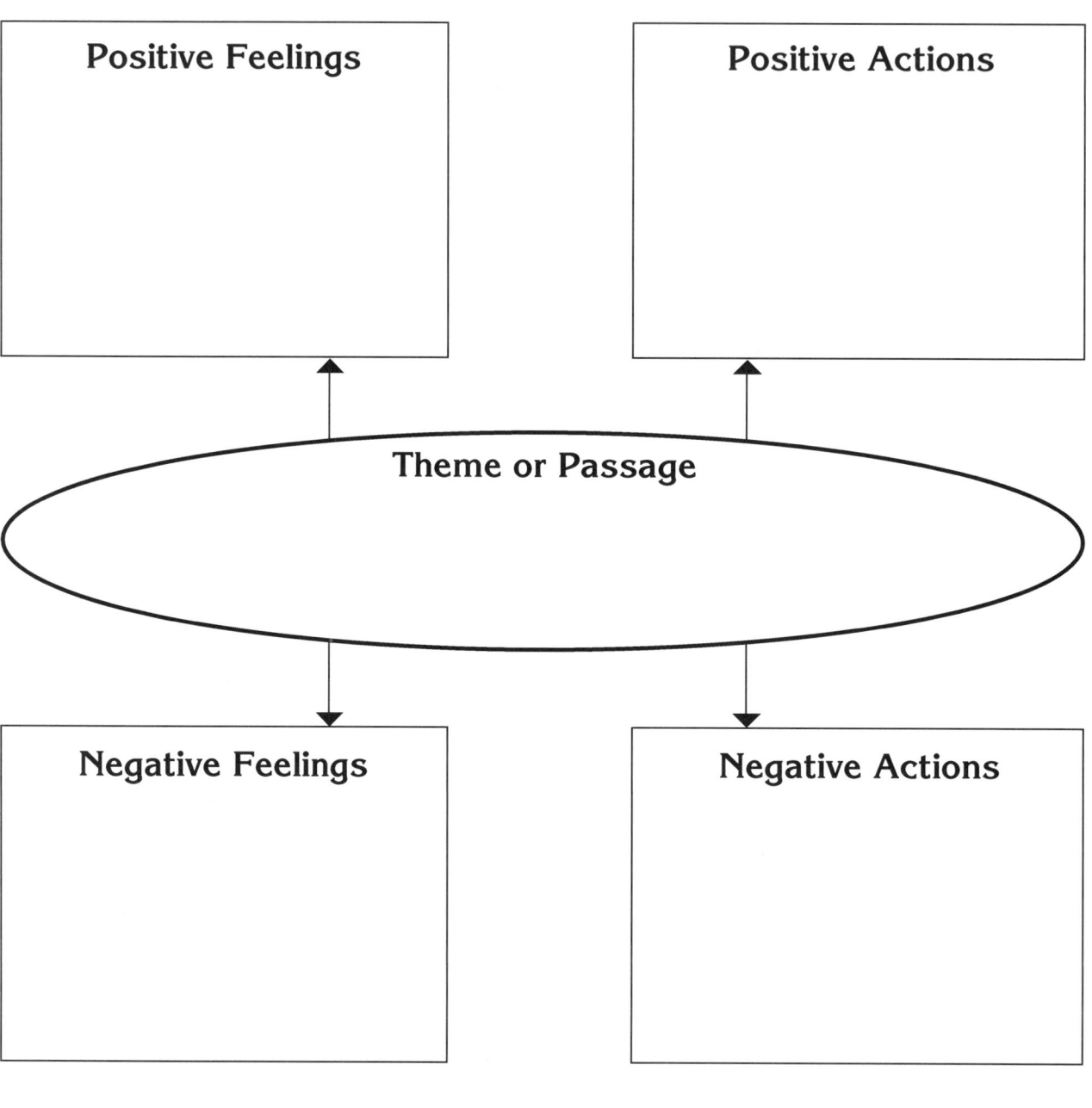

Meaning and Content (Semantics)

Unit 11: Part-Whole and Whole-Part (Metonymy) Metaphors

Educational Levels

Upper elementary through secondary

Objectives

(1) Understand the structure and words used to create underlying, implied meanings in part-whole and whole-part metaphors; (2) analyze part-whole and whole-part metaphors in speech and text; and (3) construct novel examples of part-whole and whole-part metaphors

Completed Maps

The first map uses metaphors from the speech *I Have a Dream* by Martin Luther King, Jr. Students in Grade 7 completed the map after identifying part-whole and whole-part metaphors in the speech.

Show the Completed Map to students and say, for example:

> *This map shows examples of metaphors that use the name of a part for the whole or the name of the whole for a part. These metaphors are from the speech* I Have a Dream *by Martin Luther King, Jr. Let's look at the expressions he used and identify part-whole and whole-part metaphors.*

The second map shows examples of part-whole and whole-part metaphors that students in Grade 4 created. The students made up metaphors that related to the phrase, "He drives an eighteen-wheeler."

Map It Out

Work Map

Select a text or poem with part-whole and whole-part metaphors. Show the Work Map to students and say, for example:

> *This map is empty. Let's find and write down the part-whole and whole-part metaphors in this piece of writing.*

Extended Activities

1. Ask students to remember and write down part-whole and whole-part metaphors they hear in school, at home, or on TV. Provide a written collection of the expressions, and then ask students to analyze and interpret them.

2. Ask students to make up part-whole or whole-part metaphoric expressions about a topic of their choice. As an example, ask them to create part-whole and whole-part metaphors about computers or people who use computers.

3. Select some commonly used part-whole or whole-part metaphors for analysis. Discuss the underlying relationship, help students determine why the name of the part or whole was used as the reference, and discuss the effect of the metaphor.

4. Select some names for parts of commonly used objects and ask students to use the words in making up part-whole metaphors.

Meaning and Content (Semantics)

| Master Map | **Part-Whole and Whole-Part (Metonymy) Metaphors** |

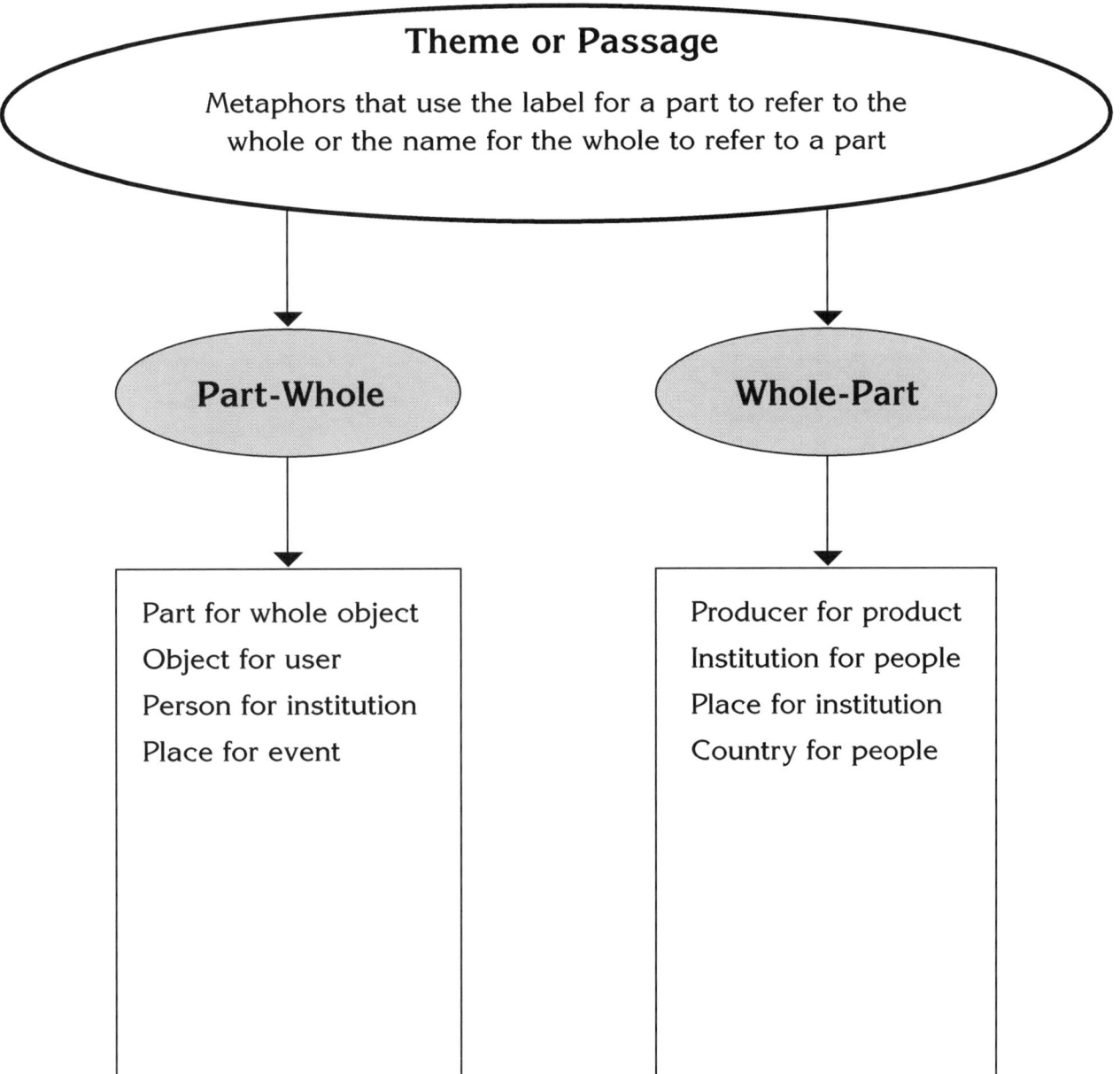

Theme or Passage
Metaphors that use the label for a part to refer to the whole or the name for the whole to refer to a part

Part-Whole
- Part for whole object
- Object for user
- Person for institution
- Place for event

Whole-Part
- Producer for product
- Institution for people
- Place for institution
- Country for people

SUMMARY: Interpretation and paraphrase of the metaphors in the theme or passage

Map It Out

| Completed Map | **Part-Whole and Whole-Part (Metonymy) Metaphors** |

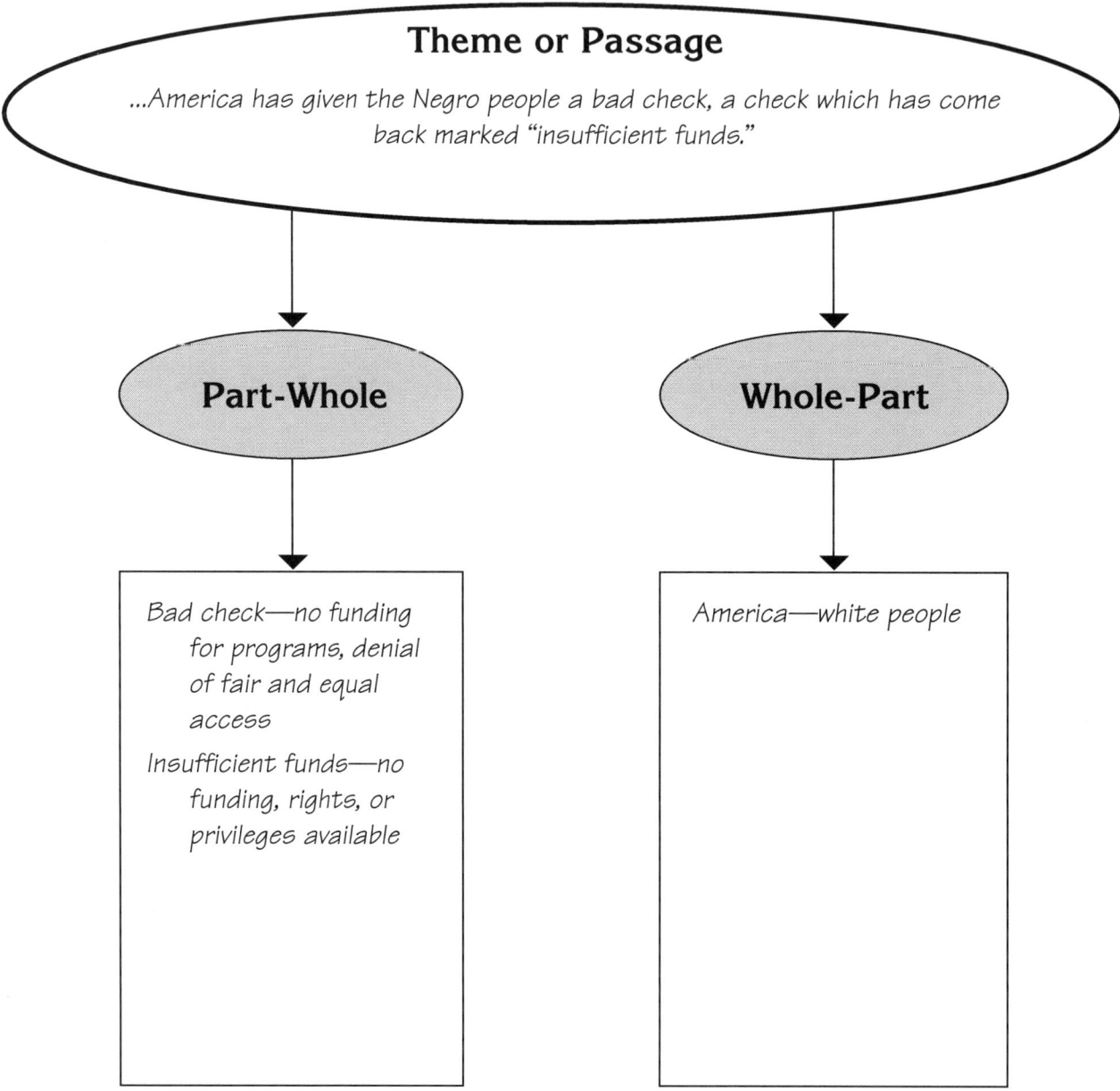

Theme or Passage

...America has given the Negro people a bad check, a check which has come back marked "insufficient funds."

Part-Whole

- Bad check—no funding for programs, denial of fair and equal access
- Insufficient funds—no funding, rights, or privileges available

Whole-Part

America—white people

SUMMARY

The majority in the United States gave a promise to the African American citizens but did not keep it, saying that the cost would be too high.

Meaning and Content (Semantics)

| Completed Map | **Part-Whole and Whole-Part (Metonymy) Metaphors** |

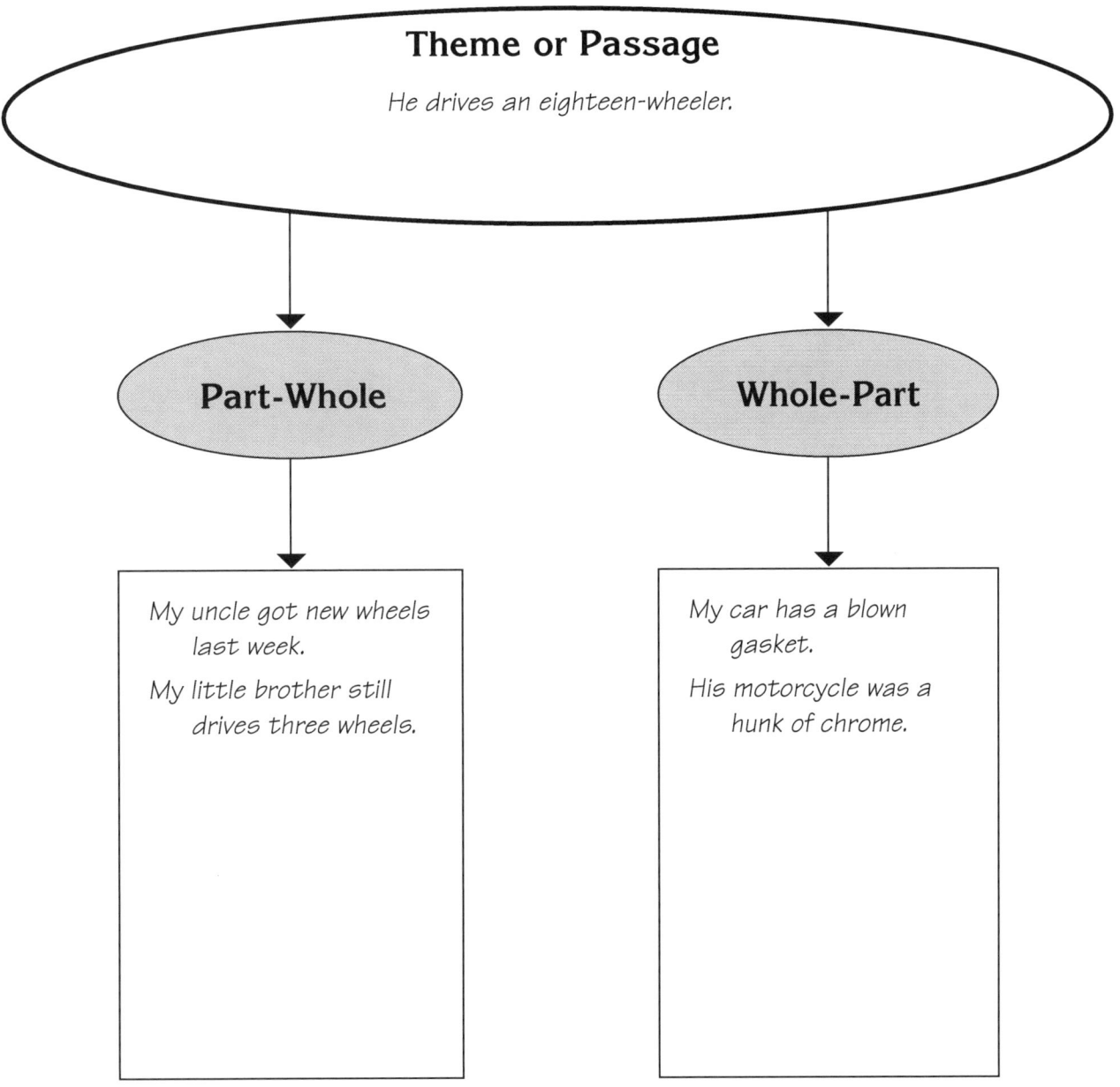

SUMMARY

We thought of all the part-whole and whole-part metaphors we could that related to "He drives an eighteen-wheeler." Each example had a part of something and a connection to a whole group or the other way around. Some of the expressions were really common. We were surprised!

Map It Out

| Work Map | Part-Whole and Whole-Part (Metonymy) Metaphors |

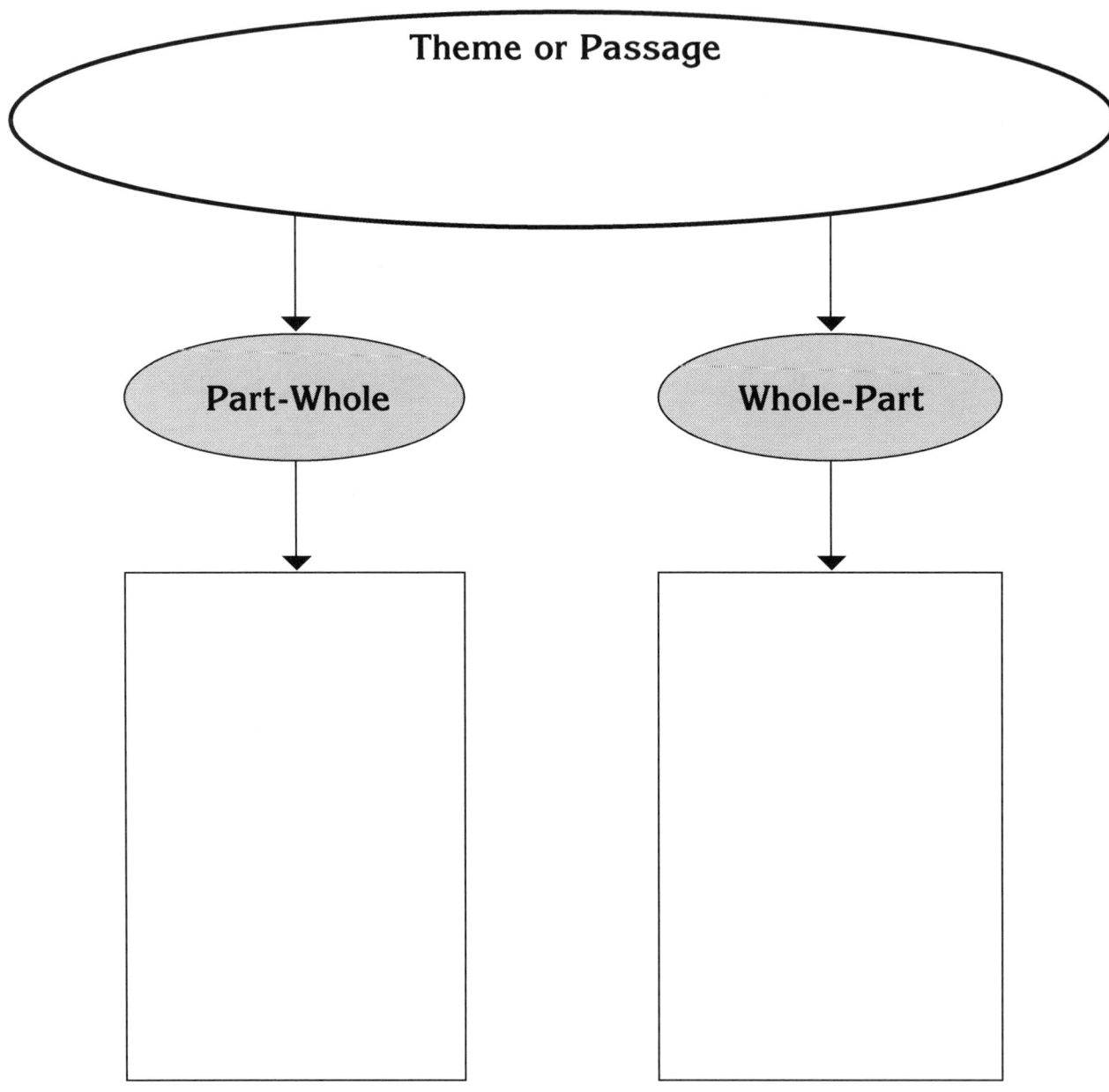

106 © 2001 by E.H. Wiig and C.C. Wilson
Duplication permitted for educational use only.

Meaning and Content (Semantics)

Unit 12: Conceptual (Ontological) Metaphors

> **Educational Level**
>
> Secondary
>
> **Objectives**
>
> (1) Understand the structures, formats, and concepts used to create conceptual (ontological) metaphors; (2) analyze and interpret conceptual metaphors in text and poetry; and (3) construct novel examples and imagery using conceptual metaphors

Completed Maps

The first map shows how students in Grade 7 analyzed and interpreted the conceptual metaphors featured in the speech *I Have a Dream* by Martin Luther King, Jr.

Show the Completed Map to students and say, for example:

> *This map shows a part of the speech* I Have a Dream. *Students were asked to analyze it to find and interpret metaphors with general concepts. Let's look at the concepts the student found and their explanations of them.*

The second map shows the conceptual metaphors created by students in Grade 10 in response to a social studies assignment comparing the industrial and technological revolutions. The teacher asked the students to apply the conceptual metaphor "time is money" to the lesson and explain the theme-related concepts.

Work Map

Select a piece of writing that has conceptual metaphors. Show the Work Map to students and say, for example:

> *This map is empty. Let's read this piece of writing and find conceptual metaphors. Then we'll interpret them.*

Map It Out

Extended Activities

1. Ask students to analyze a list of conceptual metaphors that are used in daily life.

2. Ask students to use a concept of their choice or that you provide to make up conceptual metaphors.

3. Ask students to use a condition (e.g., being in a hurry to complete a project) to create conceptual metaphors that describe the intentions associated with it.

4. Ask students to analyze or create conceptual metaphors about a state or condition of their choice or that you provide.

Meaning and Content (Semantics)

| Master Map | **Conceptual (Ontological) Metaphors** |

Explanation

Explanation

Concept

Concept

Theme or Passage

Metaphors that use a generally known or universal concept (e.g., money) to refer to specific entities, objects, actions, or events

Concept

Concept

Explanation

Explanation

SUMMARY: Interpretation or summary of the metaphors in the theme or passage

Map It Out

| Completed Map | **Conceptual (Ontological) Metaphors** |

Explanation

Riches that are more important than money, freedom, and justice

Concept

Funds

Explanation

Attitudes held by people
Places to hold valuable information

Concept

Vaults

Theme or Passage

...we refuse to believe that the bank of justice is bankrupt. We refuse to believe that there are insufficient funds in the vaults of opportunity of this nation. So we have come to cash this check—a check that will give us upon demand the riches of freedom and the security of justice.

Concept

Check

Concept

Explanation

Something earned, valuable

Explanation

SUMMARY

The Constitution promises freedom, equality, and opportunity for all. The white majority did not keep these promises. We refuse to believe that there is no justice or equal opportunity for us in America. We will get the freedom that will give us equality and riches and the justice that will give us equal opportunities.

Meaning and Content (Semantics)

| Completed Map | **Conceptual (Ontological) Metaphors** |

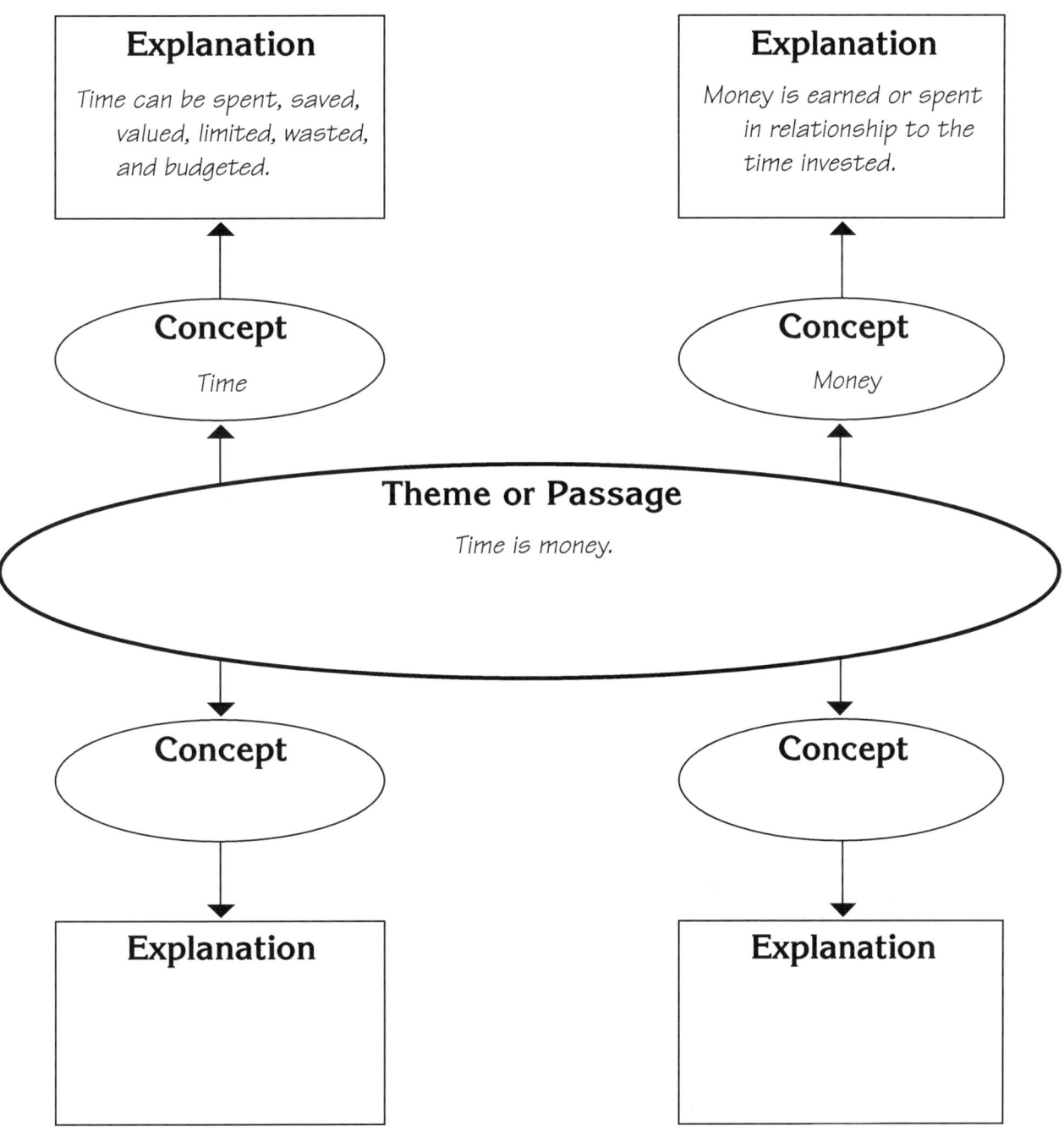

Explanation
Time can be spent, saved, valued, limited, wasted, and budgeted.

Concept
Time

Explanation
Money is earned or spent in relationship to the time invested.

Concept
Money

Theme or Passage
Time is money.

Concept

Concept

Explanation

Explanation

SUMMARY
During the Industrial Revolution, time was equated with money in many ways: workers spent their time; time was budgeted for everyone; machinery saved time for workers; and no time was wasted in the new industries. The time that was saved on work could be used by workers for something else.

© 2001 by E.H. Wiig and C.C. Wilson
Duplication permitted for educational use only.

Map It Out

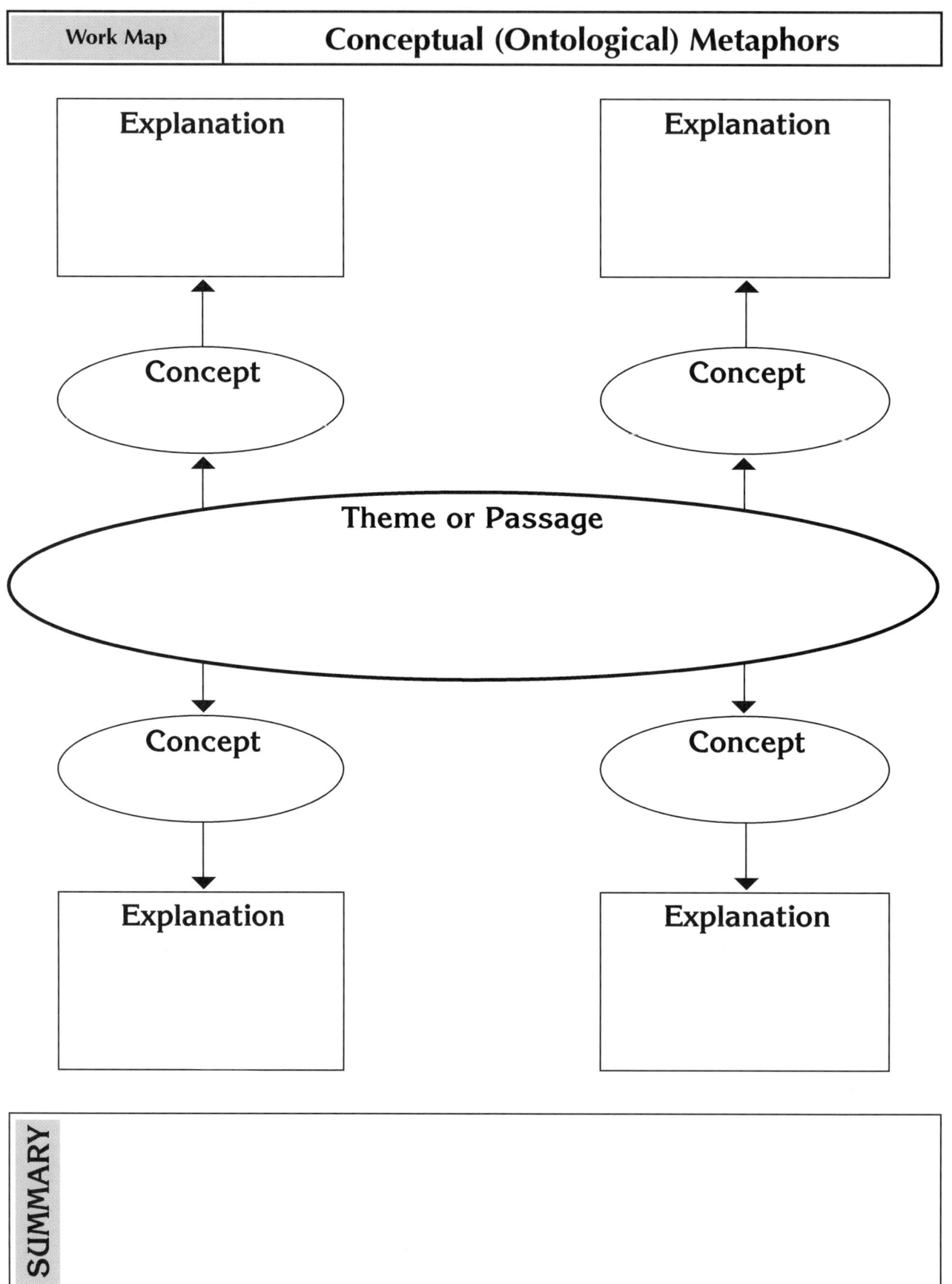

Section 2
Text Comprehension

Unit 13: Interpreting Text Titles 115

Unit 14: Story Organizer..120

Unit 15: Themes and Concepts Analysis 125

Unit 16: Story Pentad 130

Unit 17: *Who*—Story Analysis 135

Unit 18: *Where*—Story Analysis 140

Unit 19: *When*—Story Analysis 145

Unit 20: *How*—Story Analysis for Causes and Effects................................150

Unit 21: *How*—Story Analysis for Relationship Changes 155

Unit 22: *Why*—Story Analysis of Reasons
and Rationales for Actions 160

Unit 23: Dynamic Characterization 165

Unit 13: Interpreting Text Titles

> **Educational Levels**
>
> Elementary through secondary
>
> **Objectives**
>
> (1) Select, classify, and define keywords in text titles; (2) understand figurative language usage in titles; and (3) make predictions about the content of texts based on their titles

Completed Map

This map was developed by students in Grade 4. The students identified and classified the keywords in the title *Why Mosquitoes Buzz in People's Ears* by Verna Aardema. The meaning of each word and its contribution to the title were discussed, and related figurative expressions were introduced.

Show the Completed Map to students and say, for example:

> *This map shows how a group of students found and interpreted the keywords in the title* Why Mosquitoes Buzz in People's Ears. *Let's talk about the important words in the title beginning with the word* mosquitoes.

Work Map

Select a text title. Show the Work Map to students and say, for example:

> *This map is empty. Let's talk about this title. Then we'll analyze each word. When you understand the title, we will make guesses regarding what the story is about.*

Map It Out

Extended Activities

1. Bring a daily newspaper to class and select an article title. Ask students to analyze the keywords in the title and predict what the article will be about. Then read the article and compare the predicted and actual content.

2. Bring a TV guide to class and ask students to identify their favorite weekly show that subtitles each individual program. Ask students to analyze the keywords in the title of this week's show and predict what it will be about. Then tell students to watch the show and see if their predictions were close to the actual content.

3. Read a story without giving its title. Then guide students in finding keywords and phrases that can capture the theme and content of the story. After they have identified possible keywords and phrases, guide students in creating one or more titles for the story. Then compare their titles to the actual story title and discuss similarities and differences.

4. Write the titles of two or more stories, novels, or plays students can select from. Show the students each title in turn. Ask them to find and interpret keywords and phrases in the title and summarize what the text might be about. Then ask each student to select a text from the list of titles and explain why that text title appeals to him or her. You can then read a summary of the text and compare and contrast this summary with the students' predictions.

Text Comprehension

| Master Map | **Interpreting Text Titles** |

Content Words

Action Words

Title

Modifiers

Adverbial Phrases

Figurative Expressions

SUMMARY: Summary of the title and brief prediction of possible content

© 2001 by E.H. Wiig and C.C. Wilson
Duplication permitted for educational use only.

Map It Out

| **Completed Map** | **Interpreting Text Titles** |

Content Words
Mosquitoes
Ears

Action Words
Buzz

Title
Why Mosquitoes Buzz in People's Ears

Modifiers
People's

Adverbial Phrases
Why mosquitoes buzz

Figurative Expressions
Buzz—a bug in your ear

SUMMARY

The story will tell about funny reasons why and descriptions about how mosquitoes make the whining or buzzing sound that people hear.

© 2001 by E.H. Wiig and C.C. Wilson
Duplication permitted for educational use only.

Text Comprehension

| Work Map | Interpreting Text Titles |

Content Words

Action Words

Title

Modifiers

Adverbial Phrases

Figurative Expressions

SUMMARY

© 2001 by E.H. Wiig and C.C. Wilson
Duplication permitted for educational use only.

119

Map It Out

Unit 14: Story Organizer

> **Educational Level**
>
> Elementary
>
> **Objectives**
>
> (1) Identify story characters, settings, problems, and solutions; (2) organize topics within stories to form a narrative plan; and (3) retell stories

Completed Map

The map shows how students in Grade 2 analyzed and organized the content of *Goldilocks and the Three Bears*.

Show the Completed Map to students and say, for example:

> *This map shows what some students thought was important in the story* Goldilocks and the Three Bears. *Let's look at and talk about the important parts of the story beginning with the characters.*

You may want to follow up by asking, for example:

> *What else do you remember about Goldilocks? What else do you remember about the three bears? What else do you remember about the bears' house? What would you have done if you were Goldilocks?*

Work Map

Select a story. Show the Work Map to students and say, for example:

> *This map is empty. Let's read and talk about this story. Then we'll identify the characters, settings, problems, and solutions. When we have done that, I will ask you to retell the story by using this information.*

Extended Activities

1. Lay out four large colored-paper squares (e.g., green for characters and red for solutions) on the floor to simulate a narrative plan. The plan can move from left to right or from beginning to end. Then ask students to retell a part of a familiar children's story as they stand in the colored box for that story segment. You can walk one student through all squares or place a different student on each square (i.e., several students share the task of retelling the story).

2. Give students a picture of a familiar context (e.g., a circus scene). Ask them to make up characters, events, problems, and solutions to go with the picture. Enter the students' responses and then ask them to create their own stories in response to the picture and story components.

3. Read a fable to students and guide them in analyzing it for characters, settings, problems, solutions, and morals.

4. Ask students to analyze a familiar children's story (e.g., *The Three Little Pigs*). Then ask them to make up their own story with the same characters and similar events but set in today's world (e.g., the wolf might have used a bulldozer to level the houses).

5. Fill in a map's response boxes for characters, settings, and problems. Have each student to use the information to make up a story. Compare the stories the students create and discuss similarities and differences.

Map It Out

| Master Map | Story Organizer |

Characters

Who was the story about?

Who else was in the story?

Settings

Where did the story happen?

What other places were in the story?

When did the story happen?

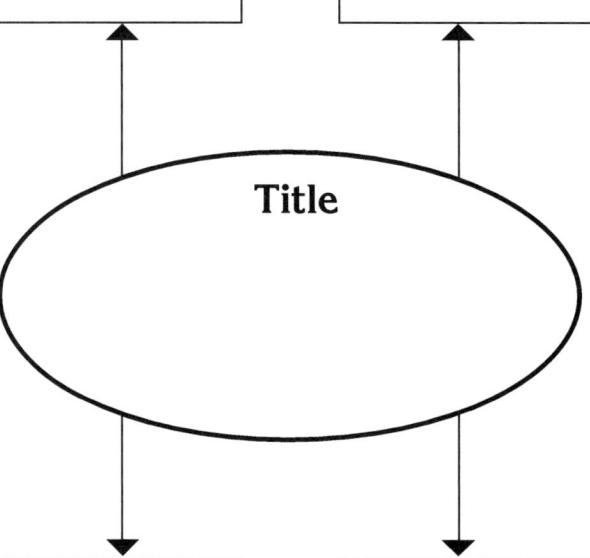

Title

Problems

What were the problems in the story?

Solutions

How were the problems solved?

SUMMARY — Record of the story events

Text Comprehension

| Completed Map | Story Organizer |

Characters

Goldilocks—a little girl who liked to explore

Papa Bear—a very large male bear

Mama Bear—a medium-sized female bear

Baby Bear—a small bear

Settings

In the three bears' house

In the woods

In spring or summer

Title

Goldilocks and the Three Bears

Problems

Goldilocks went into the bears' house and used their things without permission.

Goldilocks got very frightened by the three bears.

Solutions

Goldilocks ran home.

After she told her mother what happened, Goldilocks promised she would never again go into someone's house without permission.

SUMMARY

Goldilocks went for a walk in the woods and saw a house. She went inside, ate some porridge, sat on three nice chairs, and went upstairs to take a nap. Then the three bears who lived in the house returned. They looked at the porridge bowls and chairs and knew someone was there. They went upstairs and found Goldilocks. She woke up, got scared, and ran home. Her mom told her never to go into strangers' houses.

© 2001 by E.H. Wiig and C.C. Wilson
Duplication permitted for educational use only.

Map It Out

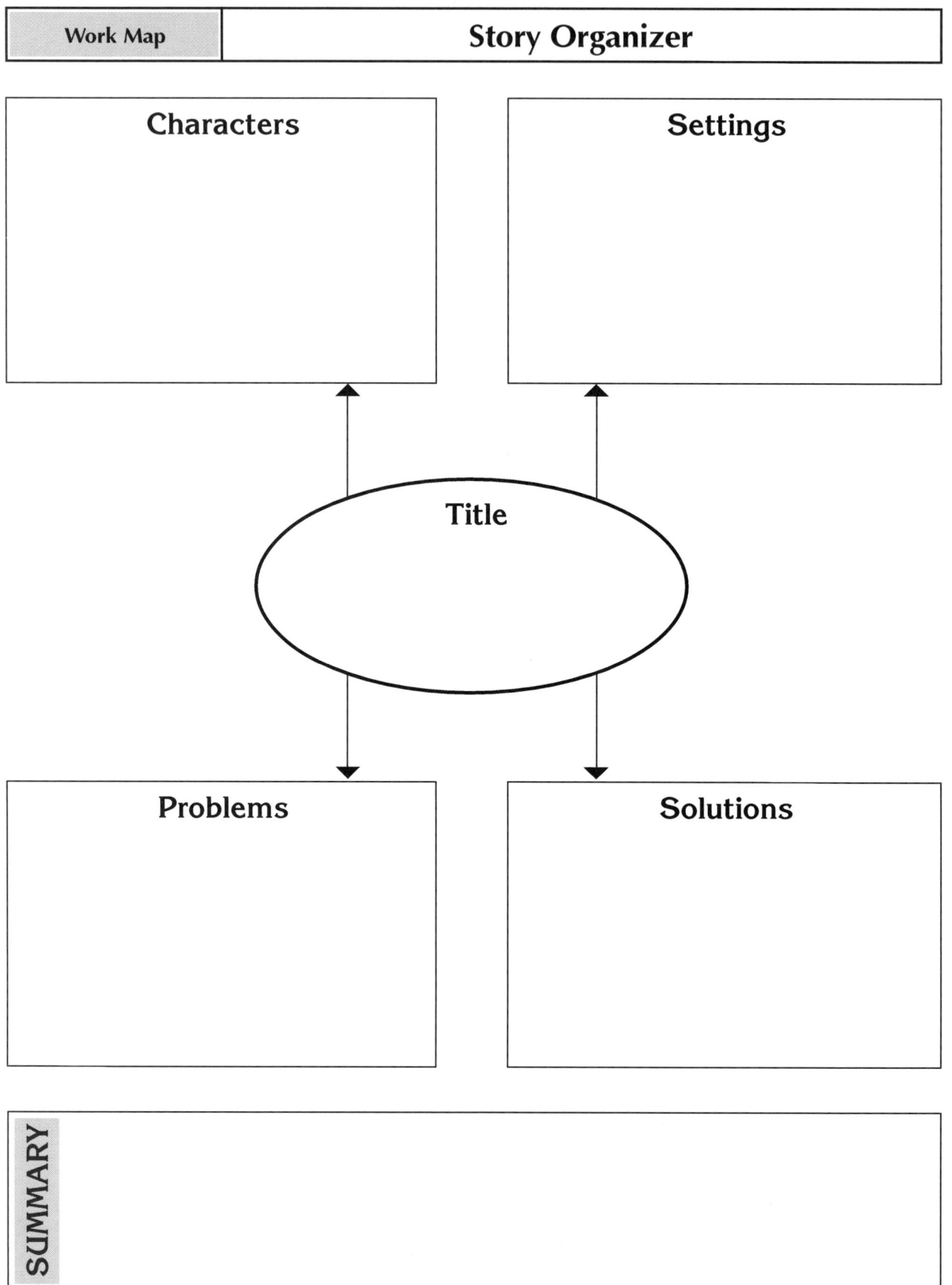

Text Comprehension

Unit 15: Themes and Concepts Analysis

> **Educational Levels**
>
> Upper elementary through secondary
>
> **Objectives**
>
> (1) Identify major and secondary themes in texts; (2) identify and categorize important words and concepts associated with those themes; and (3) interpret and define the identified words and concepts

Completed Map

The map shows how students in Grade 5 analyzed an assigned lesson on deserts. To begin, they identified the major and then the secondary theme. Then they found, categorized, and wrote down the important words and concepts associated with each theme. The class then discussed the elements of deserts and how they related to each other.

Show the Completed Map to students and say, for example:

> *This map shows how students described the themes in a social studies lesson about deserts. Let's talk about the themes and the important words and concepts that go with them.*

You may want to follow up for facts and details by asking, for example:

> *Do you know anything else about deserts that is not on this map?*

Work Map

Select a text. Show the Work Map to students and say, for example:

> *This map is empty. Let's read and talk about this text and identify the major and secondary theme. Then I will ask you to find important words and concepts related to the themes in the text. When you have grouped the words and concepts, we will discuss what they tell about the theme and talk about their meanings.*

Map It Out

Extended Activities

1. Ask students to analyze each chapter of an assigned novel (e.g., *The Outsiders* by S.E. Hinton) by identifying the themes and associated words and concepts.

2. Bring a newspaper or magazine article on a current topic to class. Read the article, and ask students questions to identify the major and secondary themes covered and the words and concepts associated with them.

3. Assign a TV show for students to watch at home. Have each student analyze the themes in the TV show. Share the completed maps, and discuss how the responses to the same TV show are similar or different according to students' perspectives. The objective is to show that two people can see the same events and interactions and yet analyze and report on them in very different ways (i.e., take different perspectives).

4. Read a novel designated in the curriculum in which the same events are viewed and described by different characters with different perspectives. An advanced example is the *Alexandria Quartet* by Lawrence Durrell. This is a series of four novels. Each chronicles a similar set of events but is told through different perspectives and covers different themes.

Text Comprehension

Master Map	**Themes and Concepts Analysis**

Characteristics
Features
Concrete descriptions

Conditions
States of being
Static versus dynamic

Primary Theme

Causes
Causal events related to the theme, its development, or both

Effects
Outcomes of the causal events

Secondary Theme

Characteristics
Features
Concrete descriptions

Conditions
States of being
Static versus dynamic

Causes
Causal events related to the theme, its development, or both

Effects
Outcomes of the causal events

SUMMARY: Discussion of each theme and the relationship between the two themes

Map It Out

| Completed Map | **Themes and Concepts Analysis** |

Primary Theme: Deserts

Characteristics
Sand, dunes, ridges, channels, boulders, mountains, oases

Conditions
Dry, barren, cloudless, hot or cold

Causes
Extreme temperature, rare cloudbursts

Effects
Reptiles, mammals, shrubs, blossoms, cactus

Secondary Theme: Natural Resources

Characteristics
Minerals, oil, gas, gold, silver, rich soil for agriculture

Conditions
Changes, increased use

Causes
Irrigation, cultivation, mining, drilling

Effects
Agriculture, farmlands, mines, oil rigs

SUMMARY

Deserts have great potential for people of the future. Deserts can be changed from being dry and barren by providing irrigation. The soil is rich and can be cultivated to provide agricultural resources. Deserts are also rich in mineral deposits, gas, oil, gold, and silver. Drilling and mining can make these resources available for use.

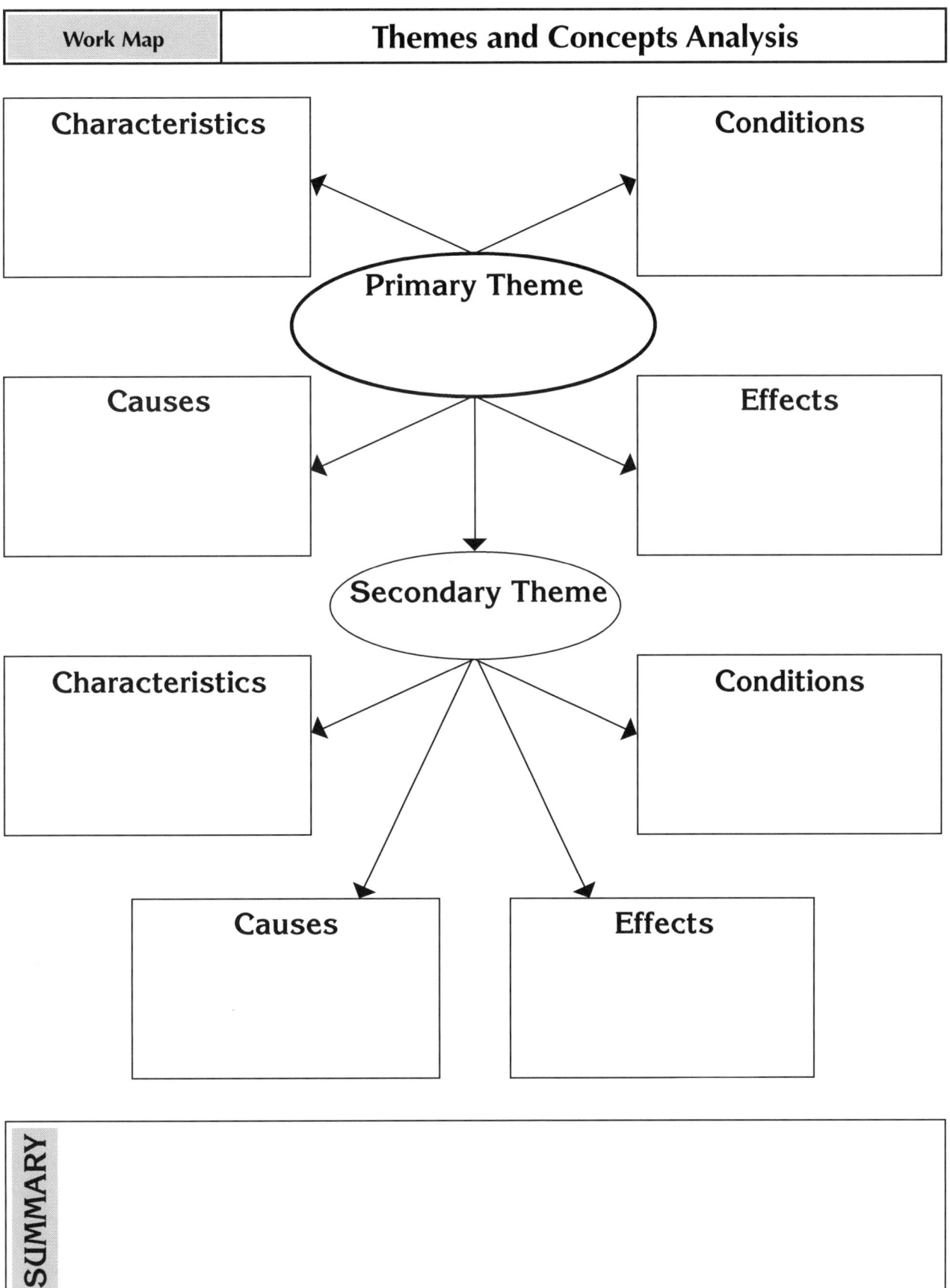

Map It Out

Unit 16: Story Pentad

Educational Levels

Upper elementary through secondary

Objectives

(1) Identify story characters, settings, and time periods; (2) list important actions and events; (3) identify and describe an author's purpose in writing a text; and (4) analyze how an author's purpose is achieved

Completed Map

The map shows how students in Grade 5 analyzed the story *Sunday for Sona* by Gladys Yessayan Cretan. The teacher guided the analysis by asking *wh*-questions to elicit responses for each box. The students' answers were recorded and discussed to make comparisons, introduce cause-effect relationships, develop an understanding of the author's purpose for writing the story, and explain how the author achieved that purpose.

Show the Completed Map to students and say, for example:

> *This map shows an example of the five main components and features identified in the story* Sunday for Sona. *Let's begin by considering the question, "Who is in the story?"*

Work Map

Show the Work Map to students and say, for example:

> *This map is empty. Let's talk about a story or chapter in a story you have read recently. Then we'll organize and analyze the text.*

Extended Activities

1. Ask students to read a story or other story-based literary work (e.g., a poem or play) from the curriculum and then analyze it in teams or independently.

2. Have each student analyze a TV show of his or her choosing that has social content. Share the maps, and discuss how they are different and how they are alike. Then ask each student to discuss how the episode he or she saw fits into the overall story of the TV series.

3. Bring a newspaper editorial to class. As a class, analyze the content of the editorial. Then guide a discussion of the students' opinions about the editor's views.

Map It Out

| Master Map | Story Pentad |

Who
Who were the major and secondary characters?

What
What were the main actions or events?

Title

Where & When
Where and when did the story take place?

Why
What was the main idea?
What was the writer's purpose?

How
How did the writer get the main idea across?
How did the writer achieve the purpose?

SUMMARY: Synopsis of the five main story components

Text Comprehension

| Completed Map | Story Pentad |

Who
Sona, Nana, Tommy, Mr. O'Brien

What
Sona longed to sail and found a way, but she disobeyed Nana by running away to sail.
In the end, Nana allowed Sona to sail.

Title
Sunday for Sona

Where & When
Nana's house, the boat, near Golden Gate bridge
Present day in spring or summer

Why
To show a person's feeling of wanting something very badly

How
By describing Sona's desire to sail and her hard work to make it happen

SUMMARY
This story was about a girl named Sona who wanted to sail very badly. She disobeyed Nana and went to help Tommy and his father prepare their boat for sailing. Sona was punished for disobeying. When Nana saw how hard Sona and Tommy had worked, she allowed Sona to continue. When the boat was ready, Nana joined Sona, Tommy, and his father for a sail.

© 2001 by E.H. Wiig and C.C. Wilson
Duplication permitted for educational use only.

Map It Out

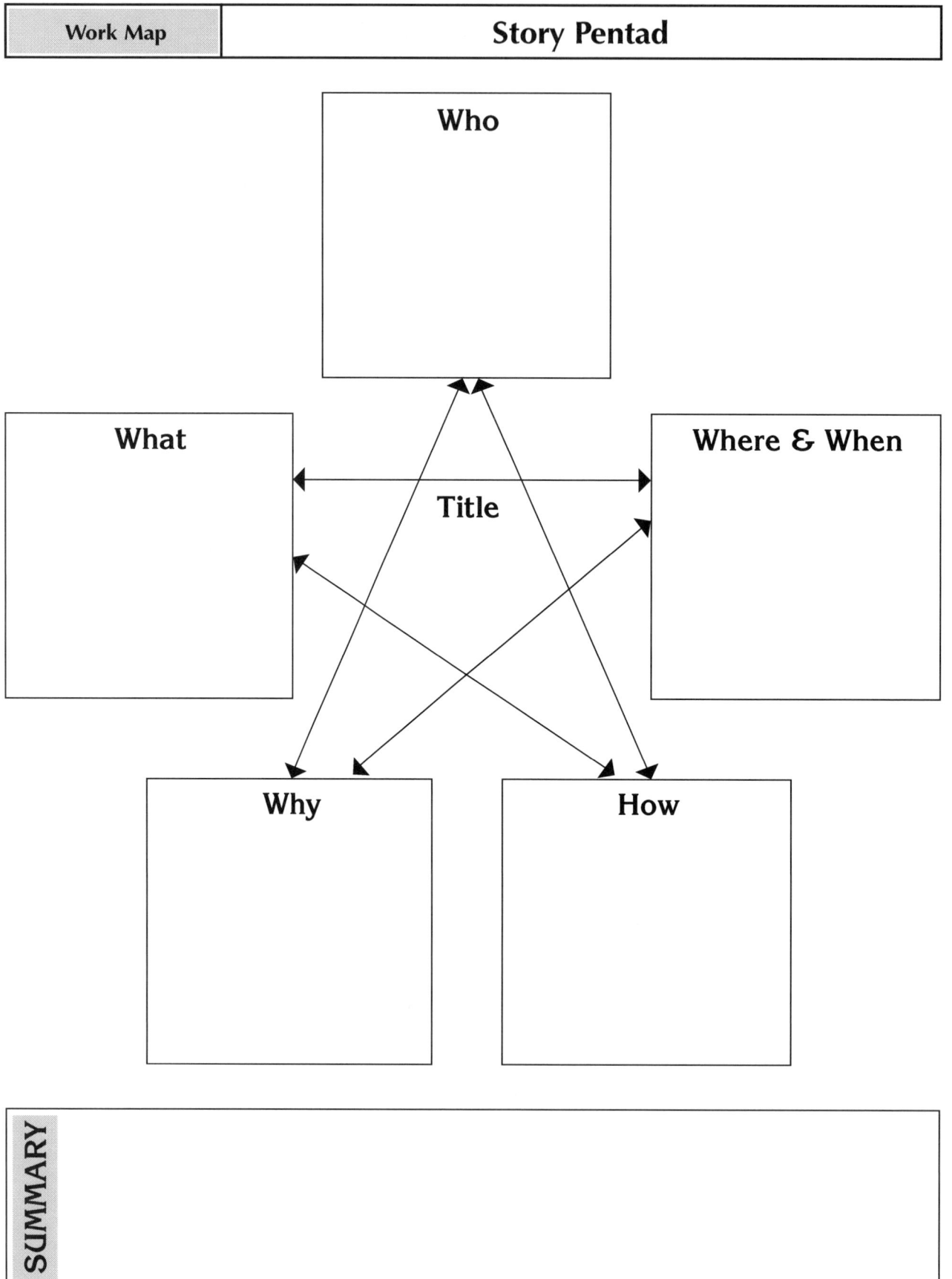

Text Comprehension

Unit 17: *Who*—Story Analysis

Educational Levels

Upper elementary through secondary

Objectives

(1) Identify and describe characters by their physical and personality traits; and (2) analyze, compare, and evaluate characters

Completed Map

This map shows an example of how students in Grade 6 analyzed the characters in *The Giver* by Lois Lowry. To begin, they analyzed the main character, Jonas. Then they analyzed the supporting characters and listed characteristics as they remembered them. The character's physical and personality traits were then compared and contrasted.

Show the Completed Map to students and say, for example:

> *This map shows an example of how a group of students described the characters in a novel called* The Giver. *Let's talk about the characters, beginning with the main character, Jonas.*

Emphasize that physical traits, typical behaviors, and personality traits can describe characters.

You may want to follow up by asking, for example:

> *What is special about Jonas? What is special about The Giver? Which characters have something in common or look alike? What other characters do you find interesting? Why?*

Work Map

Show the Work Map to students and say, for example:

> *This map is empty. Let's think of a story you have read. Then we'll name and describe each character by his or her physical traits and behaviors and personality traits.*

Map It Out

Extended Activities

1. Have each student analyze the members of his or her immediate or extended families, beginning with himself or herself as the main character.

2. Elicit descriptions from the students about you (i.e., the main character) and one or more classmates (i.e., the supporting characters). Then have each student integrate and summarize his or her perceptions. You may want to share the analyses, provided that they focus on positives and interpersonal understanding.

3. After students have read a story or novel, show them a map with descriptions but without characters' names. Ask students to identify the name of each character and add other descriptions.

4. Ask students to analyze the characters in an assigned or favorite TV series. Have them identify and describe the main character first and supporting cast members second. Discuss the relationships among the characters and how the characteristics of each play a role in the interactions (e.g., by creating humor).

5. Ask students to analyze the characters in a play assigned in the curriculum (e.g., Shakespeare's *Romeo and Juliet*). Then assign the film *West Side Story,* and ask students to analyze the characters. After the analyses are completed, compare the characters in these related dramatic works, and discuss similarities and differences.

Text Comprehension

| Master Map | *Who*—Story Analysis |

Physical Traits & Behaviors
- Looks
- Acts

Personality Traits
- Feels
- Thinks

Main Character

Title

Secondary Characters

Character
- Physical traits and behaviors
- Personality traits

Character
- Physical traits and behaviors
- Personality traits

Character
- Physical traits and behaviors
- Personality traits

Character
- Physical traits and behaviors
- Personality traits

Character
- Physical traits and behaviors
- Personality traits

SUMMARY
Summary of character interactions

© 2001 by E.H. Wiig and C.C. Wilson
Duplication permitted for educational use only.

Map It Out

| Completed Map | **Who**—Story Analysis |

Physical Traits & Behaviors
11 years old, pale eyes, dark hair, tall for age, rode a bike, went to learning center

Personality Traits
Did many volunteer jobs, was careful about language, had "depth," received memories

Main Character
Jonas

Title
The Giver

Secondary Characters
The Giver, Gabe, Lily, Mom, Dad

Character
The Giver—Very old, pale eyes, kept memories, used books, gave memories to Jonas

Character
Dad—Nurturer, good-natured, patient, quiet, cared for babies

Character
Gabe—Under 1 year old, pale eyes, happy

Character
Mom—Worked for Department of Justice, enforced rules

Character
Lily—7 years old, talked a lot

SUMMARY

The most important character was called Jonas. He was a very likable boy, and he had pale eyes, which was important in this story. The Giver was another important person. He was old and wise and kept the memories of the pain and pleasure of life. He had the pale eyes that went with the wisdom of a Giver. Jonas was chosen to receive the memories from The Giver.

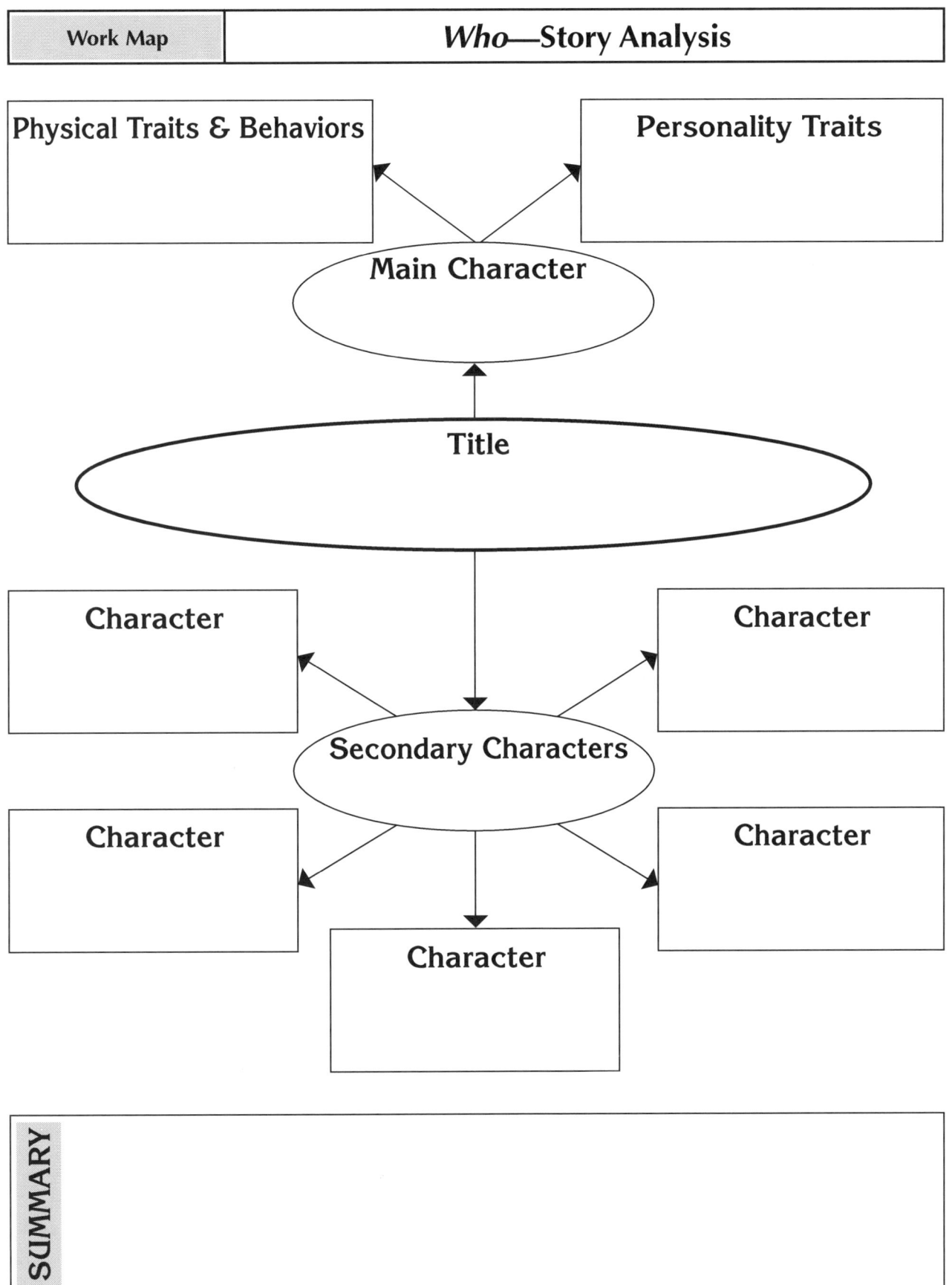

Map It Out

Unit 18: *Where*—Story Analysis

> **Educational Levels**
>
> Upper elementary through secondary
>
> **Objectives**
>
> (1) Organize and understand primary and secondary settings in texts; and (2) compare and contrast features of settings

Completed Map

This map came from students in Grade 6. They were asked to analyze the settings featured in *The Giver* by Lois Lowry. They were asked to enter the names and characteristics of settings and the characters and events associated with the settings. The teacher then guided a compare and contrast activity in which the students identified the important similarities and differences between settings.

Show the Completed Map to students and say, for example:

> *This map shows an example of how students described the settings in a novel called* The Giver. *Let's talk about the settings, beginning with the most important one—the Community.*

Emphasize that name, location, physical characteristics, and components can describe settings.

You may want to follow up by asking:

> *What is special about the Community? What is special about Elsewhere? How is the Community the same as or different from where you live? Where would you prefer to live? Why?*

Work Map

Show the Work Map to students and say, for example:

This map is empty. Let's use a story you have read recently and name and describe the settings in it.

Extended Activities

1. Ask students to describe and analyze one or more familiar settings, such as school and home. Follow up with a compare and contrast activity between the home setting and school setting.

2. Select two or more communities the students are exploring in social studies. The communities can be local, regional, national, or international. Have each student analyze and describe the selected settings. Guide an activity where students share and compare their findings.

3. Have each student select two or more popular TV comedy or drama series; view an episode of each series; and analyze, compare, and contrast the two settings. Prepare students to share and discuss their findings.

4. Have each student analyze two or more settings featured in a novel or a play that is part of the curriculum. Share the maps, and discuss the differences in what the students found important.

5. Ask students to analyze each of the settings in two related works (e.g., *Julie of the Wolves* by Jean Craighead George and *White Fang* by Jack London or *Romeo and Juliet* by William Shakespeare and *West Side Story* by Irving Shulman). Then guide a compare and contrast activity.

Map It Out

| Master Map | *Where*—Story Analysis |

Primary Setting

Components (name, location)
Characteristics
Reasons for importance (functions)

Title

Secondary Setting

Components (name, location)
Characteristics
Reasons for importance (functions)

Secondary Setting

Components (name, location)
Characteristics
Reasons for importance (functions)

SUMMARY — Discussion of the significance of and interaction among settings

Text Comprehension

| **Completed Map** | *Where*—Story Analysis |

Primary Setting
The Community

Jonas's house—exactly like all other houses in the Community; House of the Old and Annex—where The Giver lived and had his books; the Nurturing Center—where Dad worked taking care of the children; Department of Justice—where Mom worked enforcing the rules; House of the Elders—where ceremonies took place; the Learning Center—where Jonas went to school

Title
The Giver

Secondary Setting

The River

The river runs on the outskirts of the Community.

It separates the Community from Elsewhere.

Secondary Setting

Elsewhere

Elsewhere is on the other side of the river and far away.

Everyone has memory and can make choices in Elsewhere.

SUMMARY

There were three different settings in the story. The most important one was called the Community. It was futuristic and everyone had and did the same. Only The Giver could make choices because he had the memories of the true pains and pleasures of life. The river separated the Community from Elsewhere. In Elsewhere, things were not ruled and regulated and everyone had memory and could make choices.

© 2001 by E.H. Wiig and C.C. Wilson
Duplication permitted for educational use only.

Map It Out

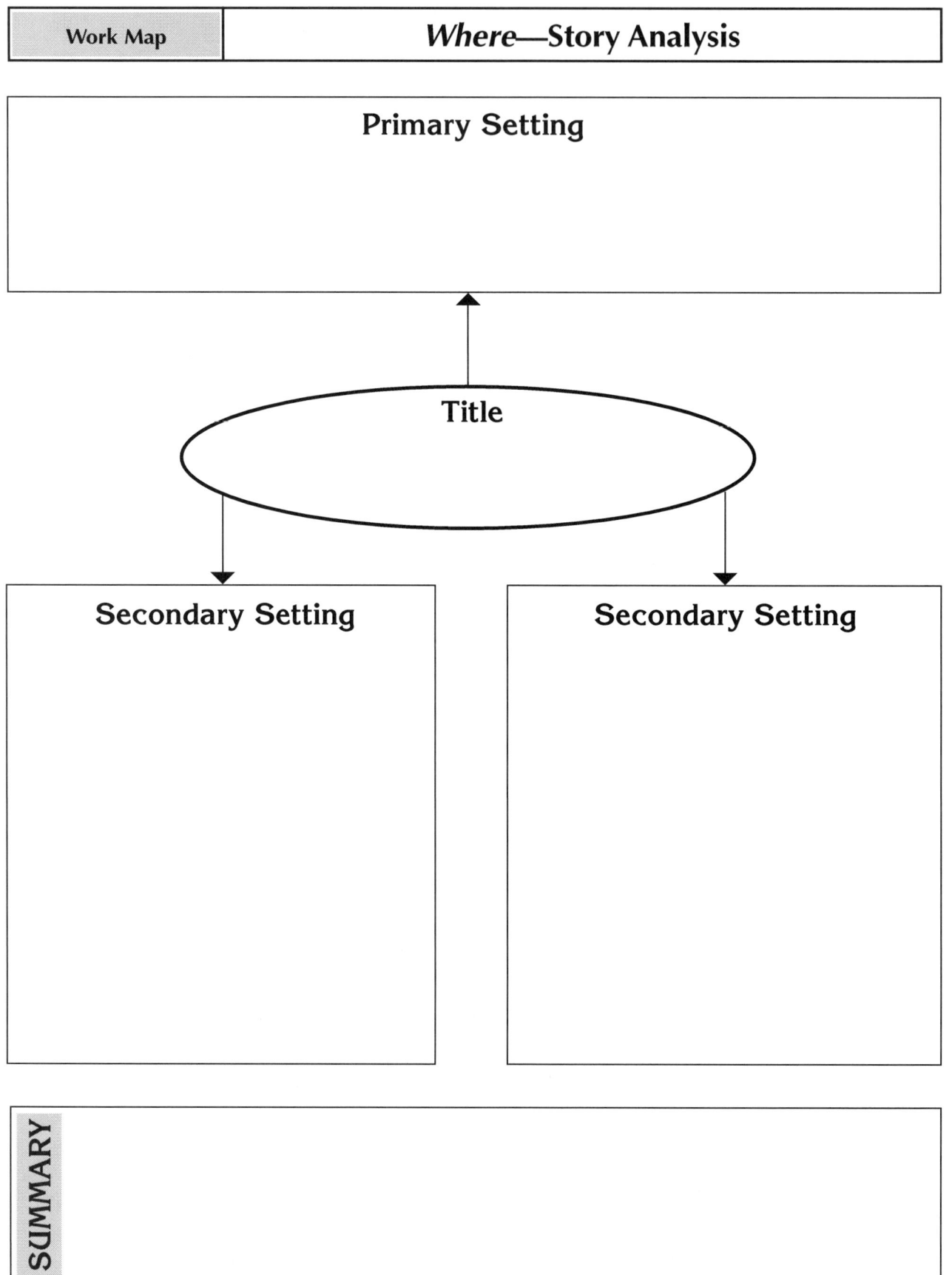

Unit 19: *When*—Story Analysis

> ### Educational Levels
> Upper elementary through secondary
>
> ### Objectives
> (1) Identify major time periods; (2) identify major events; (3) associate time periods with events; and (4) connect events and time periods in a dynamic visual representation

Completed Map

This map shows how students in Grade 6 analyzed the relationships between events and time periods in *April Morning* by Howard Fast. The students first analyzed and recorded the events in the story in chronological order. Then they identified the major time period during which the events happened.

Show the Completed Map to students and say, for example:

> *This map shows an example of how students organized the time periods and events in the novel* April Morning. *Let's talk about the events and the time each occurred.*

Emphasize that each of the smaller time periods was part of one large time period that consisted of only one day.

You may want to extend the introduction by asking questions, such as:

> *How could you organize important time periods in your life in blocks on a time line? What events do you associate with each of the major time-period blocks of your life time line?*

Map It Out

Work Map

Select a story. Show the Work Map to students and say, for example:

This map is empty. Let's read and talk about this story. Then we'll organize the events and time periods in the story.

Extended Activities

1. Have each student analyze an event (e.g., a car accident) that happened in his or her life and indicate the time periods when the subevents (e.g., got in the car and drove too fast) occurred. Students may select ages or stages as indicators of the time of events.

2. Select a lesson from social studies that deals with historical events and times. Ask students to analyze the order of major historical events and the times when they occurred.

3. Ask students to analyze a story, single chapter in a novel, or complete novel for the major events described and the times they occurred.

4. Divide students into teams to analyze the major events and times that occur in two related texts (e.g., *Julie of the Wolves* by Jean Craighead George and *White Fang* by Jack London or *Romeo and Juliet* by William Shakespeare and *West Side Story* by Irving Shulman). Share and compare the map produced for each text. Discuss similarities and differences in the relationships between events and times in the two texts.

Text Comprehension

| Master Map | *When*—Story Analysis |

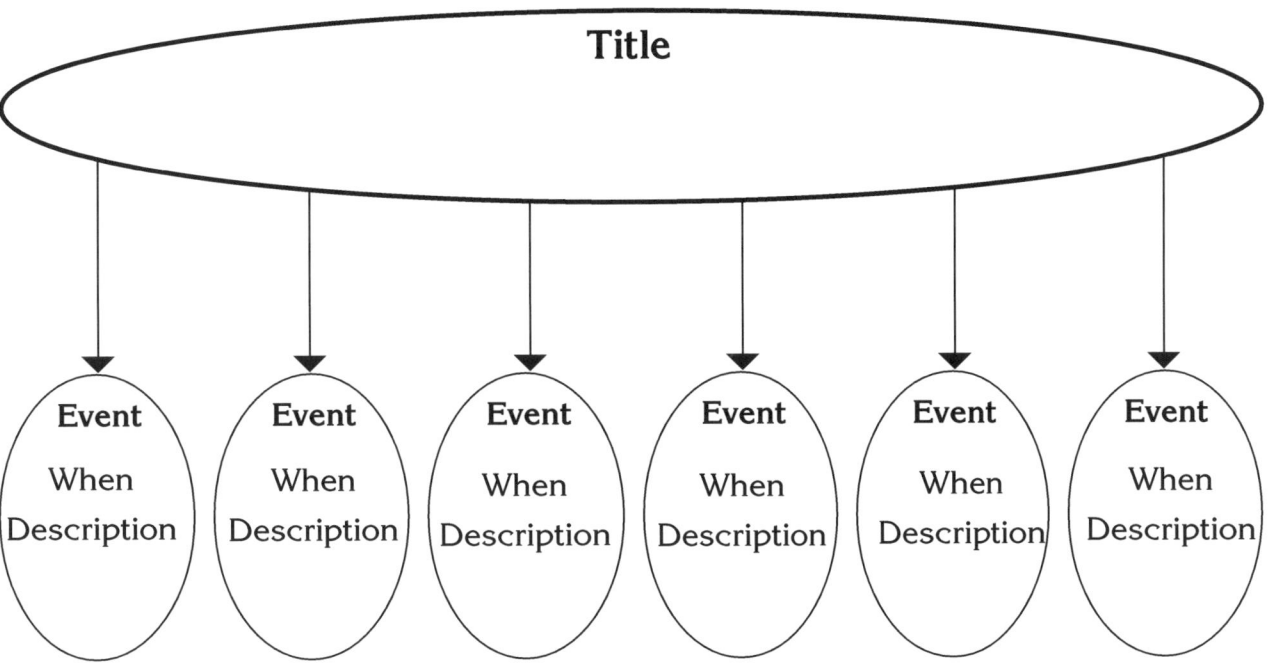

Beginning ———————————————————————→ End

Blocks of Time

| Dates/Time period
Name of block | → | Dates/Time period
Name of block | → | Dates/Time period
Name of block |

SUMMARY: Overview of the story in time-element periods

© 2001 by E.H. Wiig and C.C. Wilson
Duplication permitted for educational use only.

147

Map It Out

| Completed Map | *When*—Story Analysis |

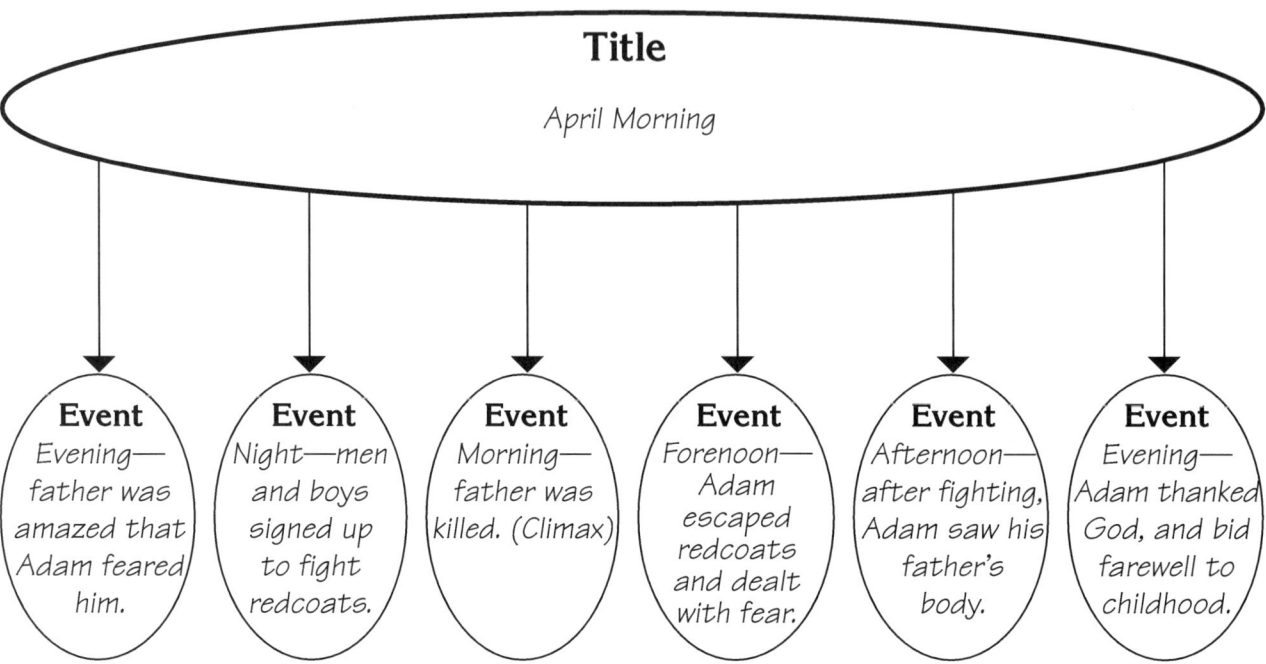

Title: April Morning

Event: Evening—father was amazed that Adam feared him.

Event: Night—men and boys signed up to fight redcoats.

Event: Morning—father was killed. (Climax)

Event: Forenoon—Adam escaped redcoats and dealt with fear.

Event: Afternoon—after fighting, Adam saw his father's body.

Event: Evening—Adam thanked God, and bid farewell to childhood.

Beginning →→→ End

Blocks of Time

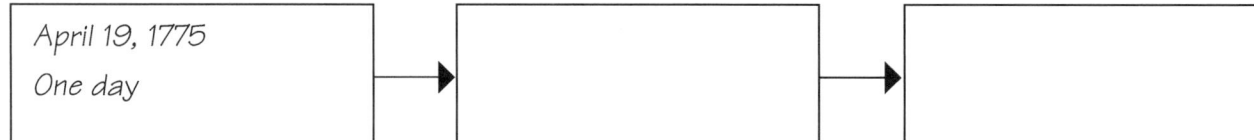

April 19, 1775
One day

SUMMARY

The events in this story happened in a single day in April 1775. The evening before, Adam was a boy who feared and hated his father. During the night, he and his father signed up to fight the redcoats. Adam's father was killed in the early morning, but Adam escaped. Adam saw his father's body in a casket that afternoon. That evening, he thanked God for his escape and knew that his childhood was over. He had become a man.

Text Comprehension

| Work Map | *When*—Story Analysis |

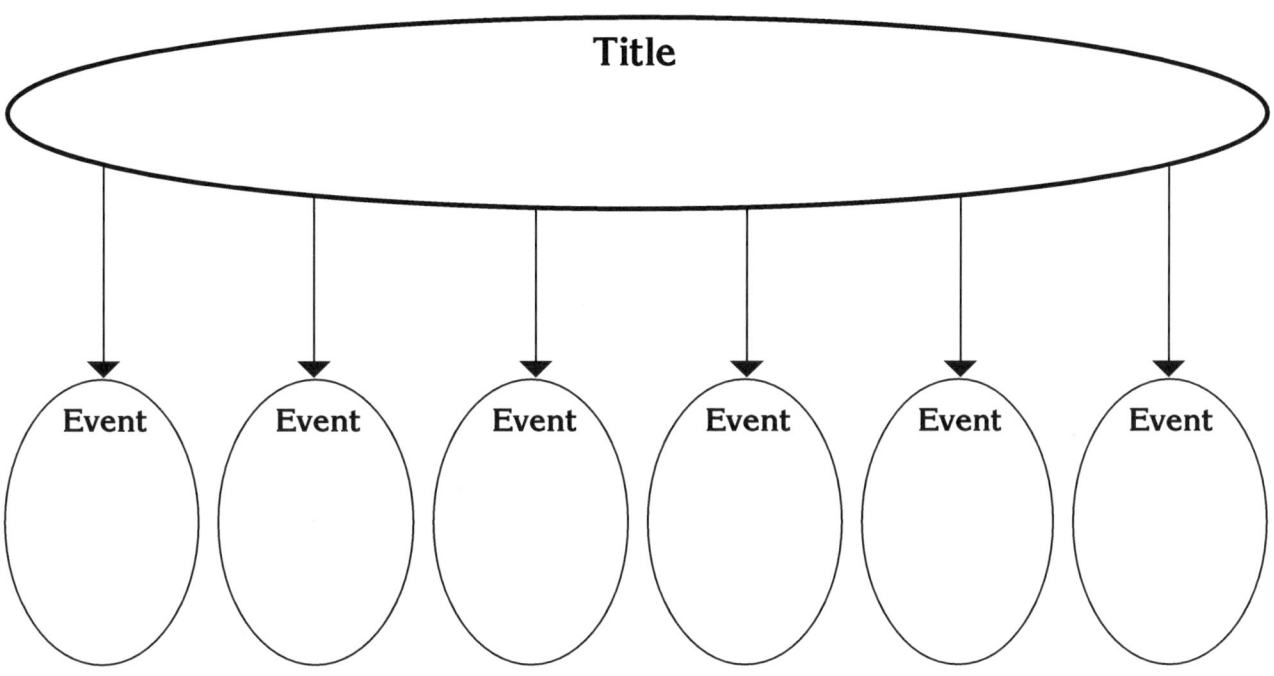

Beginning → **End**

Blocks of Time

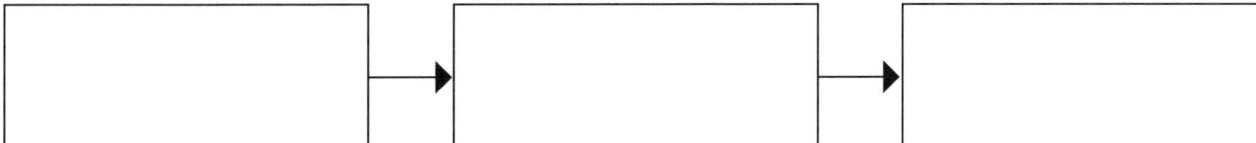

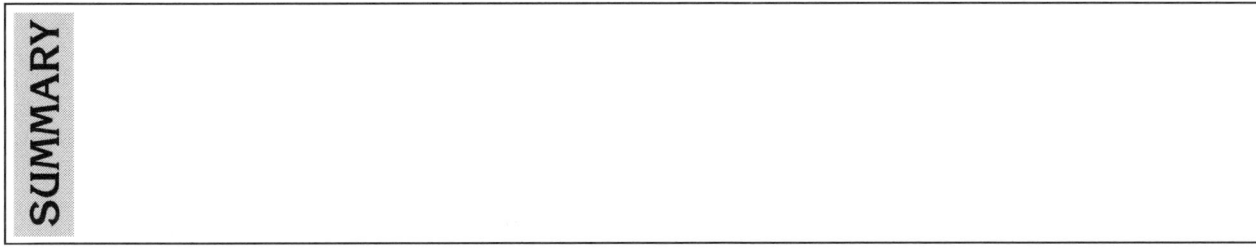

SUMMARY

Map It Out

Unit 20: *How*—Story Analysis for Causes and Effects

> **Educational Levels**
>
> Upper elementary through secondary
>
> **Objectives**
>
> (1) Identify objectives, intents, major reasons, and driving forces; (2) record specific causes and effects; and (3) connect causes and effects to understand dynamic relationships

Completed Map

This map shows how students in Grade 6 analyzed and integrated causes and effects in *April Morning* by Howard Fast. They focused on what happened and how it affected Adam's life on the day of the battle with the redcoats. They discussed which cause-effect relationships were based on actions by Adam or others and which were based in Adam's emotions and reactions on that day.

Show the Completed Map to students and say, for example:

> *This map shows an example of how students described the relationships among events in the novel* April Morning. *Let's talk about the causes for events, the effects of events, and how the causes and effects are related.*

You may want to extend the introduction by asking, for example:

> *How could you analyze an important event in your life to show the causes and effects and the relationships between them?*

Work Map

Select a story. Show the Work Map to students and say, for example:

> *This map is empty. Let's read and talk about this story and the major events in it. Then we'll analyze and evaluate the important events for the cause-effect relationships in the story.*

Extended Activities

1. Have each student identify, analyze, and describe the cause-effect relationships in a major event or change in his or her life. Possible events include (1) the first day of school, (2) the arrival of a younger sibling, (3) a religious ceremony, or (4) moving into a different house. Prepare students to share their work.

2. Select a current event reported by newspaper, magazine, or TV news sources. Ask students to identify causes and effects and discuss the possible relationships between them.

3. Ask students to analyze a short story or novel that is part of the curriculum for cause-effect relationships. Because causes are often implied and not explicitly stated in fiction, students should be asked to identify the stated causes versus those that they inferred.

4. Select a play that is assigned in the curriculum (e.g., Shakespeare's *Romeo and Juliet*), and ask students to analyze and relate major outcomes with their stated or implied causes. You may want to ask guided questions to support the activity.

5. Ask students to read two related stories, novels, or plays that are part of the curriculum (e.g., *Julie of the Wolves* by Jean Craighead George and *White Fang* by Jack London). Ask students to analyze the causes and effects in each text. Then guide a discussion to compare and contrast the causes and effects in the two texts and identify similarities and differences.

Map It Out

| Master Map | *How*—Story Analysis for Causes and Effects |

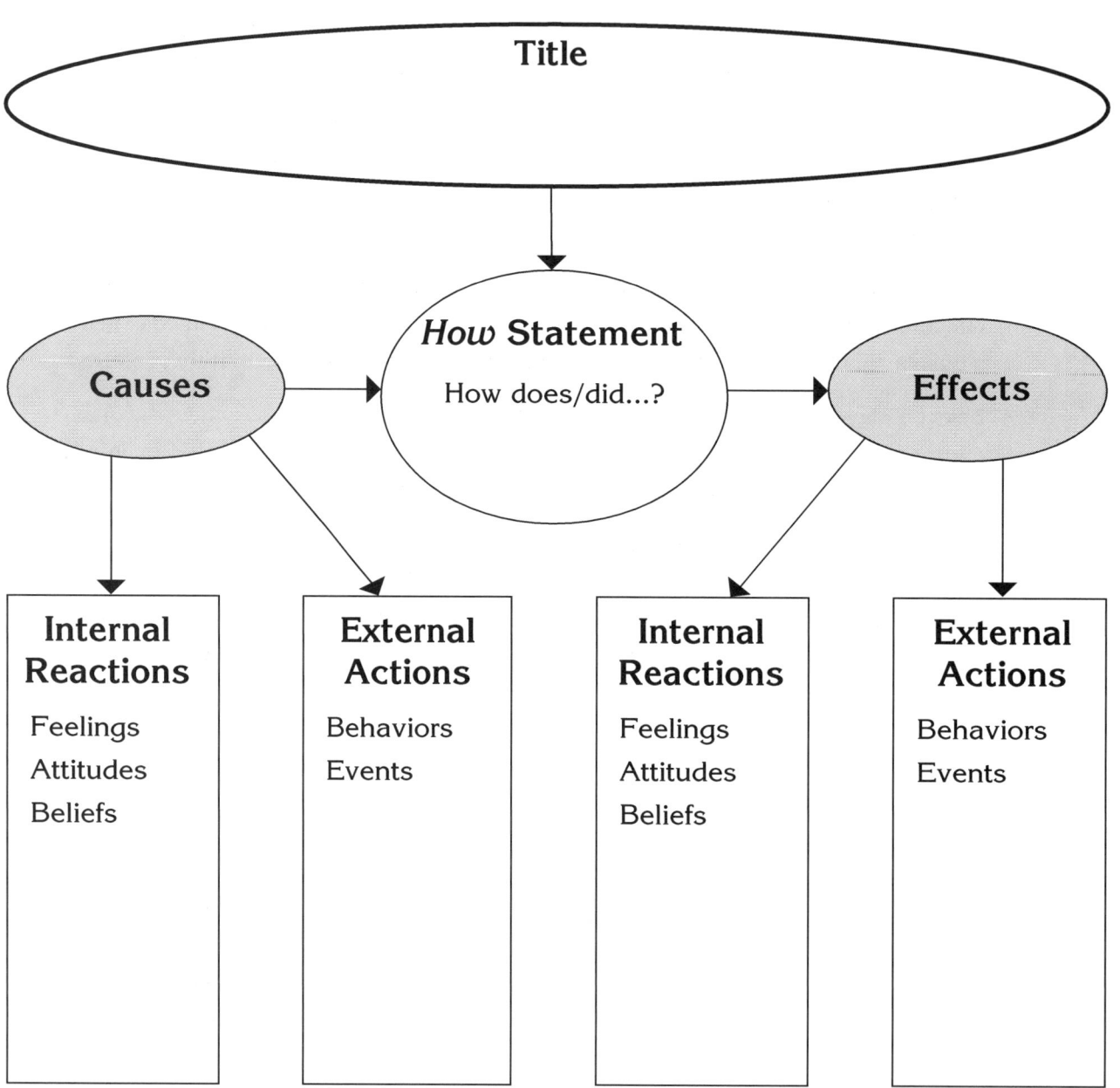

152 © 2001 by E.H. Wiig and C.C. Wilson
Duplication permitted for educational use only.

Text Comprehension

Completed Map | *How*—Story Analysis for Causes and Effects

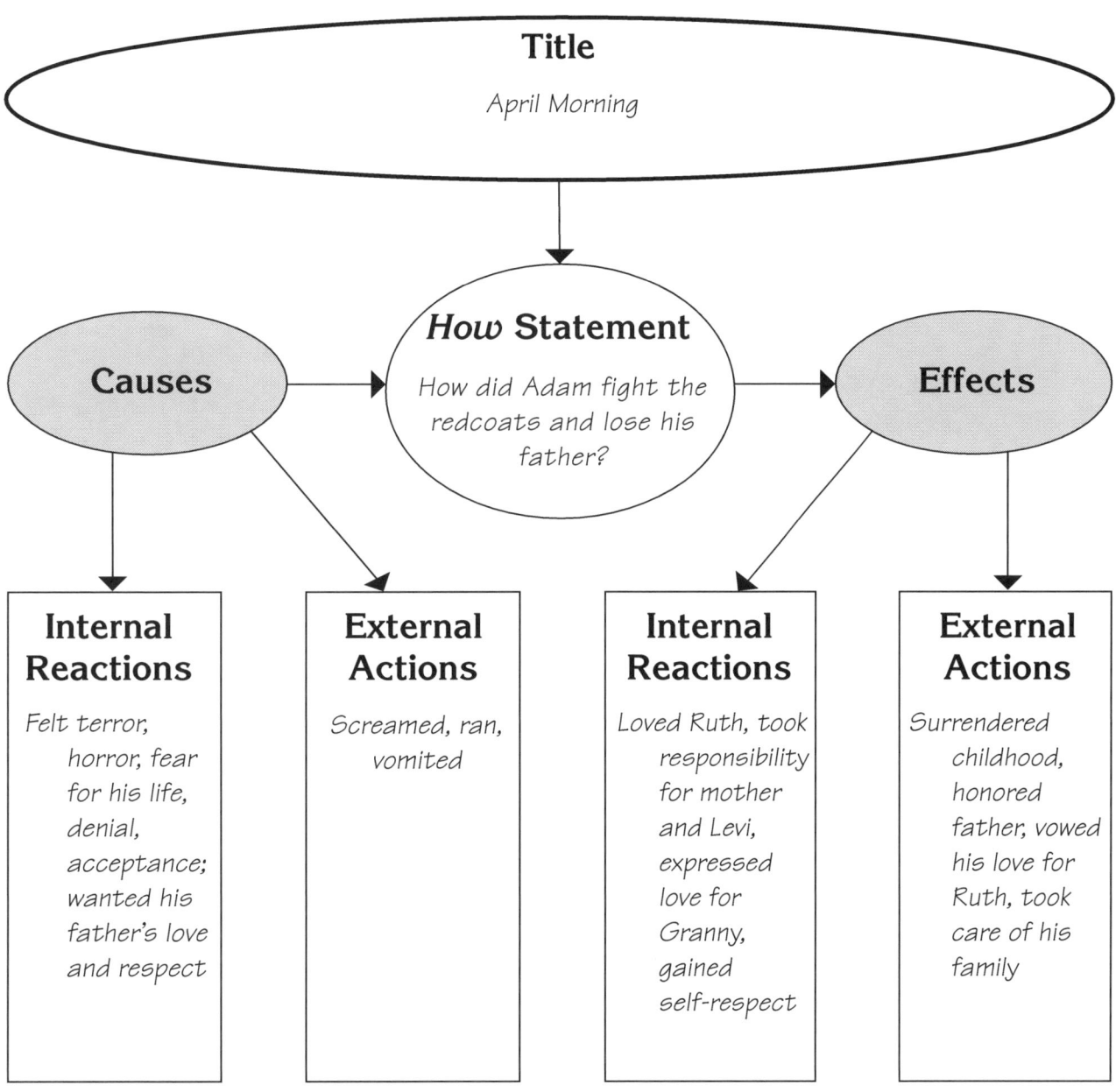

SUMMARY

Before the battle with the redcoats, Adam very much wanted to gain his father's love and respect, even though he feared his father. During the battle, Adam showed that he was only a boy. He was horrified, screamed, and ran away. After the battle, Adam changed from boy to man. He found his father's body in a coffin and honored him. He recognized that he loved Ruth and took on the responsibility of supporting his family.

Map It Out

| Work Map | *How*—Story Analysis for Causes and Effects |

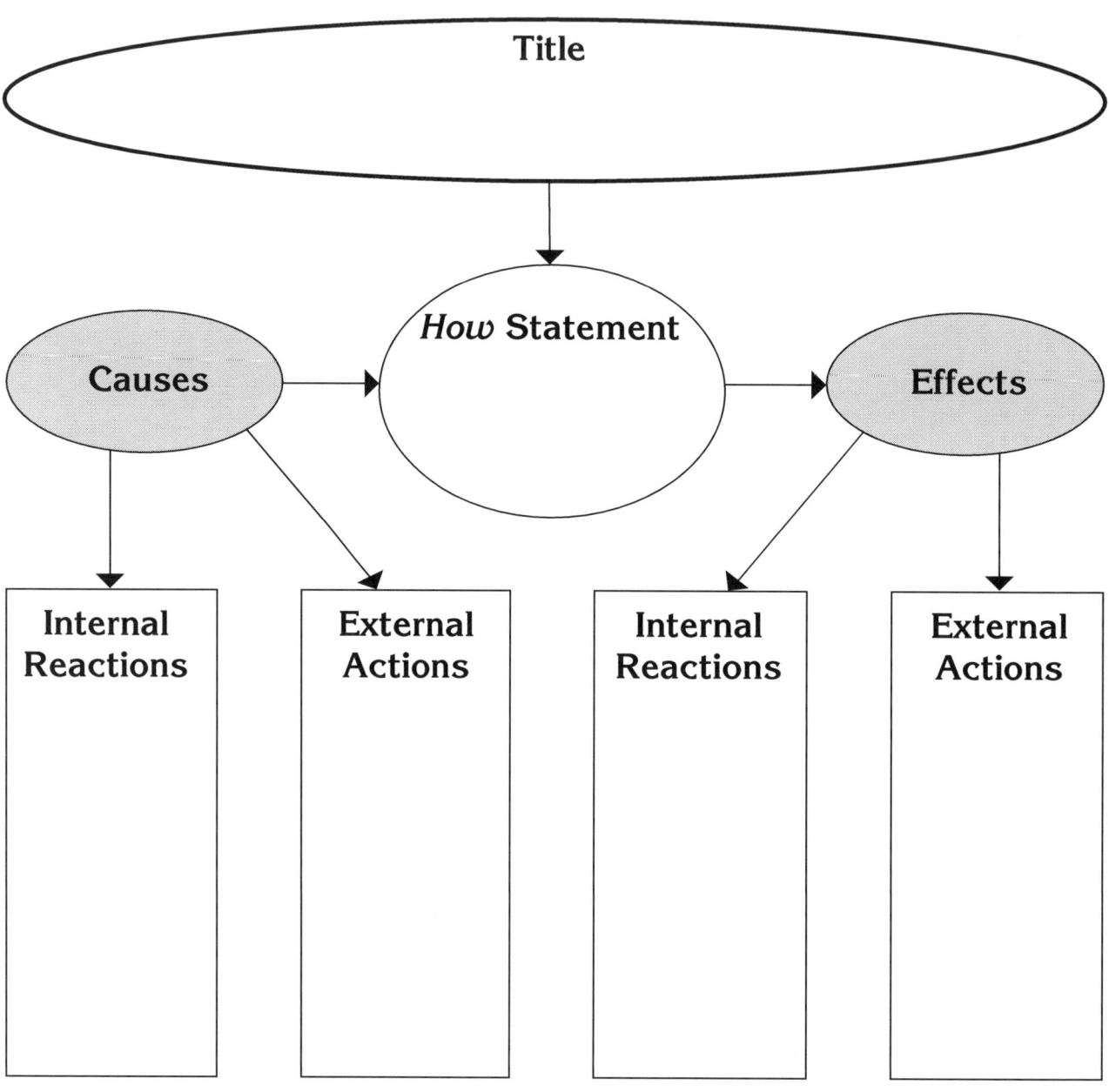

154

© 2001 by E.H. Wiig and C.C. Wilson
Duplication permitted for educational use only.

Unit 21: *How*—Story Analysis for Relationship Changes

Educational Levels

Upper elementary through secondary

Objectives

(1) Identify major driving forces in character relationships; (2) compare and contrast features of relationships before and after major changes occur; and (3) relate causes and effects to gain a dynamic view of the changes that often occur in character relationships over time

Completed Map

This map was constructed by students in Grade 8 who were assigned *Master Harold and the Boys* by Athol Fugard. To begin, they identified and recorded characteristics of the major characters involved in the relationship between a white boy (Sam) and an African servant (Halley). Then they analyzed the social forces and conditions that existed in the community before and after the turning point (i.e., when the relationship changed).

Show the Completed Map to students and say, for example:

> *This map shows an example of how students analyzed the relationship between two people in the novel* Master Harold and the Boys. *Let's talk about the relationship before and after the turning point. Then we'll look at the conditions before and after the change, the causes for the change, and how they are related.*

You may want to extend the activity by asking, for example:

> *Have you ever been in a friendship that suddenly changed? What were some of the driving forces and outside influences that changed the relationship?*

Map It Out

Work Map

Select a story. Show the Work Map to the students and say, for example:

This map is empty. Let's read and talk about this story. Then we'll analyze important changes in one of the relationships in the text and talk about the factors that caused the changes.

Extended Activities

1. Select a relationship between two characters in a popular comedy or drama series on TV. Ask students to discuss changes that have occurred in the relationship between the characters. Then ask them to identify and record causes and effects for the changes. When they have finished, ask students to predict and discuss possible relationship changes in the future.

2. Ask students to analyze a relationship between characters in a short story or novel that is part of the curriculum. Because causes for changes in character relationships are often implied and not explicitly stated, ask students to identify the causes that are stated and those that they infer.

3. Select a play that is assigned in the curriculum (e.g., Shakespeare's *Romeo and Juliet* or *Julius Caesar*). Ask students to analyze the relationship between two characters or groups and how the relationship changed. You may want to ask guided questions to support the activity.

4. Ask students to analyze an existing relationship between individuals or groups that is covered by newspaper, magazine, or TV news sources. Ask students to analyze the relationship as it existed in the past and as it exists today. If major changes have occurred, ask students to identify and discuss turning points and explicit or implied causes for the changes.

Text Comprehension

| Master Map | *How*—Story Analysis for Relationship Changes |

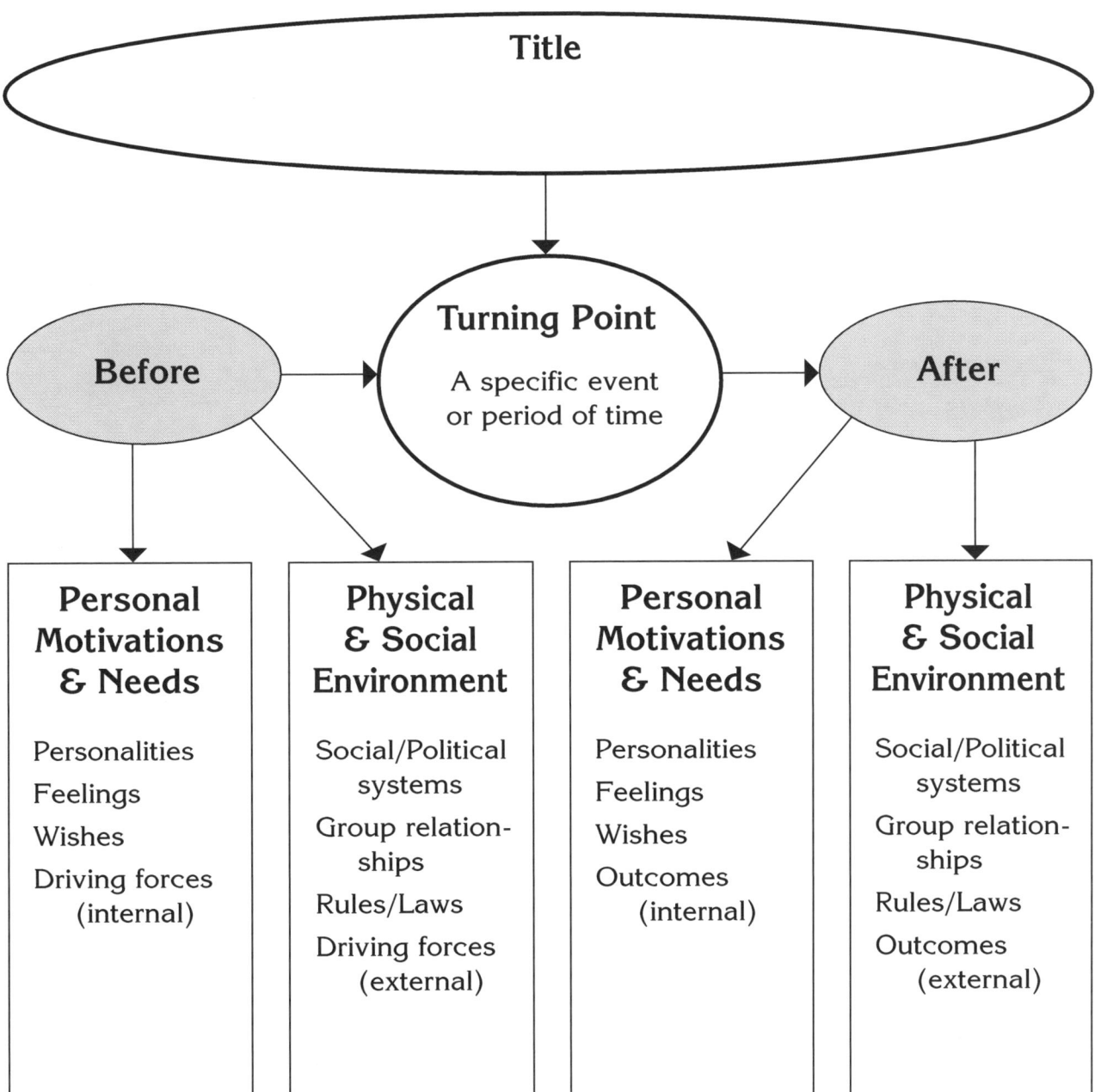

© 2001 by E.H. Wiig and C.C. Wilson
Duplication permitted for educational use only.

157

Map It Out

| Completed Map | *How*—Story Analysis for Relationship Changes |

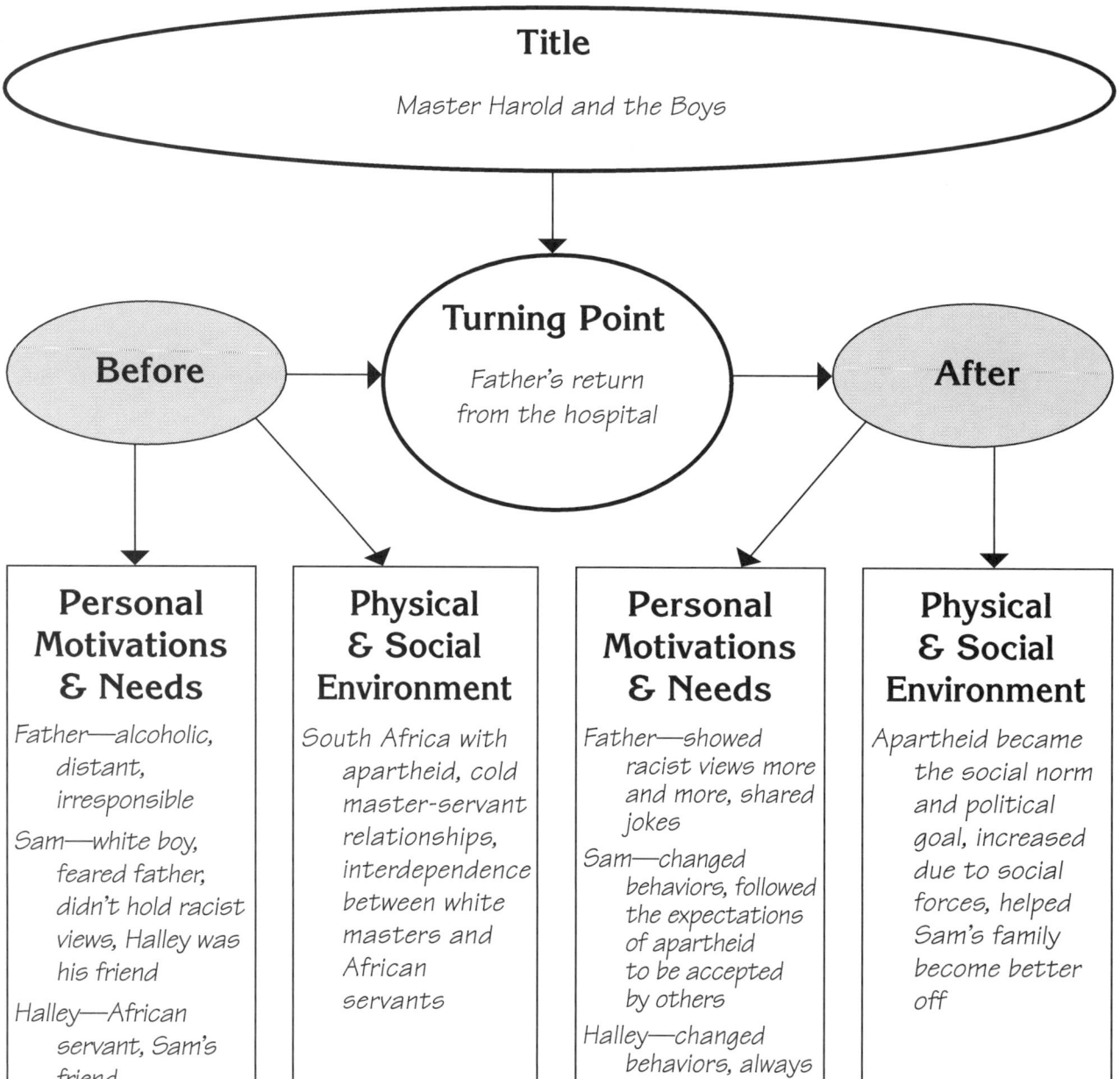

Text Comprehension

| Work Map | *How*—Story Analysis for Relationship Changes |

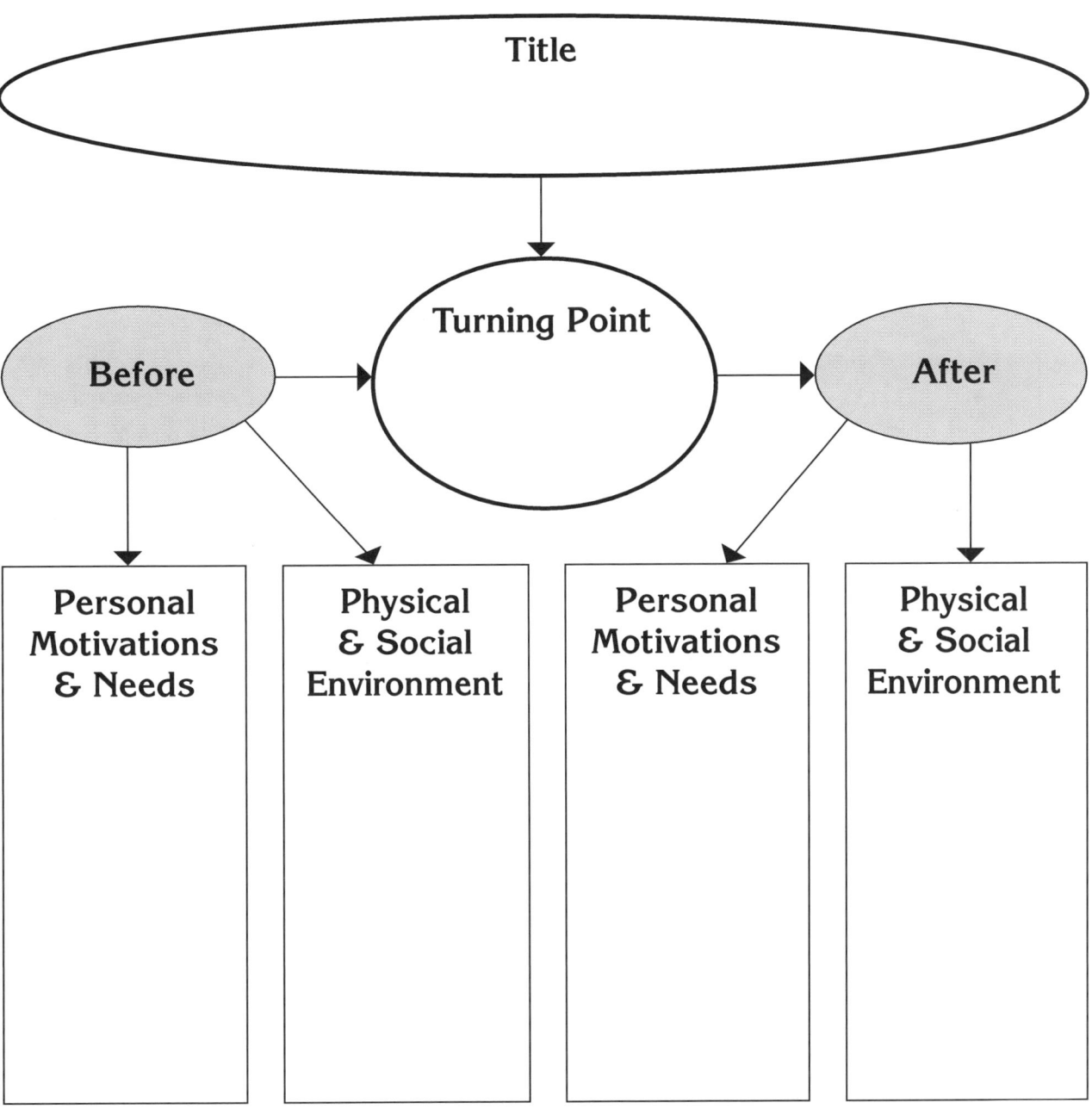

© 2001 by E.H. Wiig and C.C. Wilson
Duplication permitted for educational use only.

159

Map It Out

Unit 22: *Why*—Story Analysis of Reasons and Rationales for Actions

> **Educational Levels**
>
> Upper elementary through secondary
>
> **Objectives**
>
> (1) Identify feelings, reactions, and motives that are created by past events; (2) identify important external reasons and internal rationales for actions; and (3) relate causes and effects to gain a dynamic view of the action-reaction chains and the evolution of forces that cause positive (e.g., heroes) or negative (e.g., villains) actions and outcomes

Completed Map

This map was constructed by students in Grade 12 who analyzed the reasons and rationales for major characters' actions in *Tell Me a Tale* by James McEachin. Students were asked to identify and analyze the external causal events and internal feelings, motives, and actions for Moses's actions in the novel. They were asked to analyze and describe what caused the trusting and lovable boy—Moses—to turn into a calculating, revengeful adult. After completing the map, students shared and discussed their own feelings towards Moses and his act of revenge.

Show the Completed Map to students and say, for example:

> *This map shows an example of how students analyzed the reasons for and effects of a character's actions in the novel* Tell Me a Tale. *Let's talk about the events, feelings, and motives that caused the character to act. Then we'll look at the reactions and actions that followed and how the reasons and outcomes are related.*

Work Map

Select a story. Show the Work Map to students and say, for example:

> *This map is empty. Let's read and talk about this story. Then we'll analyze and organize important reasons and rationales for a character's actions in the text. Then we'll discuss and evaluate what the character did and what the outcomes were.*

Extended Activities

1. Have each student analyze the causes and effects of something he or she did in the past that was either good or bad. Ask students to volunteer to share what they did and what the driving forces and motives were that caused them to act the way they did.

2. Select a hero and a villain in a popular drama series on TV. Ask students to identify and record external events and internal reactions and discuss changes that could have influenced the characters and their actions. Then ask students to predict possible changes in the characters and their actions in the future.

3. Have each student analyze the driving forces and motives for characters' actions in a short story or novel that is part of the curriculum. Since motives for characters' actions are often implied and not explicitly stated, ask students to identify the motives that they infer.

4. Select a play that is assigned in the curriculum (e.g., Shakespeare's *Julius Caesar*). Ask students to analyze the driving forces and motives behind the actions of one or more main characters.

5. Ask students to analyze a current, negative event (e.g., a political conflict) that is reported by newspaper, magazine, or TV news reports. Ask students to analyze the explicit external and the implicit internal causes and driving forces that could have determined the actions. Have students identify and discuss how explicit or implied causes for negative acts might be changed.

6. Ask students to analyze a current difference in personal or political opinion (e.g., regarding health care or violence on TV) that is discussed in the news. Have them identify explicit external events that caused the news to focus on the difference or conflict. Then ask them to speculate and draw inferences about implicit internal forces and motives for the differences. You may want to ask students to debate with each other about the different opinions.

Map It Out

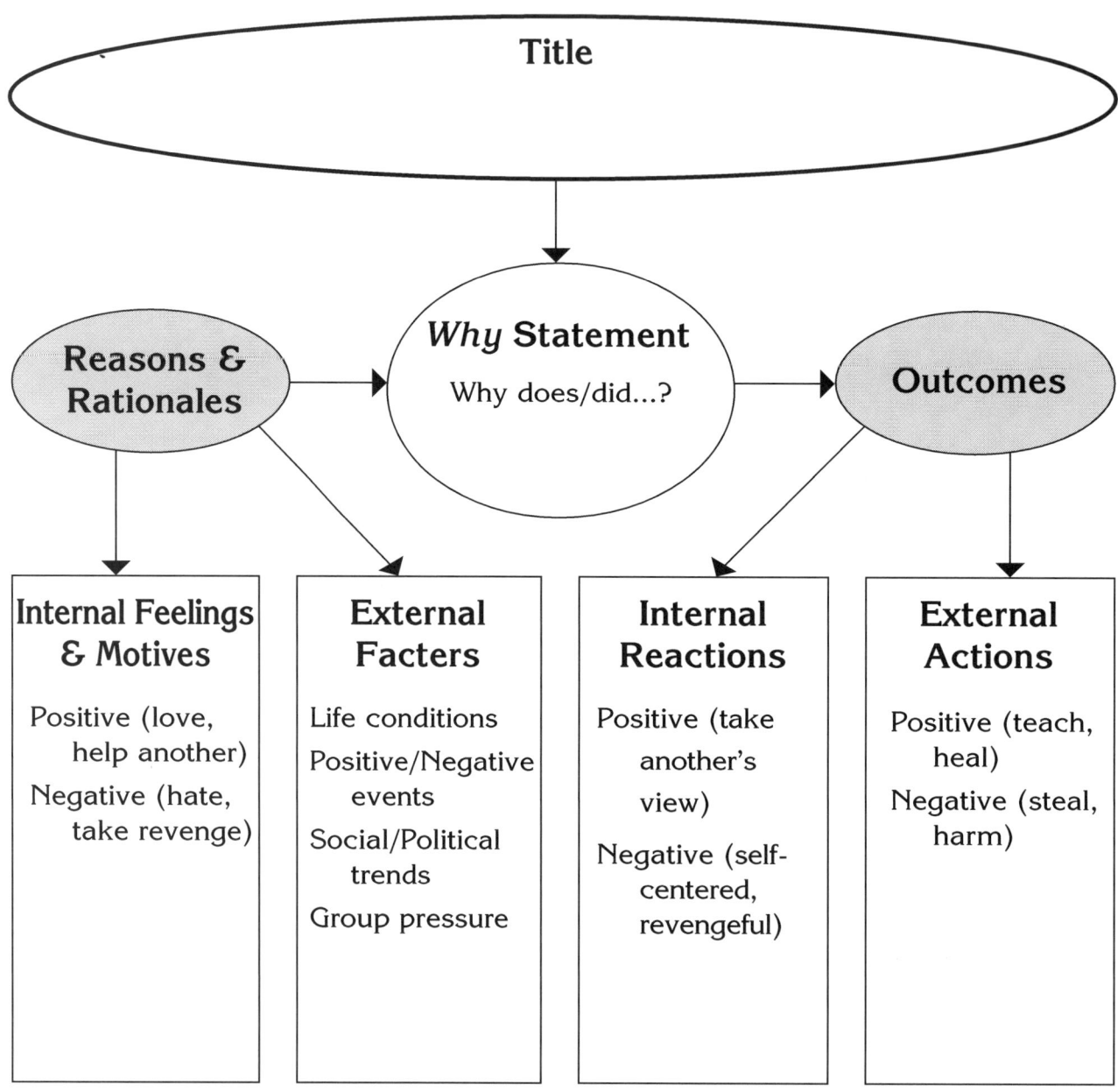

Text Comprehension

| Completed Map | **Why—Story Analysis of Reasons and Rationales for Actions** |

Title
Tell Me a Tale

Why Statement
Why did Moses change from a loving boy to a calculated killer?

Reasons & Rationales

Outcomes

Internal Feelings & Motives
Rejected by white father, loved by uncle, feared for his life, grieved the loss of his family, wanted revenge, wanted the killers to confess and say they were sorry

External Facters
Saw his father and uncle tortured and killed by four white men, because they had disobeyed rules set for slavery by acknowledging kinship

Internal Reactions
Feared for his life, felt loss of protection, felt powerless to do anything for himself, turned inward and became lonely and secretive, relied on himself for everything

External Actions
Escaped to freedom, educated himself, planned to return to his home, faced the killers, told his story, listened to their abuse of him, saw no regret

SUMMARY

Moses was the son of a slave and her master. He was a loving boy and was loved by his mother and her brother. His father rejected him, and this confused him. After his mother's death, Moses saw his father and uncle tortured and killed by four white men. He feared for his life and escaped. He never forgot the killers and planned revenge. He returned home, faced the killers in a general store, and tried to make them show regret and ask for forgiveness. They abused Moses instead, so he proceeded with his plan for revenge.

© 2001 by E.H. Wiig and C.C. Wilson
Duplication permitted for educational use only.

Map It Out

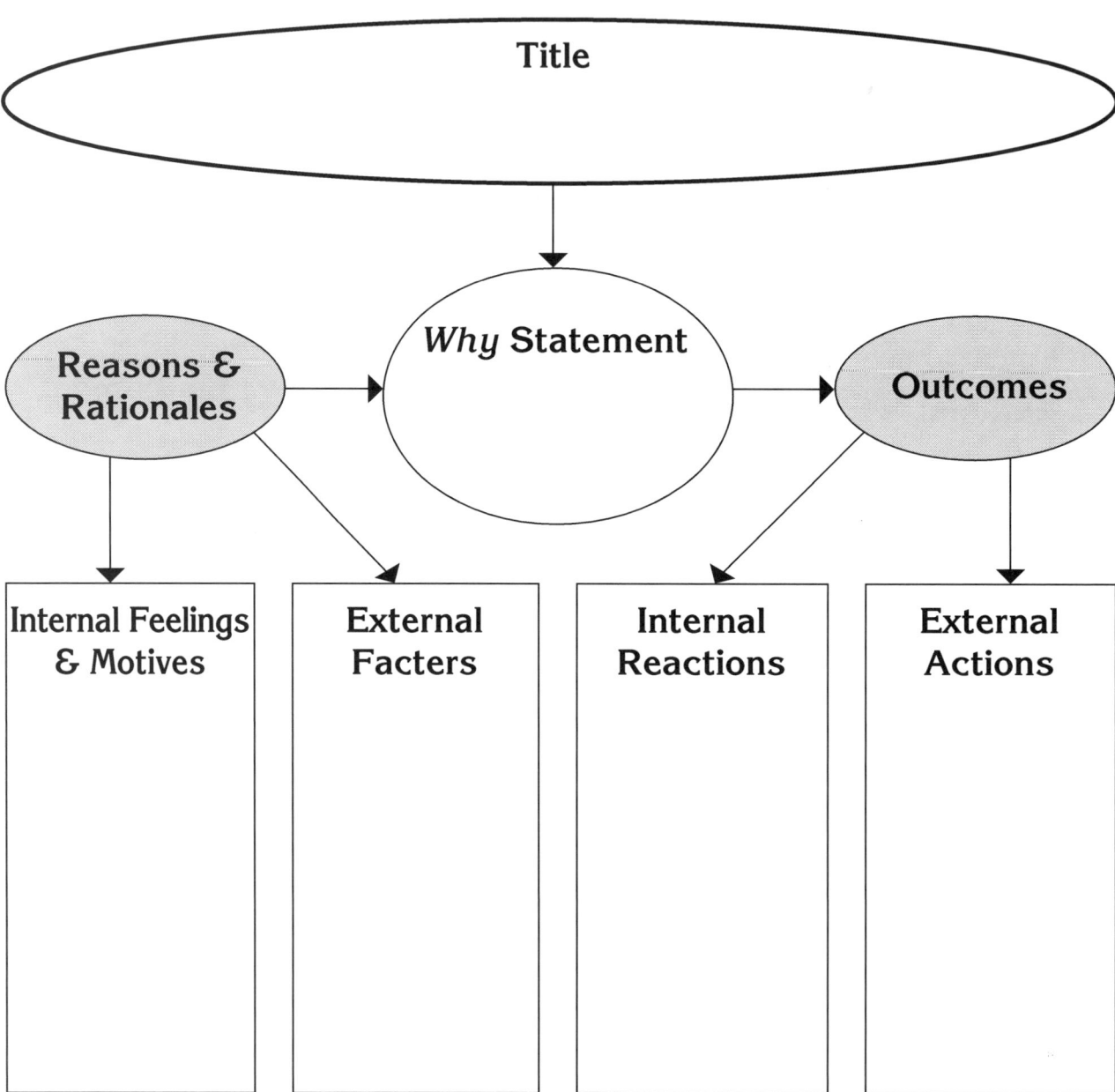

Text Comprehension

Unit 23: Dynamic Characterization

Educational Levels
Upper elementary through secondary

Objectives
(1) Identify major traits of and motivating forces in characters; (2) analyze and discuss the nature of interactions between characters; and (3) relate the driving forces in characters to the interactions between them

Completed Map

This map shows how students in Grade 6 analyzed the two major characters, Adam and his father, in *April Morning* by Howard Fast. Students worked in two teams to analyze the characteristics of the two characters. Each team focused on a character (i.e., father or son) and the character's traits (e.g., physical, behavioral, or social). Afterward they combined and refined the results of their analyses on one map.

Show the Completed Map to students and say, for example:

> *This map shows an example of how students analyzed character interactions in the novel* April Morning. *Let's talk about the traits of each character. Then we'll look at the factors that can influence and determine the quality of interactions between characters.*

Work Map

Select a story. Show the Work Map to students and say, for example:

> *This map is empty. Let's read and talk about this story. Then we'll analyze and evaluate important traits of and driving forces in the characters and the effects these elements had on their relationships and interactions.*

Map It Out

Extended Activities

1. Have each student analyze two important people in his or her immediate environment (e.g., parents or friends). Ask students to volunteer to share what they found and discuss how the people's traits might influence the interactions between them.

2. Select two characters that are opposites (e.g., a funny character and a serious character) in a popular comedy or drama series on TV. Ask students to identify and record the traits of each character and analyze and discuss the nature and dynamics of interactions between them. Then ask students to predict possible changes in the characters and their interactions in the future.

3. Ask students to analyze and record the traits of two characters in a short story or novel that is part of the curriculum. Have students discuss the traits and how they could influence the nature of interactions between the characters.

4. Select a play that is part of the curriculum (e.g., *Julius Caesar* by William Shakespeare or *Who's Afraid of Virginia Woolf* by Edward Albee). Have each student analyze the traits of two characters in the play. Afterwards ask students to share and discuss their analyses and relate personal traits of the characters to features of their interactions using examples from the play.

5. Ask students to analyze a current interaction between nonpublic or public figures that is reported by newspaper, magazine, or TV news sources. Have students identify the personal traits that might influence the nature of interactions.

6. Ask students to identify and discuss how explicit or implied personality traits of individuals or groups can determine positive or negative interactions between them. Elicit suggestions for how the nature of negative interactions between individuals or groups might be changed.

Text Comprehension

| Master Map | Dynamic Characterization |

Knowledge & Skills
Ideas/Thoughts
Experiences

Communication
Style
Positive/Negative

Personality & Behavior
Attitudes
Feelings

Appearance
Gender
Age

Character

Social Status
Titles
Possessions

Nature of Interaction

Appearance
Gender
Age

Social Status
Titles
Possessions

Knowledge & Skills
Ideas/Thoughts
Experiences

Character

Communication
Style
Positive/Negative

Personality & Behavior
Attitudes
Feelings

SUMMARY — Highlight of similarities and differences

© 2001 by E.H. Wiig and C.C. Wilson
Duplication permitted for educational use only.

167

Map It Out

| Completed Map | **Dynamic Characterization** |

Character: Adam's Father

- **Knowledge & Skills**: Books, farming, leadership, debate, responsibility
- **Communication**: Fluent and flamboyant, can arouse others to action, can be abusive
- **Personality & Behavior**: Mean, proud, hardworking, didn't show love
- **Appearance**: Middle-aged, strong, commanding
- **Social Status**: Respected by the community, self-educated, accomplished citizen

Nature of Interaction
Tense; based on fear, not love

Character: Adam

- **Appearance**: Age 15, normal teenage features
- **Social Status**: Had a well-known and highly respected father, educated like other teens of the time, gained friendships and love
- **Knowledge & Skills**: Books, school life, chores, games, responsibility
- **Communication**: Respectful, smart mouth, less fluent than father
- **Personality & Behavior**: Impulsive, defiant, active

SUMMARY

It is easy to understand why Adam feared his father and thought he did not love him. The father was not one to show or tell about his feelings. He was silent and assumed others knew he loved them. The father probably often had to reprimand Adam when he was defiant or disrespectful toward others. The differences in their personalities interfered with their love.

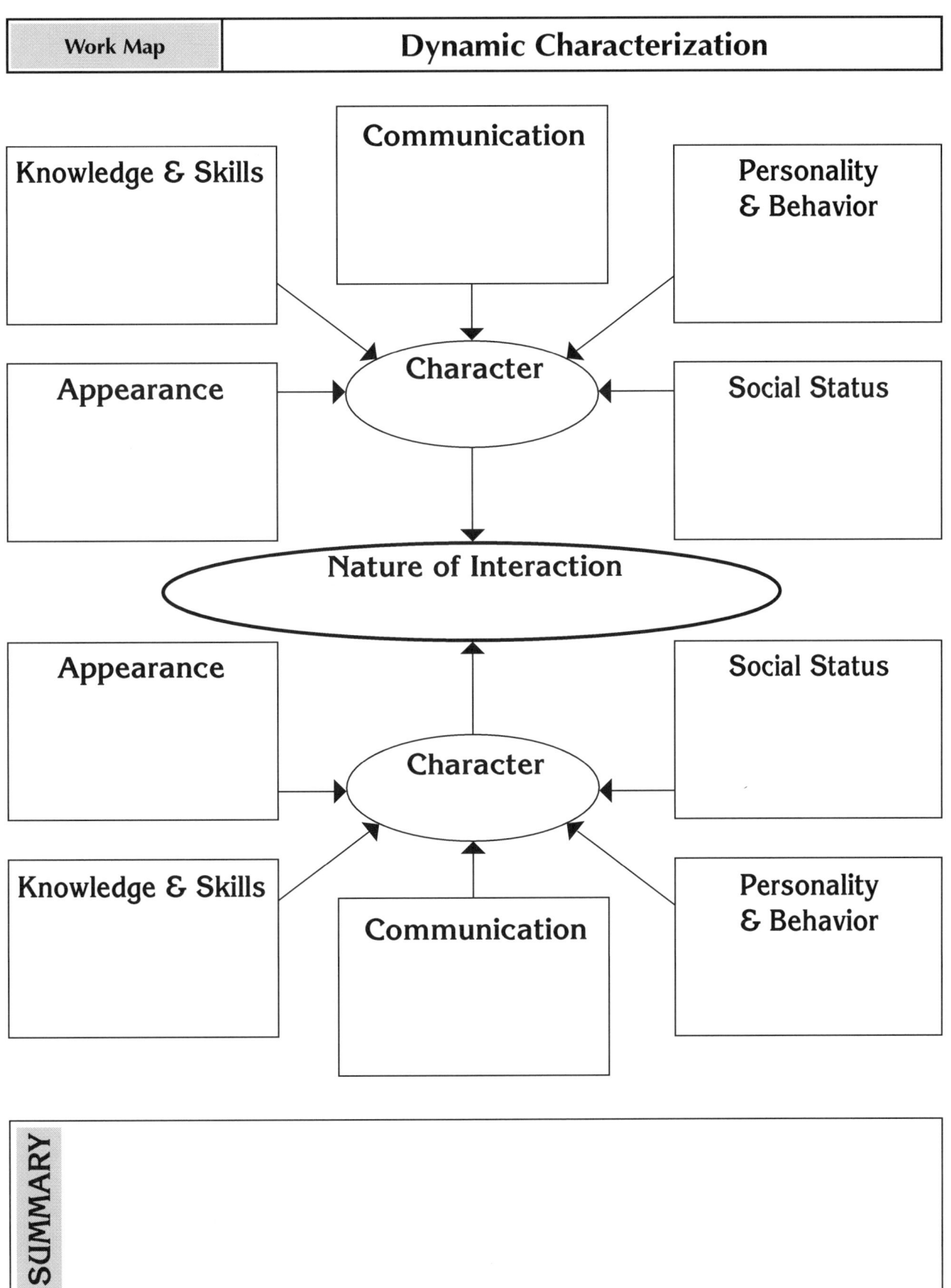

Section 3
Context (Pragmatics)

Unit 24: Dimensions of Verbal Communication 173

Unit 25: Dimensions of Nonverbal Communication 178

Unit 26: Controlling Variables for Pragmatics 183

Unit 27: Decision-Making for Pragmatics 188

Unit 28: Communication Breakdown and Clarification 193

Unit 29: Requests for Clarification 198

Unit 30: Requests for Actions and Favors 203

Unit 31: Cultural Features of Communication 208

Unit 32: Pragmatic Characterization 213

Unit 33: Perspective Taking 218

Unit 34: Sharing, Borrowing, and Exchanging 223

Unit 35: Negotiating Terms 228

Unit 36: Establishing Better Relationships 233

Unit 37: Developing Trust 238

Unit 38: Causes for Conflict or Disagreement 243

Unit 39: Ongoing Conflict Resolution 248

Unit 40: Understanding Relationship Changes 253

Unit 41: Preparing for Role-Playing 258

Unit 24: Dimensions of Verbal Communication

> **Educational Levels**
>
> Elementary through secondary
>
> **Objectives**
>
> (1) Analyze dimensions of verbal communication in people or characters in texts, films, or plays; (2) describe an actual situation and interaction; and (3) apply these skills to new situations

Completed Map

For this map, students in Grade 10 were asked to identify and write down how the tree and the boy communicated in *The Giving Tree* by Shel Silverstein. The teacher and students discussed the content and form dimensions of verbal communication. Then the teacher guided and mediated a discussion to make students aware of the author's use of words, sentence and word structure, and formality and politeness features.

Show the Completed Map to students and say, for example:

> *This map shows types of verbal communications a group of students found when they listened to a story called* The Giving Tree. *Let's talk about each example and what is special about it.*

Work Map

Show the Work Map to students and say, for example:

> *This map is empty. Let's read about or watch a video of some people talking. We want to find out what is special about how they communicate with words. Then we'll analyze how the people expressed themselves when they spoke to each other.*

Map It Out

Extended Activities

1. Select a story with extensive dialogue. Ask students to analyze how the characters in the story talk to each other.

2. Select a short skit or section of a play. Have each student read a character's dialogue aloud and analyze features of his or her verbal communication. After the analysis, ask students to role-play the skit or act out a scene from the play. You may want to assist students in taking on the characteristics of their character by using the maps and activities in Unit 41: Preparing for Role-Playing (see page 260).

3. Have each student analyze his or her verbal communication. Then form student pairs or small teams and have students share their analyses, give and receive peer validation, and modify their findings.

4. Have each student view an interview on television and analyze the verbal characteristics of the interviewer or, in more advanced groups, all participants in the interview. Have students share their findings and discuss the effects of different communication styles on viewers (e.g., the person seemed trustworthy).

5. Show a film or TV show that features participants from different cultural and linguistic backgrounds. Ask students to analyze the verbal characteristics of the communication of one or more participants. Guide a discussion of how the cultural and linguistic backgrounds and personalities of the participants were portrayed in the film or TV show.

6. Ask students to read a story or scene from a play and analyze how the characters communicate verbally. Then ask students to speak or write the dialogue in a different form (e.g., less formal).

Context (Pragmatics)

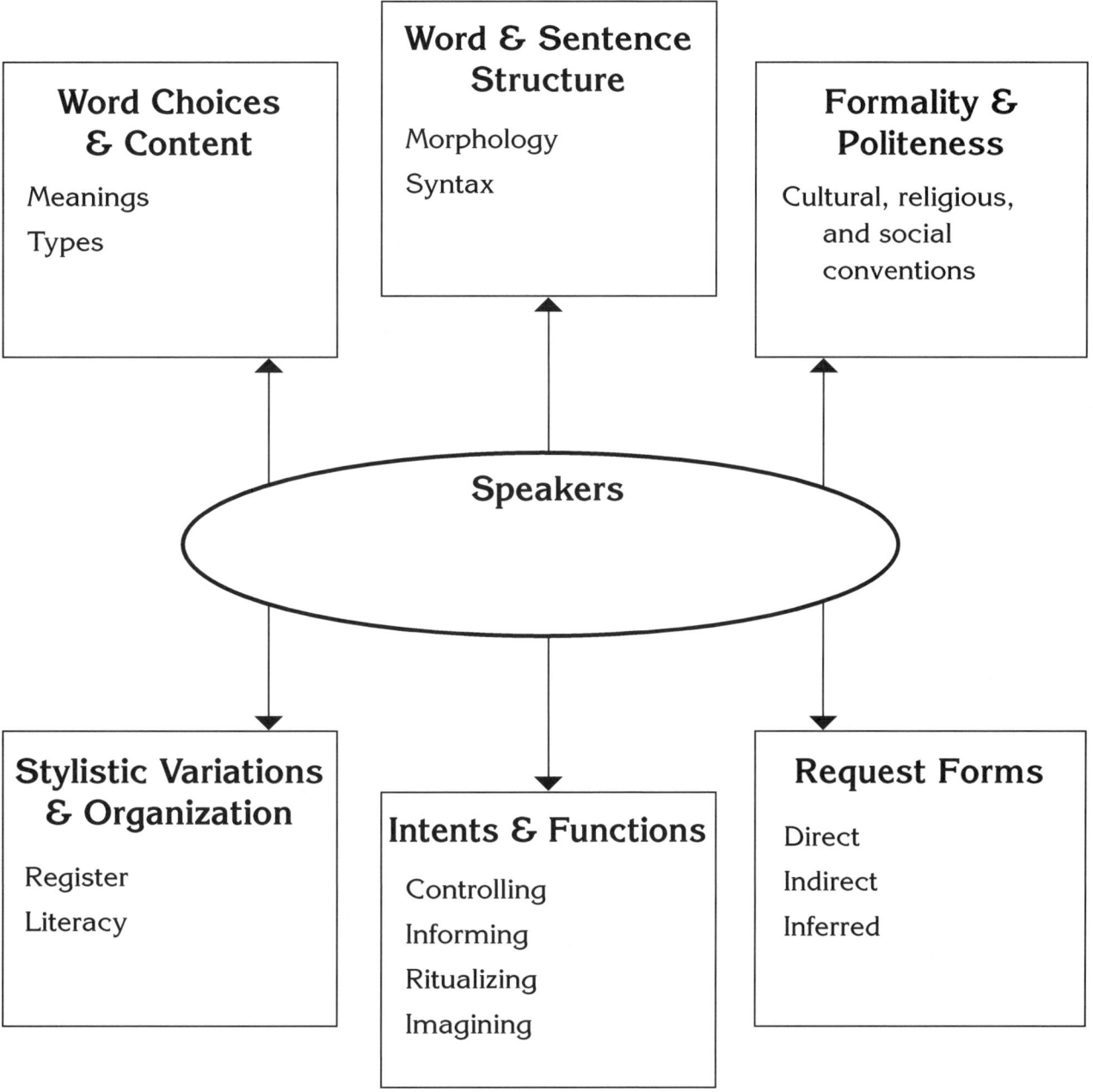

| Master Map | Dimensions of Verbal Communication |

Word Choices & Content
Meanings
Types

Word & Sentence Structure
Morphology
Syntax

Formality & Politeness
Cultural, religious, and social conventions

Speakers

Stylistic Variations & Organization
Register
Literacy

Intents & Functions
Controlling
Informing
Ritualizing
Imagining

Request Forms
Direct
Indirect
Inferred

SUMMARY: Synthesis of verbal characteristics

© 2001 by E.H. Wiig and C.C. Wilson
Duplication permitted for educational use only.

Map It Out

| Completed Map | **Dimensions of Verbal Communication** |

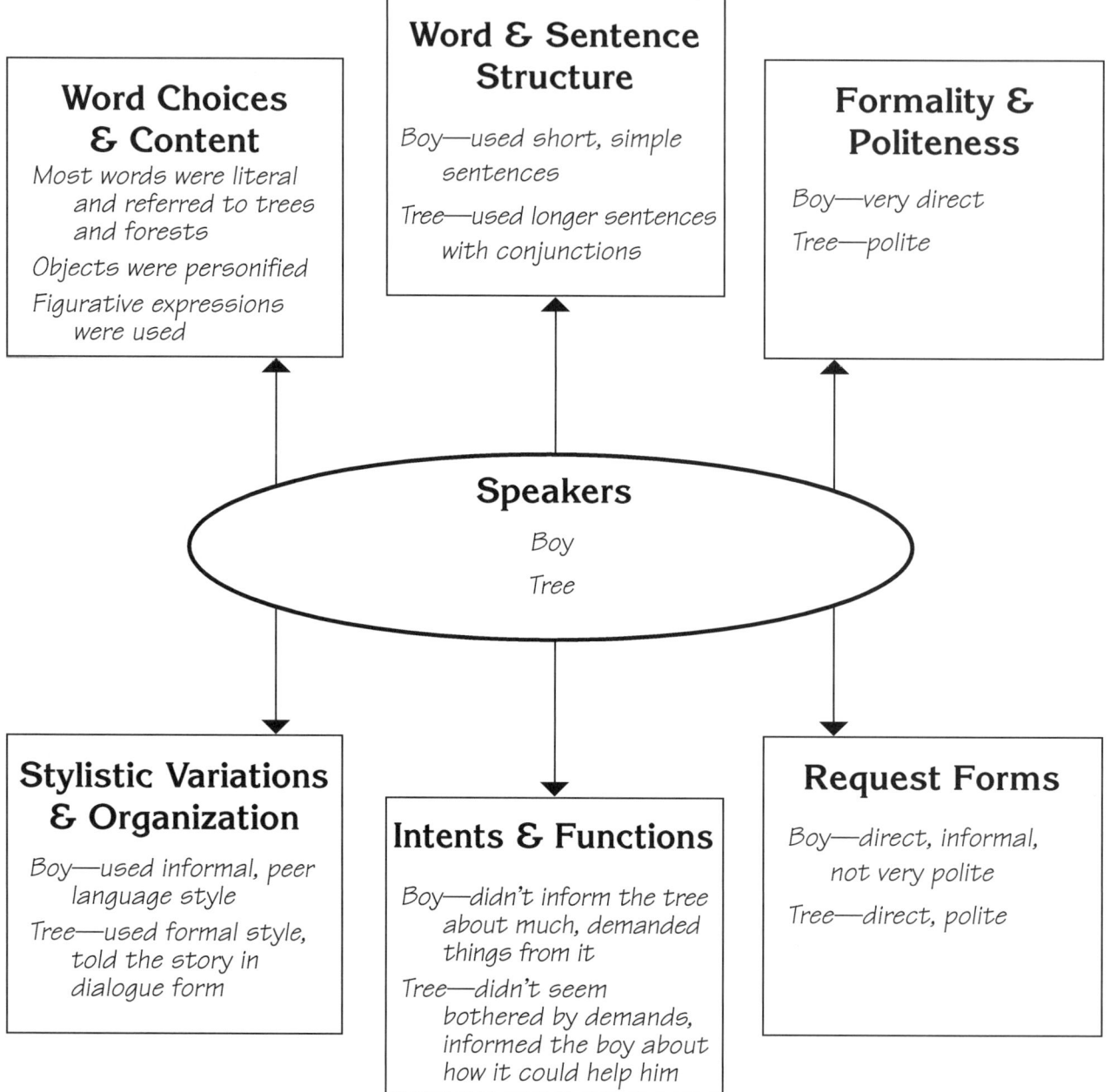

Word Choices & Content
Most words were literal and referred to trees and forests
Objects were personified
Figurative expressions were used

Word & Sentence Structure
Boy—used short, simple sentences
Tree—used longer sentences with conjunctions

Formality & Politeness
Boy—very direct
Tree—polite

Speakers
Boy
Tree

Stylistic Variations & Organization
Boy—used informal, peer language style
Tree—used formal style, told the story in dialogue form

Intents & Functions
Boy—didn't inform the tree about much, demanded things from it
Tree—didn't seem bothered by demands, informed the boy about how it could help him

Request Forms
Boy—direct, informal, not very polite
Tree—direct, polite

SUMMARY
The boy talked to the tree in a childish way, even when he became a man. He asked the tree to help him get everything important in his life. The tree was very loving in the way it talked back to the boy. It was always polite and never offended the boy. If the tree had not loved the boy, it might have talked to him in a rough way to get him off its back.

176

© 2001 by E.H. Wiig and C.C. Wilson
Duplication permitted for educational use only.

Context (Pragmatics)

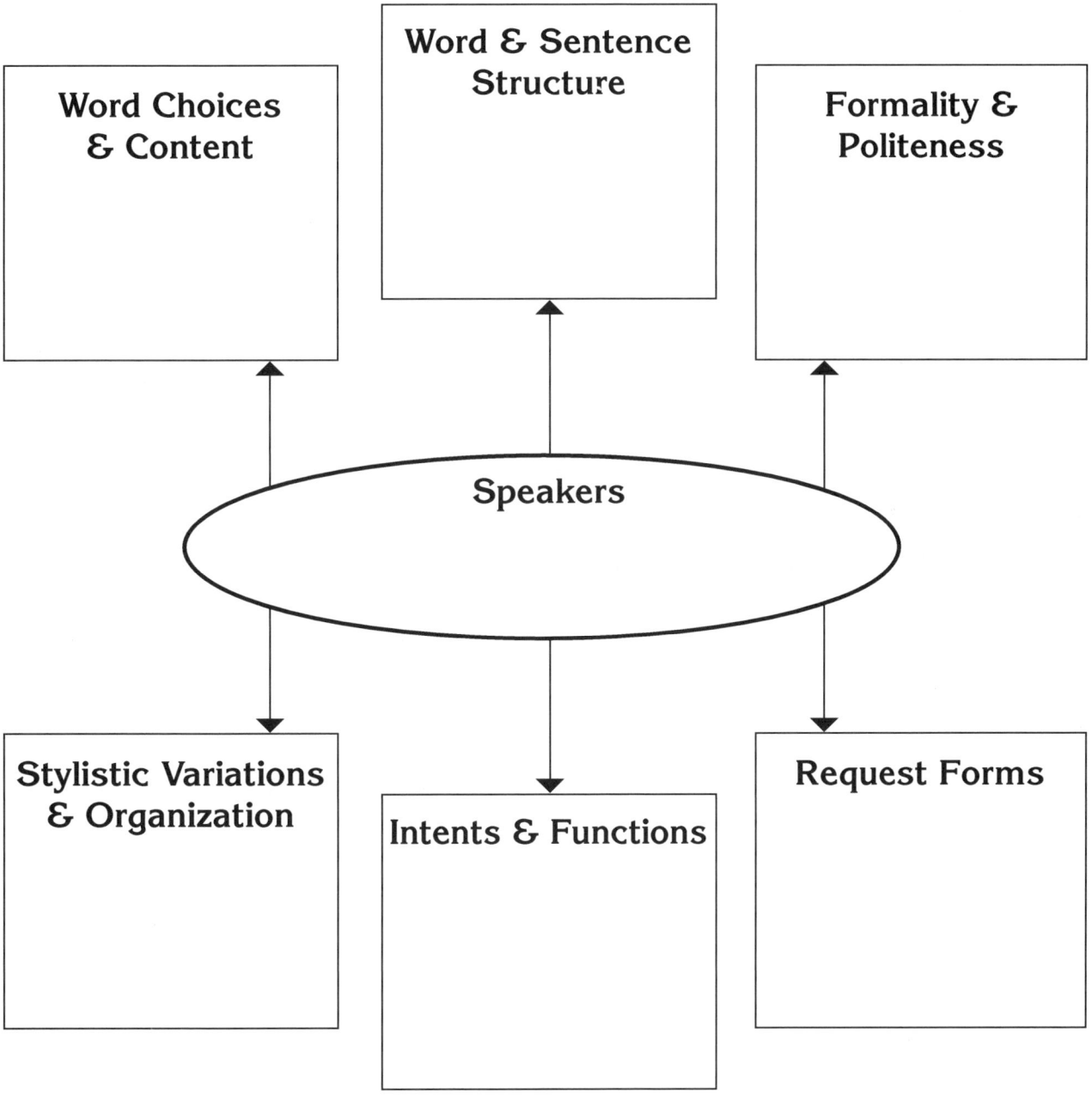

© 2001 by E.H. Wiig and C.C. Wilson
Duplication permitted for educational use only.

177

Map It Out

Unit 25: Dimensions of Nonverbal Communication

> **Educational Levels**
>
> Elementary through secondary
>
> **Objectives**
>
> (1) Analyze dimensions of nonverbal communication in people or characters in films, plays, or true-life situations; (2) describe an actual situation and interaction; (3) understand and appreciate other cultural forms of communication; and (4) apply these skills to new situations

Completed Map

This map was completed by students in Grade 8. Students were asked to give some examples of body talk. One student gave the example of someone who looked angry during a fight. The students were asked to identify how anger is expressed physically.

Show the Completed Map to students and say, for example:

> *This map shows examples of how people might express anger. Let's talk about each of the ways anger could be expressed.*

You may want to extend the activity by asking, for example:

> *What happens to make people angry? What words do you think people say to express their anger?*

Work Map

Show the Work Map to students and say, for example:

> *This map is empty. Let's talk about a situation. Then we'll analyze how the person involved expressed feelings and attitudes.*

Extended Activities

1. Select a story with illustrations or photographs of interactions. Ask students to analyze how the characters in the pictures express themselves with body talk.

2. Select a short skit or section of a play. Ask students to read the dialogue. Then ask them to analyze how they think the characters would use body talk to support their feelings or reactions.

3. Have each student analyze his or her body talk. Then form student pairs or small teams and have students share their analyses, give and receive peer validation, and modify their findings.

4. Select a video, TV show, cartoon, or silent film—silent films are especially well suited for this type of analysis since nonverbal communication cues are exaggerated. Show your selection to students, and ask them to analyze the body talk of one or more of the characters.

5. Select one or more newspaper cartoons with few or no words. Ask students to analyze and interpret the body talk in each frame. Afterward ask them to talk about the content of the cartoon.

6. Ask students to role-play a skit or scene from a play. After role-playing, ask students to analyze the body talk of one or more of the characters. You may want to prepare students for role-playing by using the maps and activities in Unit 41: Preparing for Role-Playing (see page 258).

7. Have each student view an interview on TV and analyze the nonverbal characteristics of the interviewer or, in more advanced groups, all participants in the interview. Ask students to share their findings and discuss the effects of different nonverbal communication styles on viewers (e.g., the person seemed relaxed).

8. Show a film or TV show that features participants from different cultural and linguistic backgrounds. Have each student analyze the characteristics of the nonverbal communication of one or more characters. Have students share their findings. Then guide a discussion of how the cultural and linguistic background of the character and his or her personality are portrayed through body talk.

Map It Out

| Master Map | **Dimensions of Nonverbal Communication** |

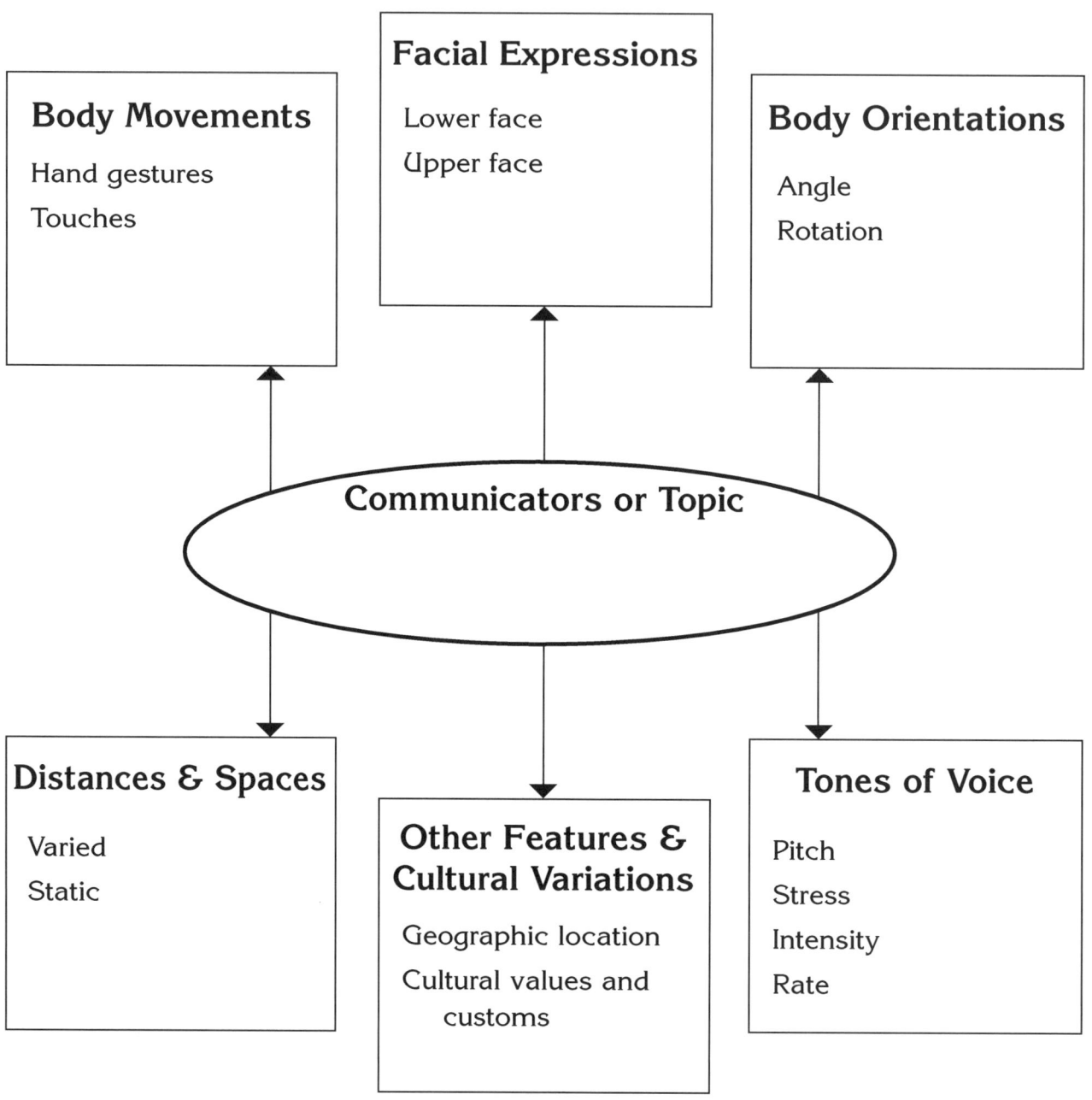

Body Movements
Hand gestures
Touches

Facial Expressions
Lower face
Upper face

Body Orientations
Angle
Rotation

Communicators or Topic

Distances & Spaces
Varied
Static

Other Features & Cultural Variations
Geographic location
Cultural values and customs

Tones of Voice
Pitch
Stress
Intensity
Rate

SUMMARY: Summary of nonverbal characteristics

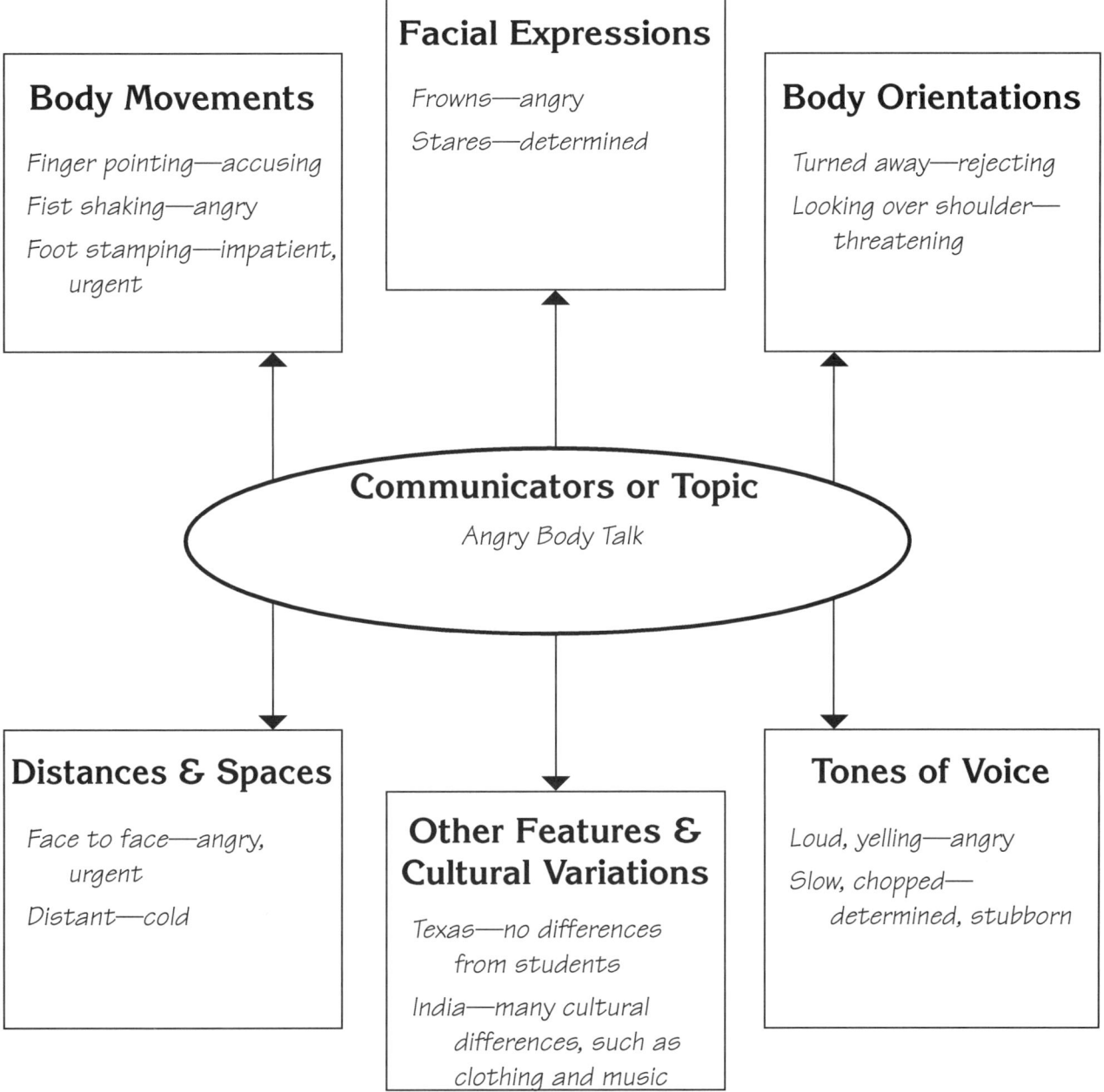

Context (Pragmatics)

Completed Map — **Dimensions of Nonverbal Communication**

Body Movements
Finger pointing—accusing
Fist shaking—angry
Foot stamping—impatient, urgent

Facial Expressions
Frowns—angry
Stares—determined

Body Orientations
Turned away—rejecting
Looking over shoulder—threatening

Communicators or Topic
Angry Body Talk

Distances & Spaces
Face to face—angry, urgent
Distant—cold

Other Features & Cultural Variations
Texas—no differences from students
India—many cultural differences, such as clothing and music

Tones of Voice
Loud, yelling—angry
Slow, chopped—determined, stubborn

SUMMARY
It is amazing how much you can tell others without saying a word. Every feeling or reaction you express with your face, tone of voice, movement, or body orientation can be understood by others. So you have to be careful about how your body talks. Your body can reveal a secret. It can turn others off. It can make others feel comfortable or uncomfortable.

© 2001 by E.H. Wiig and C.C. Wilson
Duplication permitted for educational use only.

Map It Out

| Work Map | **Dimensions of Nonverbal Communication** |

- Body Movements
- Facial Expressions
- Body Orientations

Communicators or Topic

- Distances & Spaces
- Other Features & Cultural Variations
- Tones of Voice

SUMMARY

182

© 2001 by E.H. Wiig and C.C. Wilson
Duplication permitted for educational use only.

Context (Pragmatics)

Unit 26: Controlling Variables for Pragmatics

> **Educational Levels**
>
> Upper elementary through secondary
>
> **Objectives**
>
> (1) Analyze the controlling variable for verbal and nonverbal communication in different interactions and situations; (2) describe an actual situation or interaction in a context; and (3) apply these skills to new settings, situations, or interactions

Completed Map

This map was constructed by a group of students in Grade 6 who were preparing to tell a children's story to a preschool class. First they identified and recorded the controlling variables for how they might communicate to the younger children in school. Second they discussed their choices and demonstrated some of the ways they planned to tell the story for effect.

Show the Completed Map to students and say, for example:

This map shows what a group of students came up with when they prepared themselves to tell a story to a group of younger children. Let's talk about each variable and what the students thought were important aspects.

You may want to follow up by asking, for example:

What do you think an informal setting is like? What effects do you think it could have if there are more boys than girls? What kinds of questions could you ask the children to get them to participate?

Work Map

Show the Work Map to students and say, for example:

This map is empty. Let's talk about a situation. Then we'll identify which variables should control what, when, and how the speaker would communicate.

Map It Out

Extended Activities

1. Identify and present some examples of true-life interactions, and ask students how the controlling variables would influence the what, when, how, and why of the communication. Focus students' attention on both verbal and nonverbal aspects of communication. Then ask students to analyze one of the interactions you discussed.

2. Have each student analyze the controlling variables that influenced the characters' communication styles in a short story or novel. Ask students to share their results, and mediate any additions or modifications.

3. Ask students to read selected articles in a local newspaper. Then ask them to consider how the writer of the article responded to the controlling variables for newspaper writing. Focus their attention on the readers, medium, length allowed, and perceived objectives or intents. Then give each student an article to analyze.

4. Show a segment of an episode from a current TV series. Ask students to identify and label the variables that control how the characters communicate.

5. Comedy, as we see it in TV series or late-night shows, is often created by someone violating the rules associated with one or more of the controlling variables for communication. Show an episode of a current comedy show. Have each student analyze how each character responds to the controlling variables for communication and identify a character or an interaction that violates the rules. Have each student give an oral presentation of his or her findings.

6. Select different media for communicating with others (e.g., a telephone call or an email message). Ask students to analyze which variables control communications with each of the media. Give students a message to communicate to someone else and assign a different communication medium to each student. Have each student write down what he or she would say and how he or she would support the verbal message with body talk. Then ask students to share their communication of the message.

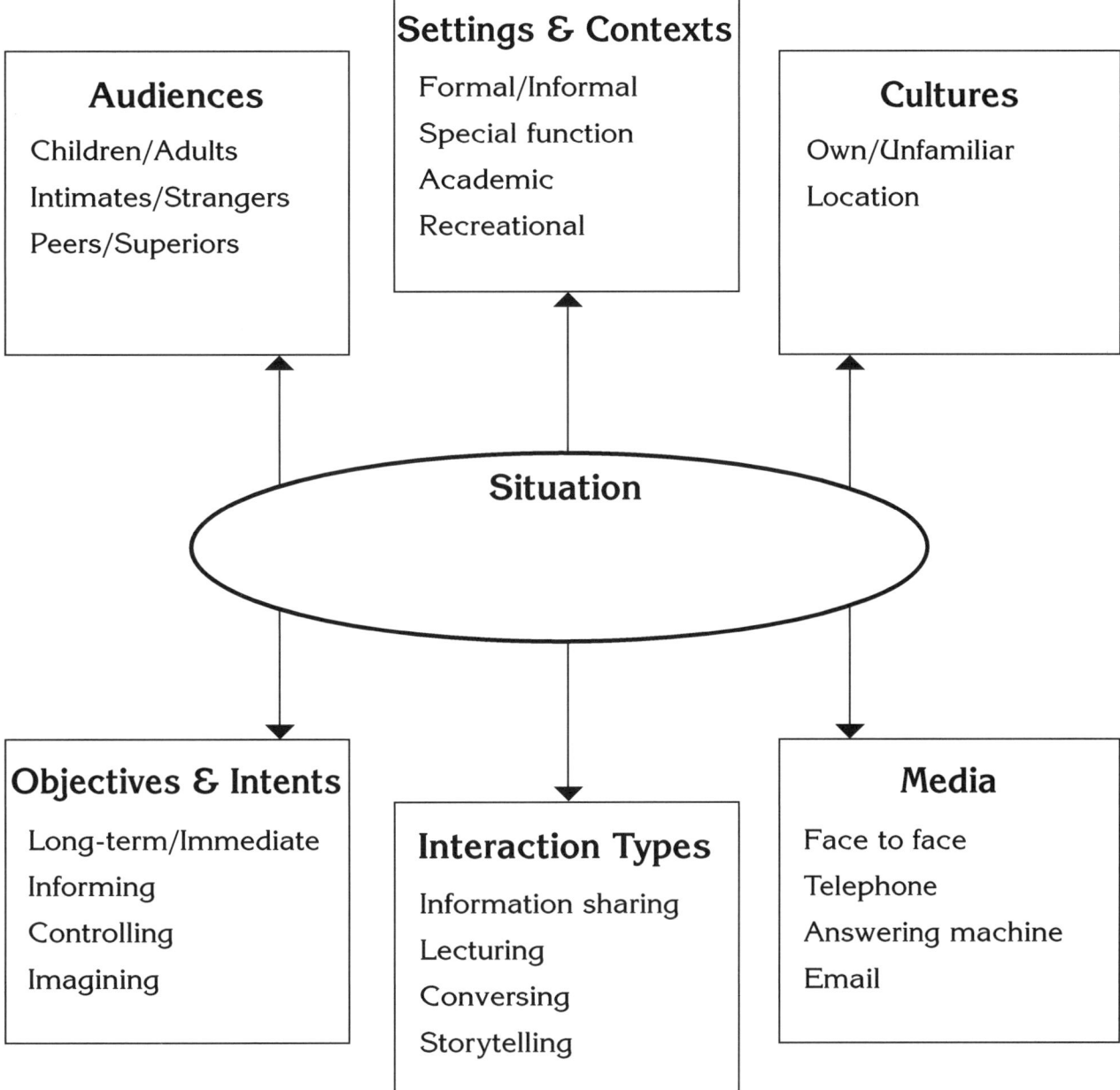

Map It Out

| Completed Map | **Controlling Variables for Pragmatics** |

Audiences
A group of about 10 preschool children (ages 4–5) with more boys than girls

Settings & Contexts
Preschool classroom with storytelling circle

Cultures
Diverse cultural and linguistic backgrounds, including African American, Asian, and Middle Eastern children

Situation
Telling a children's story to preschoolers

Objectives & Intents
Tell a children's story with exciting events to help the children imagine

Interaction Types
Informal storytelling for entertainment

Interaction with comments, questions, and answers

Face to face

Media
A picture storybook for telling the story and showing the pictures to the children

SUMMARY

We thought it was going to be easy to read a story to small children. While preparing, however, we learned that we needed to practice to make the story come alive. We learned how to show the story pictures, ask and answer questions, make sure everyone saw and heard us well, and change our tone of voice and facial expressions to make the events exciting.

Context (Pragmatics)

| Work Map | **Controlling Variables for Pragmatics** |

Audiences

Settings & Contexts

Cultures

Situation

Objectives & Intents

Interaction Types

Media

SUMMARY

Map It Out

Unit 27: Decision-Making for Pragmatics

Educational Levels

Upper elementary through secondary

Objectives

(1) Analyze the variables and stages in making decisions about what, when, and how to communicate with others; (2) describe an actual situation and communication task; and (3) apply the decision-making process to new, unfamiliar situations

Completed Map

This map was developed by a group of students in Grade 7 who were interested in interviewing for jobs in their neighborhoods. The students were given three job choices and worked in small groups. Each group presented its decision-making map and plan for one student's interview to the class. The class then discussed which approaches and strategies might work best. Afterward each team role-played their final plan for the interview.

Show the Completed Map to students and say, for example:

> *This map shows what a group of students came up with when they prepared for interviews to get jobs in their neighborhoods. Let's talk about what the students thought was important.*

You may want to follow up by asking one or more of the following:

> *What do you think the students did when they identified variables to rank priorities? What do you think was the most difficult step in planning? What choices would you select for revising your statements if you were not understood?*

Work Map

Show the Work Map to students and say, for example:

> *This map is empty. Let's talk about a situation. Then we'll plan for the interaction by making decisions about how to communicate. We'll identify which controlling variables to consider. Then we'll rank them to set priorities, decide on some choices for revising, and come up with an overall plan.*

Extended Activities

1. Have each student analyze his or her plans for interviewing for a job (e.g., newspaper deliverer). Ask students to share their plans and discuss how they made their decisions.

2. Have each student plan and engage in a decision-making process for a presentation about his or her favorite hobby. Then ask each student to give the presentation to tell other students about the hobby.

3. Prepare a message for students to deliver to someone in the school setting (e.g., a principal or janitor). Then have each student prepare to deliver the message by planning and engaging in a decision-making process. Ask each student to role-play delivering the message to the intended audience.

4. Select a skit, story with extensive dialogue, or scene from a play and have each student analyze the situation. Share and discuss the analyses and identify similarities and differences.

5. Ask students to prepare a short presentation on a theme or topic that is part of the current curriculum. Tell them that the presentation will be shared with students in a different class to prepare them for the same theme or topic. First ask students to analyze the theme or topic in small teams. Second let the teams share their maps. Third have each team write a presentation. Fourth let students read each presentation and select the one they think is best and should be presented to the other class.

Map It Out

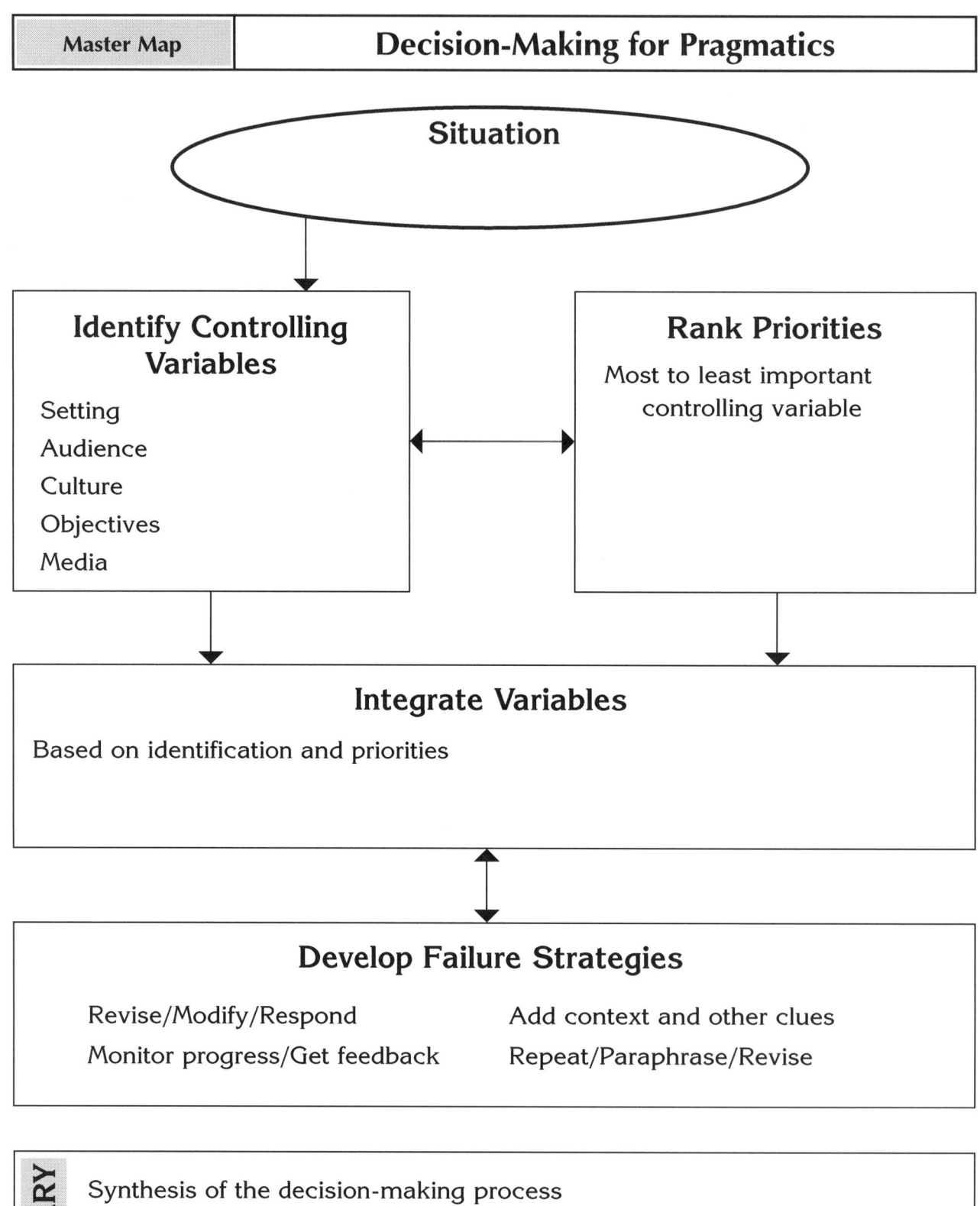

Context (Pragmatics)

| Completed Map | **Decision-Making for Pragmatics** |

Situation
Interviewing for a neighborhood job

Identify Controlling Variables

Employer—age, gender, relationship, finances

Objectives—show ability to do the job, get hired, and negotiate terms (e.g., pay, time, tools), use the right words

Rank Priorities

1. Tell about ability to do the job
2. Negotiate terms after being promised a hire
3. Use the right words and expressions to get intents across

Integrate Variables

Abilities—dependable, responsible, experienced, hired by others

Terms—pay same as others, work after school, Wednesday or Saturday best, no more than three hours at a time

Develop Failure Strategies

Abilities—make sure good points are considered (e.g., repeat, paraphrase, invite questions)

Points for negotiation—less pay, more flexible work hours

SUMMARY

I want to interview to do yard work. I have already done that job and I am good at it. Other neighbors have already hired me for the summer. I would like to work Wednesdays or Saturdays up to three hours at a time. I will negotiate for the same fee per hour that the other neighbors pay me. I will need to discuss whose tools to use for the yard work. I prefer not to carry my yard tools around.

© 2001 by E.H. Wiig and C.C. Wilson
Duplication permitted for educational use only.

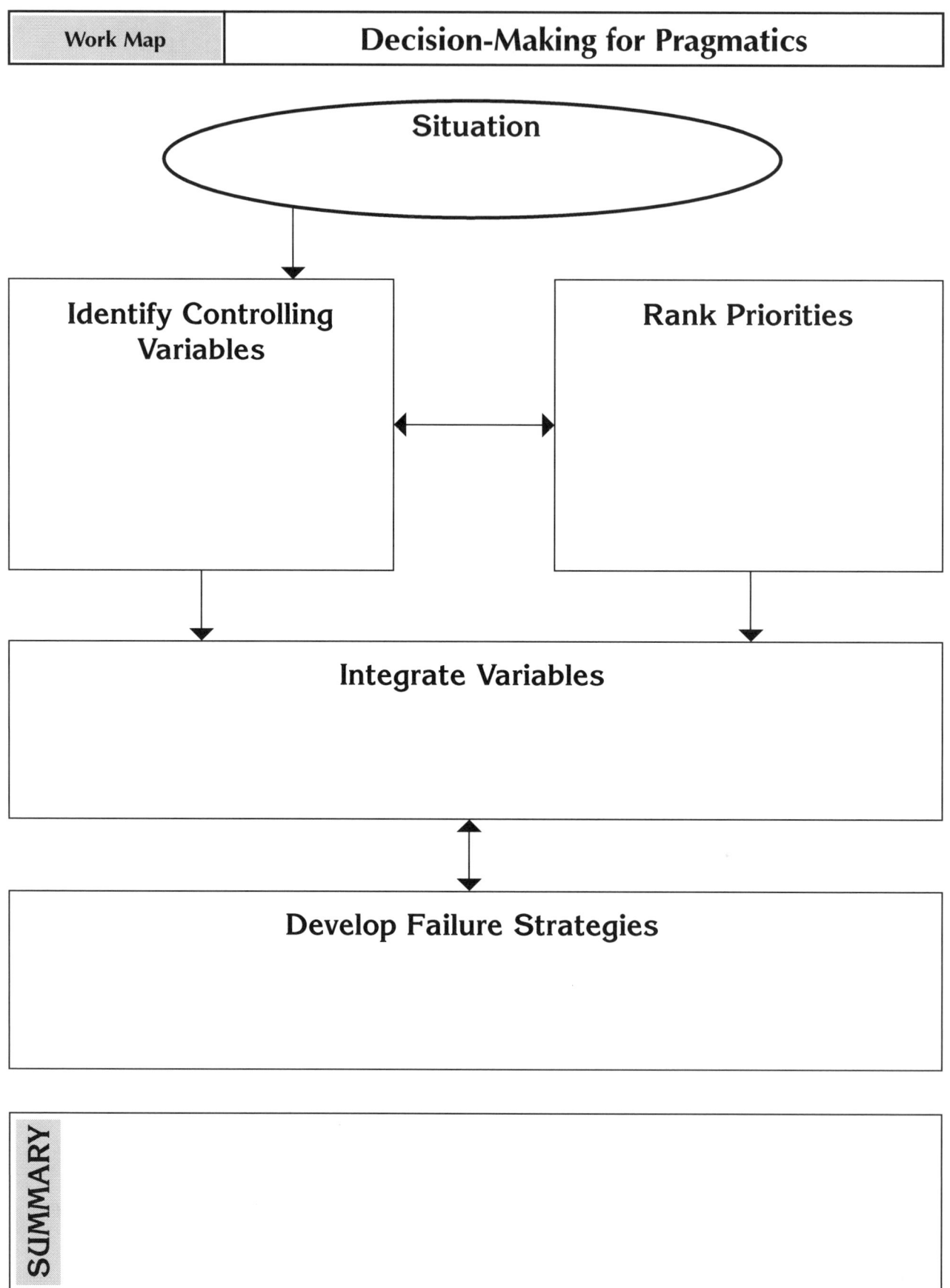

Context (Pragmatics)

Unit 28: Communication Breakdown and Clarification

> ### Educational Levels
> Upper elementary through secondary
>
> ### Objectives
> (1) Analyze causes for breakdowns in verbal communication; (2) identify ways to clarify messages and intents; (3) describe an actual situation and task; and (4) apply a process of clarification to new tasks and situations

Completed Map

This map shows how students in Grade 6 revised messages that had caused breakdowns in communication. Students were asked to imagine communication breakdowns that could be caused by something they said during interviews for neighborhood jobs. The examples they gave were recorded on the chalkboard. The teacher guided a discussion of what went wrong in each example. Each student selected an example from each type of breakdown on the map and then revised it to clarify the meaning and intent.

Show the Completed Map to students and say, for example:

> *This map shows how a student cleared up misunderstandings that could occur during an interview to get job in his neighborhood. Let's talk about the reasons for the breakdowns and look at how the student made the messages clearer to others.*

You may want to follow up by asking one or more of the following questions:

> *In what other ways could the student have made the messages clearer? How would you revise what you said if you were not understood?*

Map It Out

Work Map

Show the Work Map to students and say, for example:

> *This map is empty. Think of some situations where someone did not understand what you meant to say. We'll discuss what went wrong. Then we'll revise what you said to make the meaning of the messages clearer.*

Extended Activities

1. Prepare or find a skit or short dialogue in literature that contains communication misunderstandings. Ask students to identify what caused each misunderstanding and then revise the dialogue to make the meaning and intent clear to others.

2. Have students role-play a telephone conversation in which one speaker causes a communication breakdown. You can give participating students cue cards containing each conversational turn on their side of the phone call. Ask other students to listen for and identify unclear messages. After the role-play, ask students to revise unclear messages to make them clear and understandable.

3. Compose a letter to the class with five or six sentences that are unclear and should cause misunderstandings. Read the letter, and give each student a copy of it. Ask students to identify and analyze the sentences that are unclear and revise them.

Context (Pragmatics)

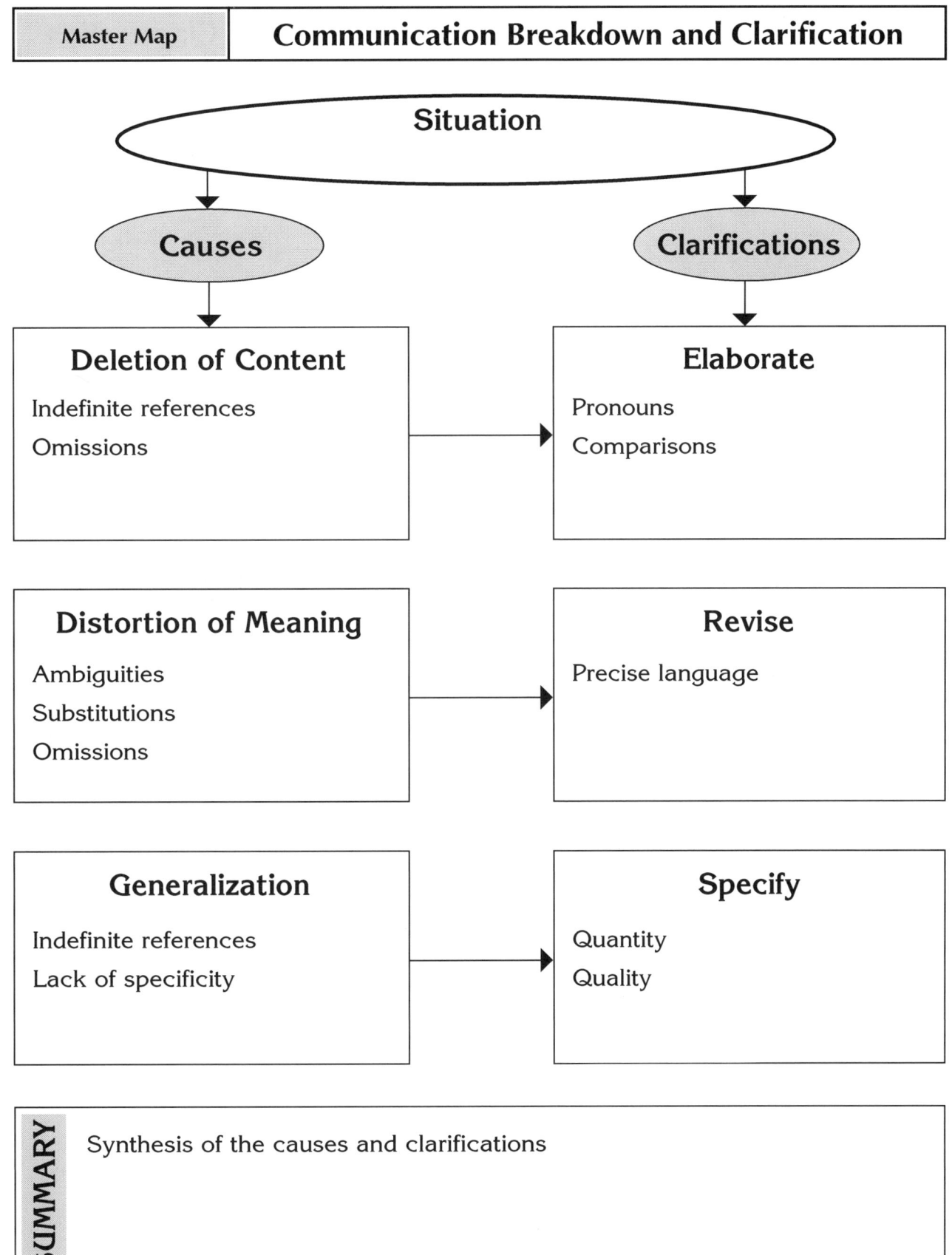

Map It Out

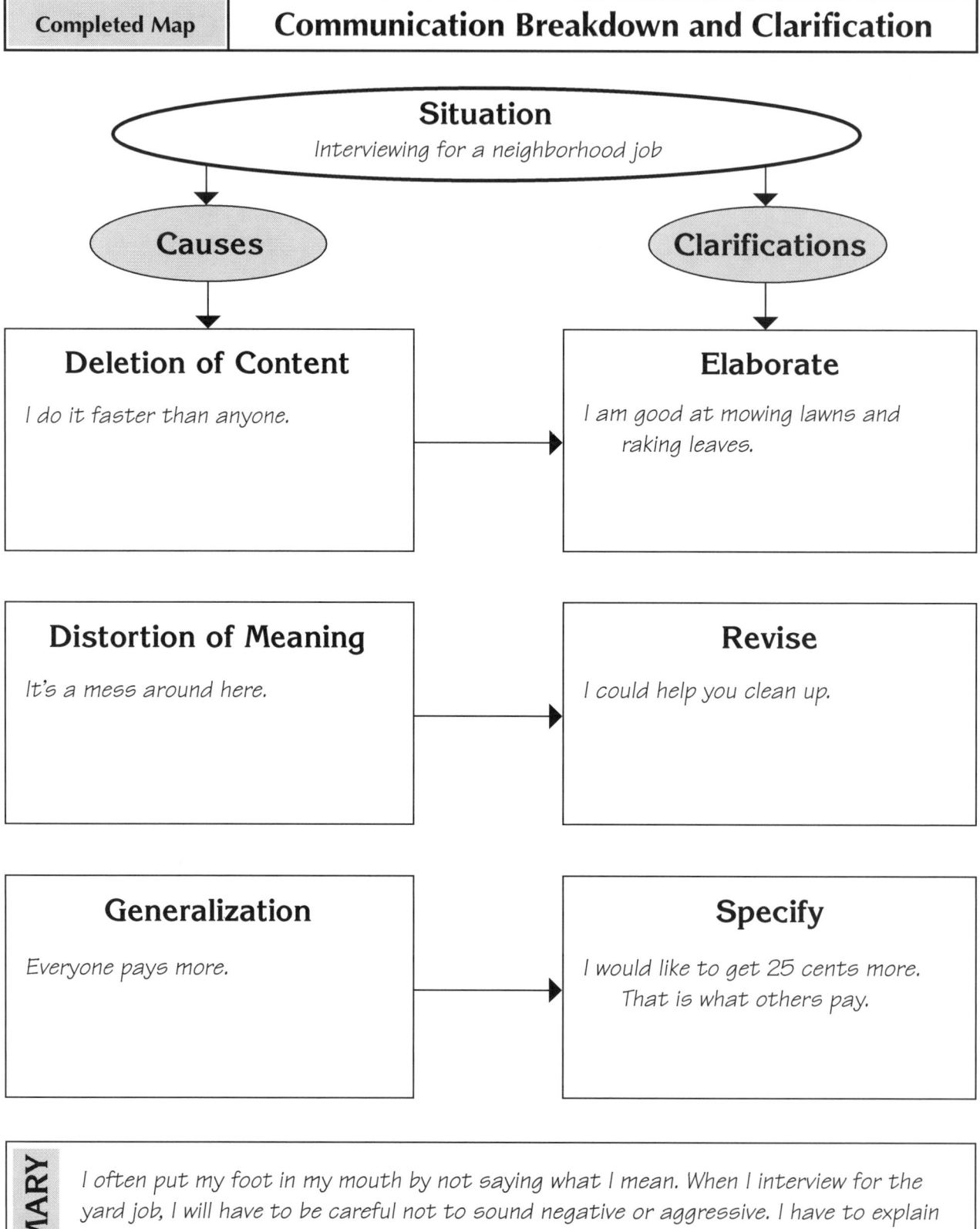

Context (Pragmatics)

| Work Map | **Communication Breakdown and Clarification** |

Situation

Causes → | **Clarifications** →

- **Deletion of Content** → **Elaborate**
- **Distortion of Meaning** → **Revise**
- **Generalization** → **Specify**

SUMMARY

Map It Out

Unit 29: Requests for Clarification

Educational Levels

Elementary through secondary

Objectives

(1) Analyze available options and appropriate forms to ask for clarification after verbal communication breakdowns; (2) describe an actual situation in which communication broke down because of misunderstandings; (3) find ways to ask for clarification; and (4) apply these skills to new situations

Completed Map

For this map, students in Grade 4 observed a skit in which the speakers communicated in ways that caused the listeners to misunderstand. In the skit, the listeners asked for clarification in inappropriate ways. Each student listened for and wrote down requests for clarification in the skit that he or she thought were inappropriate for the context. The students shared their examples and discussed what was wrong with each inappropriate request for clarification.

Show the Completed Map to students and say, for example:

This map shows how some students analyzed how characters asked for clarification. Let's talk about how the characters asked for clarification when they could not understand a message.

You may want to follow up by asking one or both of these questions:

In what other ways could the character have asked for clarification? What do you usually say when you do not understand what someone else said?

Work Map

Show the Work Map to students and say, for example:

> *This map is empty. Let's think of some situations where we might have to ask for clarification. Then we'll find some ways of asking others to clarify their verbal or written messages.*

Select examples of classroom and true-life interactions and communication breakdowns and elicit requests for clarification.

Extended Activities

1. Prepare or find a skit or short dialogue in literature with communication misunderstandings between characters. Ask students to identify what caused each misunderstanding. Then ask them to write down ways in which they might request clarifications in the situation.

2. Role-play a telephone conversation in which one speaker is difficult to understand (e.g., speaks too fast) and the other speaker asks for clarifications. You can give participating students cue cards containing each conversational turn. Ask other students to listen for and identify unclear messages and the requests for clarification that follow. After role-play, ask students to clarify and revise the requests that were not appropriate for the situation or participants.

3. Have each student write a short description of a topic of interest. Then tell students to exchange their work. Ask students to underline what they do not understand in the written description. Then return the papers to their authors, and ask authors to revise any underlined passages.

4. Write a script involving two students discussing a familiar topic. Assign roles to two students and have them read through the script in front of the class. One student should get the role of giving unclear statements and answers during the conversation. The second student can be given the role of being impatient and rudely interrupting when there is a breakdown in communication. Analyze and discuss the interactions with the class.

Map It Out

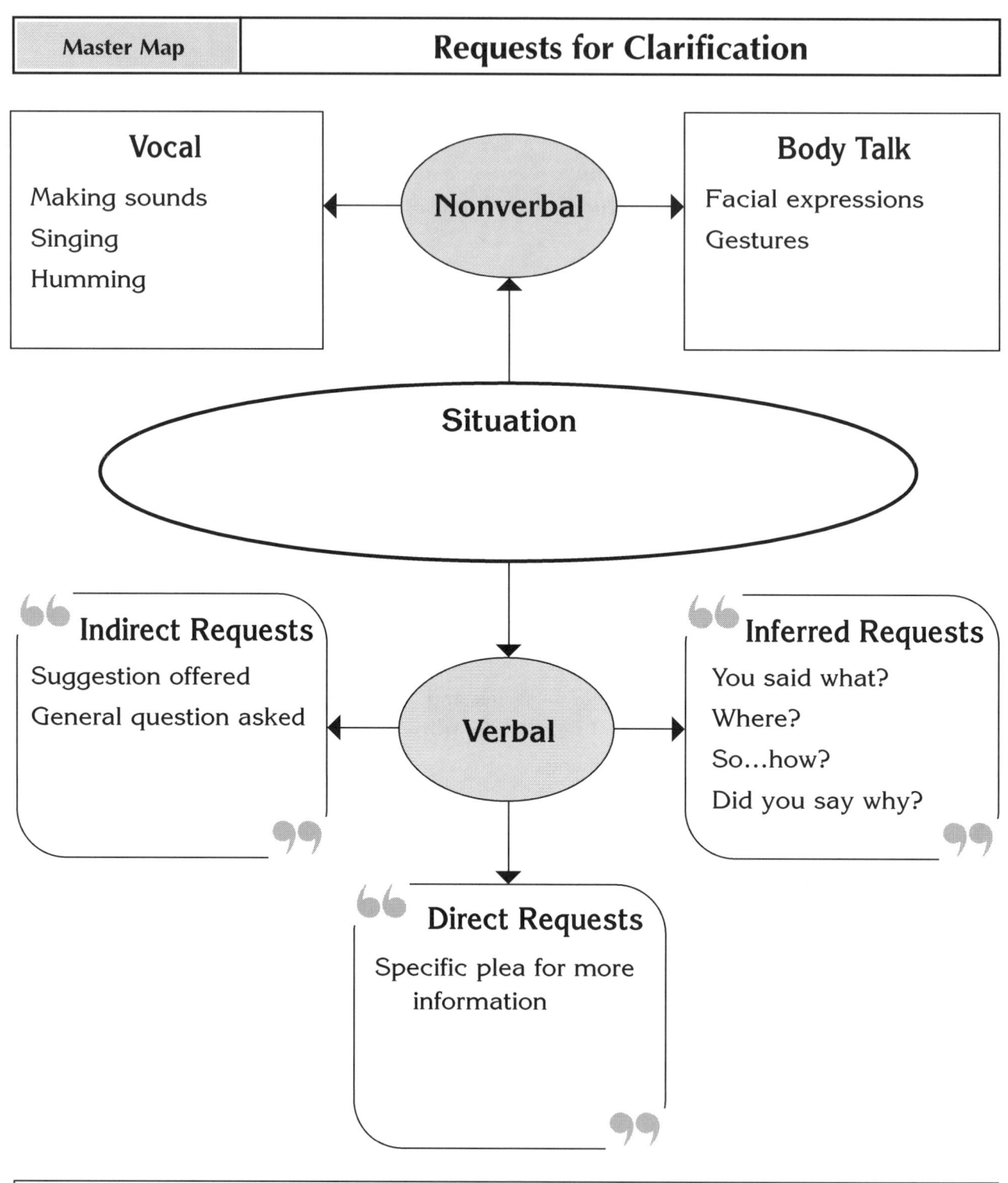

200

Context (Pragmatics)

| Completed Map | **Requests for Clarification** |

Requests for Clarification

Nonverbal

Vocal
- Hummed
- Sang

Body Talk
- Turned head and shoulders away
- Held up a sign with a question mark

Situation
Observing a skit

Verbal

Indirect Requests
"Could you speak slower now and then?
Are we supposed to hear you?"

Inferred Requests
"What? I didn't get it.
Who do you think you're talking to?"

Direct Requests
"Speak up, teacher!
Spit that gum out, so I can understand what you're saying.
Please speak more clearly. We can't hear in the back."

SUMMARY
We watched a skit and learned how to make good requests. You can ask without saying a word, but that could be rude. You can also use a direct request to tell exactly what you want done. Sometimes you want to be more polite. Then you can make an indirect or an inferred request. Indirect requests are usually polite. Inferred requests can be short and use wh-question words. Sometimes others think that inferred requests are rude.

© 2001 by E.H. Wiig and C.C. Wilson
Duplication permitted for educational use only.

Map It Out

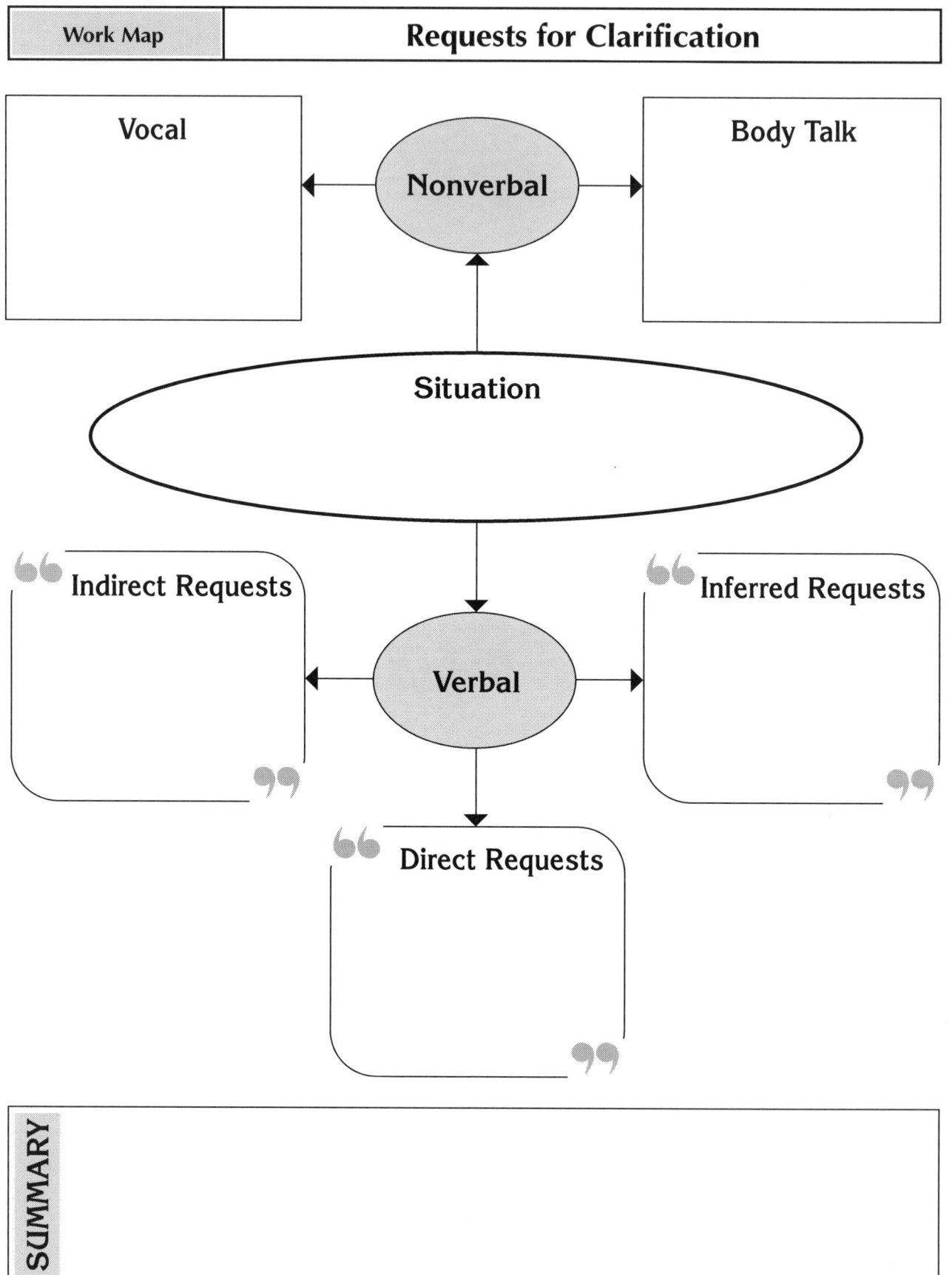

202

© 2001 by E.H. Wiig and C.C. Wilson
Duplication permitted for educational use only.

Context (Pragmatics)

Unit 30: Requests for Actions and Favors

> **Educational Levels**
>
> Elementary through secondary
>
> **Objectives**
>
> (1) Analyze available options and appropriate forms to ask others for actions or favors; (2) describe an actual situation in which actions or favors were requested; (3) find appropriate ways to ask for favors; and (4) apply these skills to new situations and tasks

Completed Map

This map was completed by students in Grade 4 who were given ambiguous requests that had been asked by characters in *Room 14* by Carolyn Wilson. The teacher asked students to analyze what was unclear about each request. After the discussion, students changed unclear verbal and nonverbal requests into clear, understandable forms. The class reviewed the clear requests and role-played situations, first with the unclear requests and then with the revised requests.

Show the Completed Map to students and say, for example:

> *This map shows how students in the book* Room 14 *asked others in their class for help. Let's talk about the verbal and nonverbal ways the students made requests.*

Ask students to judge if the requests were appropriate or not appropriate for the situation.

You may want to follow up by asking one or both of these questions:

> *In what other ways could the students have asked for a favor? What do you usually say when you want someone to do something or to do you a favor?*

Work Map

Show the Work Map to students and say, for example:

> *This map is empty. Let's think of a situation where we might have to ask others for a favor or an action. Then we'll consider how we can verbally and nonverbally make the request.*

Map It Out

Extended Activities

1. Identify a true-life situation in which students might need to leave a written message to request a favor (e.g., feed a pet or water plants). Have each student write a request. Share the requests, and guide a discussion about the appropriateness of how each request was written.

2. Have each student identify a situation in which he or she would have to ask for permission. Then have each student write down what he or she needs permission to do and from whom. Ask each student to share the situation with the class and role-play asking for permission. Guide an evaluation of the requests for permission.

3. Ask students to identify situations around school in which they might have to ask for someone's attention. Have students write a few words to describe the situation and how they would get the other person's attention. Ask students to role-play these situations, and guide a peer evaluation afterward.

4. Find or develop a skit in which some of the characters have titles or authority status. Ask students to develop a set of polite and formal requests for attention or action (e.g., "Would you please allow me get by?"). Develop replies that the characters might give. Then role-play the requests and replies.

Context (Pragmatics)

| Master Map | **Requests for Actions and Favors** |

Body Talk
Facial expressions
Gestures

Vocal
Making sounds
Humming
Singing

Signs
Exit
Yield

Nonverbal

Situation

Verbal

Indirect Requests
Suggestion offered
General question asked

Inferred Requests
A reference to a problem, but not direct

Direct Requests
Specific plea to request something

SUMMARY: Synthesis of appropriate and inappropriate requests and lessons learned

© 2001 by E.H. Wiig and C.C. Wilson
Duplication permitted for educational use only.

Map It Out

| Completed Map | Requests for Actions and Favors |

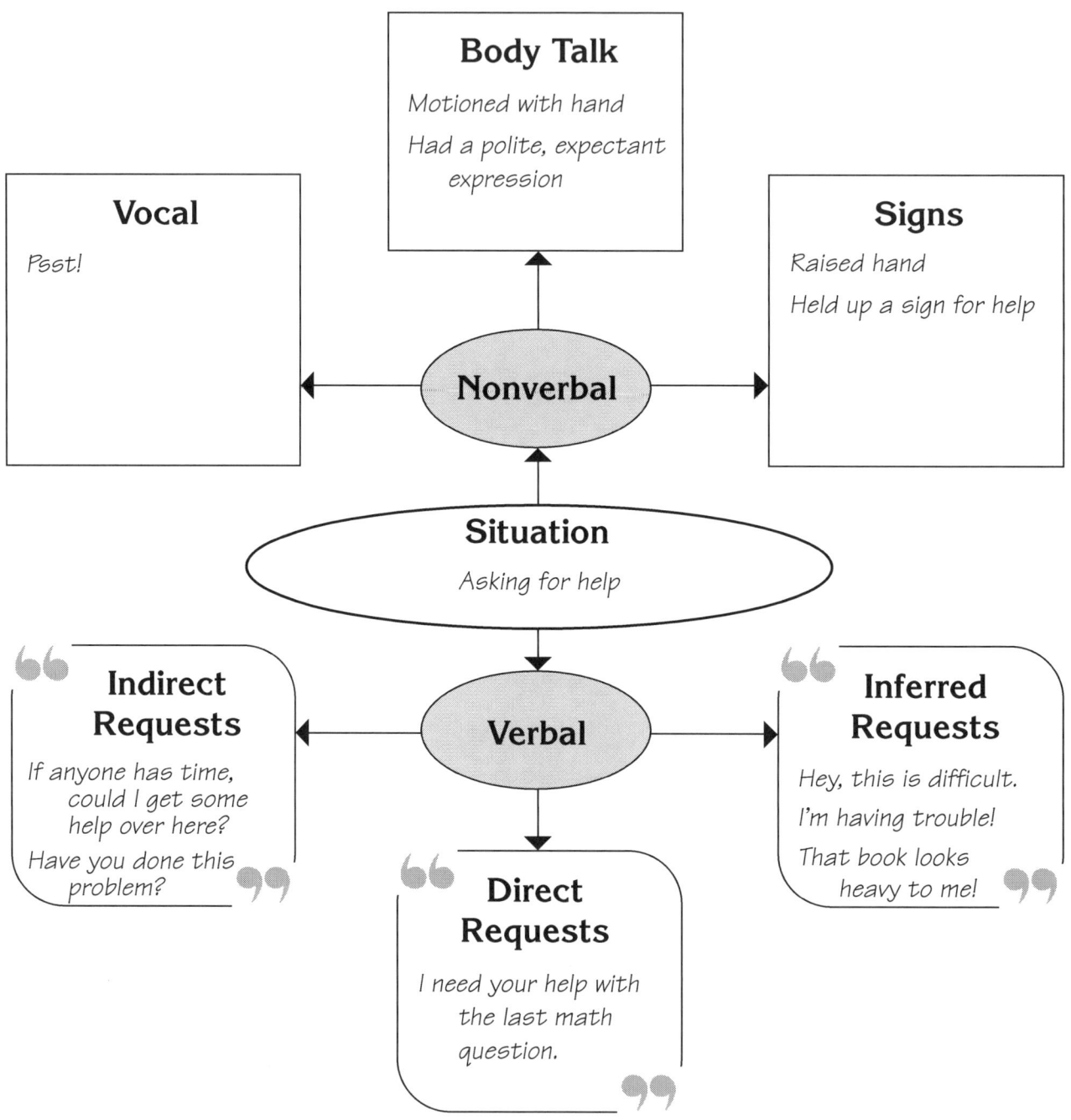

Body Talk
Motioned with hand
Had a polite, expectant expression

Vocal
Psst!

Signs
Raised hand
Held up a sign for help

Nonverbal

Situation
Asking for help

Verbal

Indirect Requests
If anyone has time, could I get some help over here?
Have you done this problem?

Direct Requests
I need your help with the last math question.

Inferred Requests
Hey, this is difficult.
I'm having trouble!
That book looks heavy to me!

SUMMARY You have to think about how to ask for help in class. Some teachers don't like you to make a sound to get their attention. They want a raised hand. Other teachers like to know what you need help with and want you to be polite. You'd better not complain in class. Don't just say, "I'm in trouble here," because that gets you nowhere.

Context (Pragmatics)

| Work Map | **Requests for Actions and Favors** |

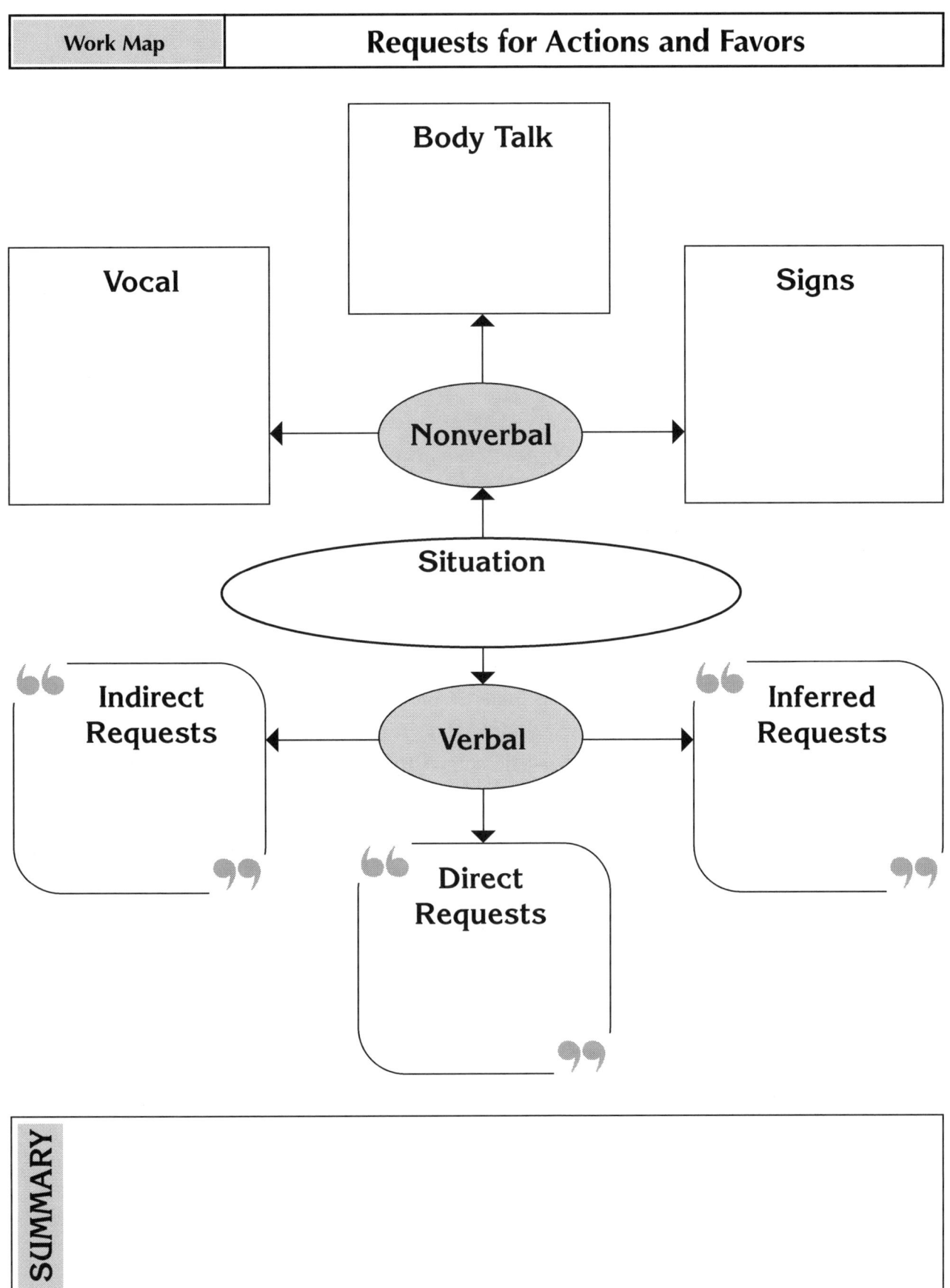

SUMMARY

Map It Out

Unit 31: Cultural Features of Communication

> **Educational Levels**
>
> Upper elementary through secondary
>
> **Objectives**
>
> (1) Analyze and compare features of verbal communication associated with variations in dialects, languages, or cultures; (2) describe an actual situation or interaction with cultural and linguistic diversity; (3) understand and respect diversity and difference; and (4) apply these skills to new instances and situations

Completed Map

This map was developed by students in Grade 10 after they had read *Tell Me a Tale* by James McEachin. The students identified and compared features of Standard American English with features of the dialect used by the local characters. Then they discussed how the differences influenced the relationships among the characters. They discussed Moses's code switching between the local dialect and educated English, what this ability meant, and how it signaled Moses's old and new identities.

Show the Completed Map to students and say, for example:

> *This map shows what a group of students found when they analyzed how the different characters in the novel* Tell Me a Tale *communicated. Let's talk about each characteristic and difference in language and communication and what features the students thought were important about them.*

You may want to follow up by asking students one or more of these questions:

> *Why do you think the main character—Moses—sometimes used Standard American English when he talked to the local men? What effect do you think this had on the local men? What impression did you get of the local men from the way they communicated?*

Work Map

Show the Work Map to students and say, for example:

> *This map is empty. Let's talk about a situation where there are differences in speakers' communication styles. Then we'll identify and discuss the differences we find.*

Emphasize the integrity, origin, and value of linguistic variations among various dialects and languages.

Extended Activities

1. Identify students who are good at code switching between Standard American English and a dialectal variation. Ask them to demonstrate examples of code switching. Then guide an analysis of the differences between the two codes.

2. Identify students who are bilingual. Ask them to answer questions about differences in the verbal and nonverbal communication features of the two languages. Then guide a discussion of what, if anything, made it difficult for them to learn and use English as a second language.

3. Select a story, novel, or play that is part of the curriculum and has characters who use different linguistic variations (e.g., dialects or languages). Have students analyze, compare, and contrast the communication features of the characters at different levels (e.g., word or structure). Ask students to read excerpts of dialogue from the text in the dialect or linguistic variation featured.

4. Have students listen to the characters in a popular TV series. Have each student identify characters who use dialects that are different from the rest of the characters and write down examples of how they talk. Share and compare the students' observations of linguistic and cultural diversity in the characters. Then discuss what effect the differences have on the viewers of the series or show.

5. Select examples of true-life interactions in school, at home, or in the community in which there are variations in dialects, languages, or communication styles. Guide a discussion of the students' reactions to the differences. Foster patience with differences, respect for individuals with differences, and tolerance of diversity.

Map It Out

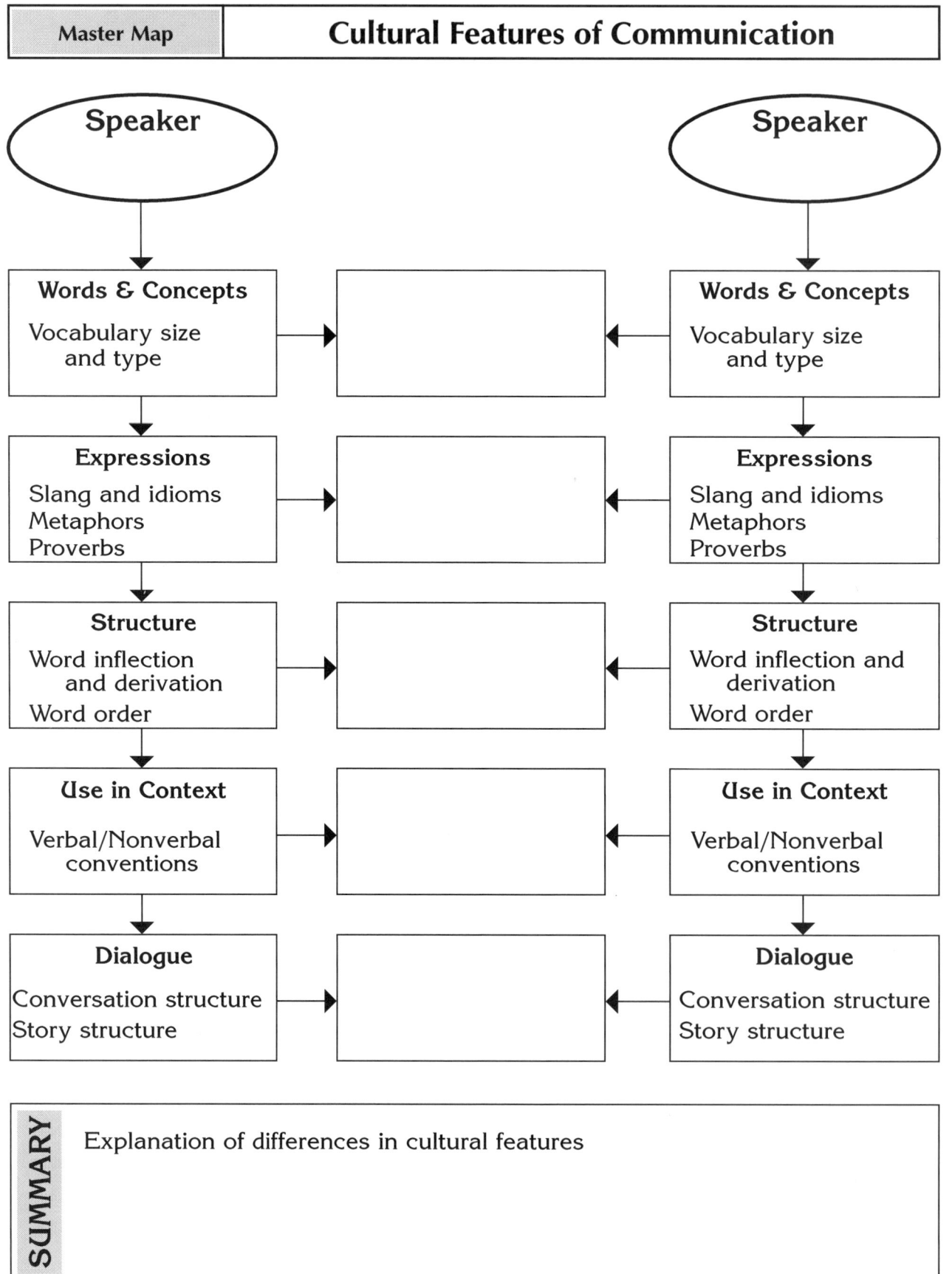

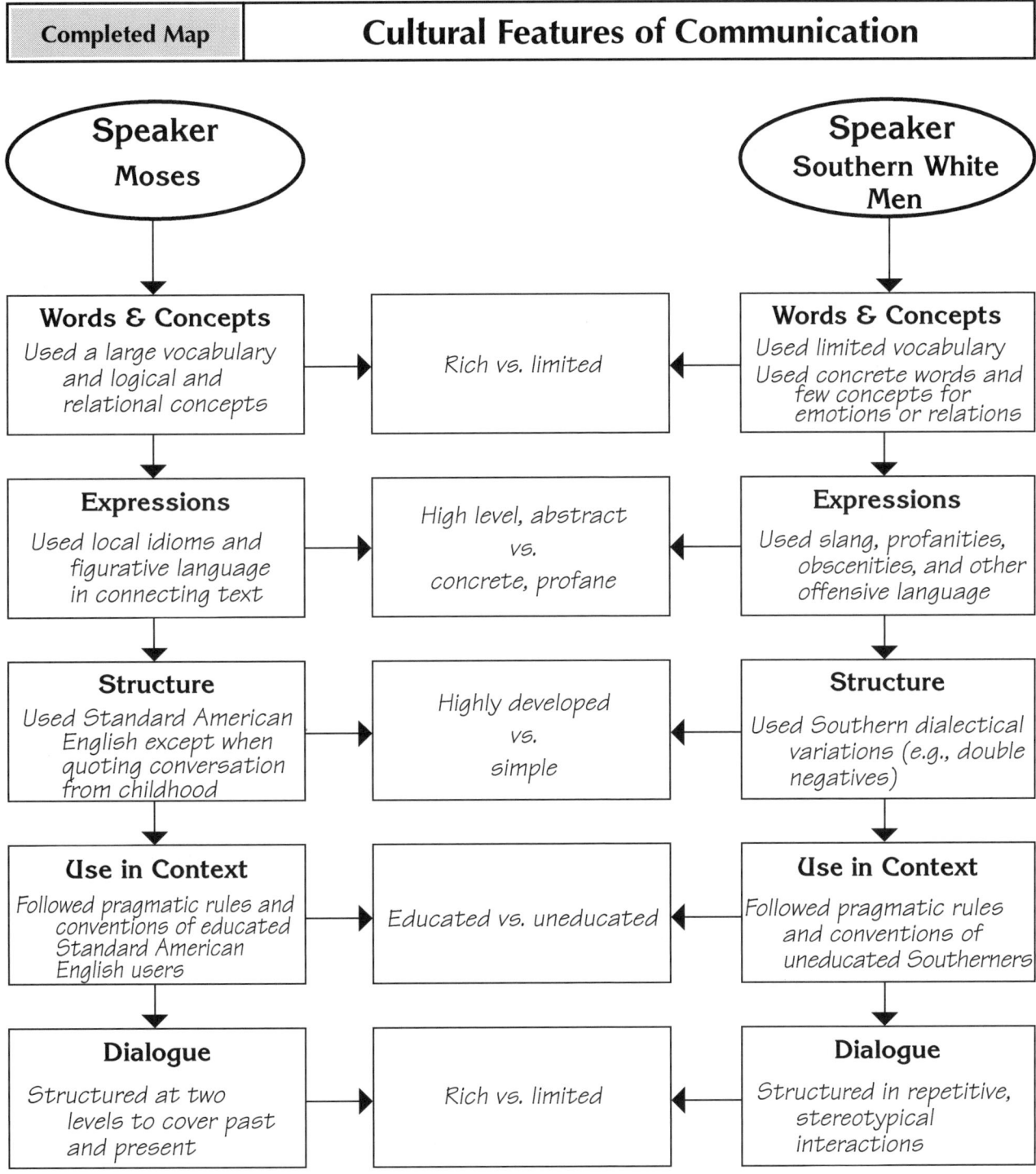

Map It Out

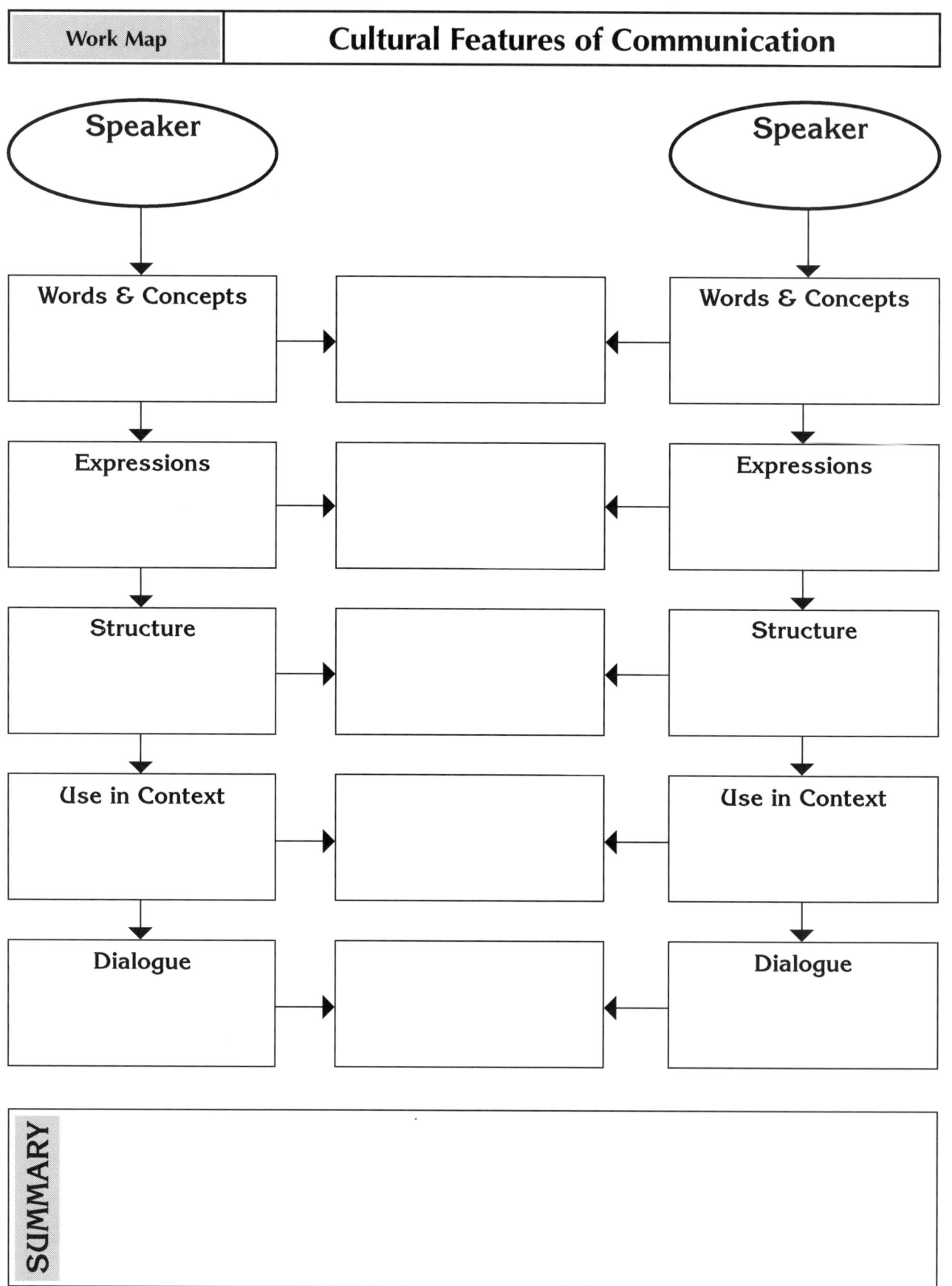

212

Context (Pragmatics)

Unit 32: Pragmatic Characterization

Educational Levels

Elementary through secondary

Objectives

(1) Identify major factors and driving forces in self and others that contribute to the quality of a relationship; (2) analyze and discuss the effects of personal characteristics on interactions in different contexts; and (3) relate features and driving forces to specific aspects or qualities of interactions

Completed Map

For this map, students in Grade 6 were asked to form teams for a geography project. Each student was given a map to record his or her personal characteristics and abilities. Then each student identified and recorded some characteristics he or she thought a good partner should have. The students posted their maps and negotiated with each other to create teams with two or three members.

Show the Completed Map to students and say, for example:

> *This map shows an example of how a student analyzed the potential interactions between himself and potential teammates. Let's talk about what the student brought to the interaction and what teammates should bring to best complement the student.*

You may want to follow up by asking one or both of the following questions:

> *How could you analyze interactions between yourself and another student in your class using this method? What characteristics in a person seem to create good interactions with others?*

Map It Out

Work Map

Show the Work Map to students and say, for example:

> *This map is empty. Let's talk about how you interact with another person. Then we'll analyze your traits and the other person's traits to gain an understanding of the interaction.*

Extended Activities

1. Have each student select two friends or siblings and analyze some of their personal characteristics. Ask students to analyze the relationship among the characteristics. Have students share their analyses. Guide a discussion of the characteristics that either made for a good relationship or a bad one.

2. Write some personal characteristics of two "imaginary" people (e.g., characters in a play). Then ask students to analyze and compare the characteristics and draw inferences about the quality of the relationship and how the characters interact with each other.

3. Select a TV series in which the relationship between two main characters is featured. Ask the students to view an episode of the TV series and prepare to analyze, compare, and contrast the personal characteristics of the two characters. Then ask them to discuss the nature of the relationship and describe which characteristics clash and which complement.

4. Have each student interview two people in a relationship (e.g., parents or siblings). Ask students to develop questions that will elicit answers to fill in the characteristics in each response box on a map (e.g., "What do you think is special about your looks?" or "How do you communicate your feelings to others?"). Then ask students to conduct the interview and record answers.

5. Ask students to form pairs. Have each student analyze the personality characteristics of his or her partner. Also have each student analyze his or her personality characteristics. Then ask the student pairs to compare the two versions and discuss any differences in perceptions.

Context (Pragmatics)

Master Map	**Pragmatic Characterization**

Knowledge
- Conceptual
- Experiential
- Procedural

Communication
- Style and register
- Attitudes
- Objectives

Behaviors
- Styles
- Attitudes
- Reactions

Appearance
- Gender and age
- Size and weight
- Unique features

What Others Bring

Social Status
- Belongings
- Family
- Education

Interaction

Appearance
- Gender and age
- Size and weight
- Unique features

Social Status
- Belongings
- Family
- Education

What You Bring

Knowledge
- Conceptual
- Experiential
- Procedural

Communication
- Style and register
- Attitudes
- Objectives

Behaviors
- Styles
- Attitudes
- Reactions

SUMMARY: Discussion of the interaction

© 2001 by E.H. Wiig and C.C. Wilson
Duplication permitted for educational use only.

Map It Out

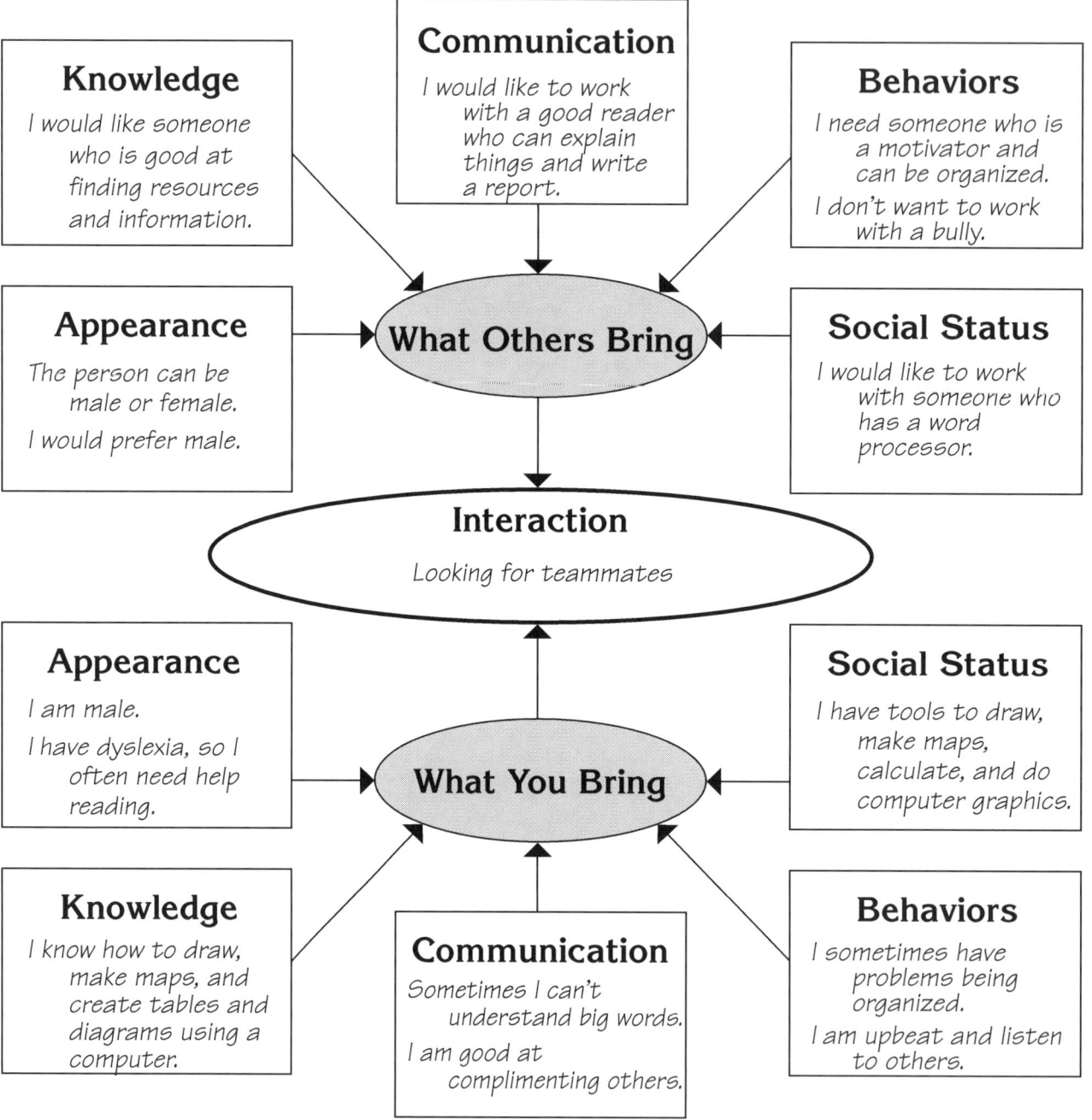

216

Context (Pragmatics)

| Work Map | **Pragmatic Characterization** |

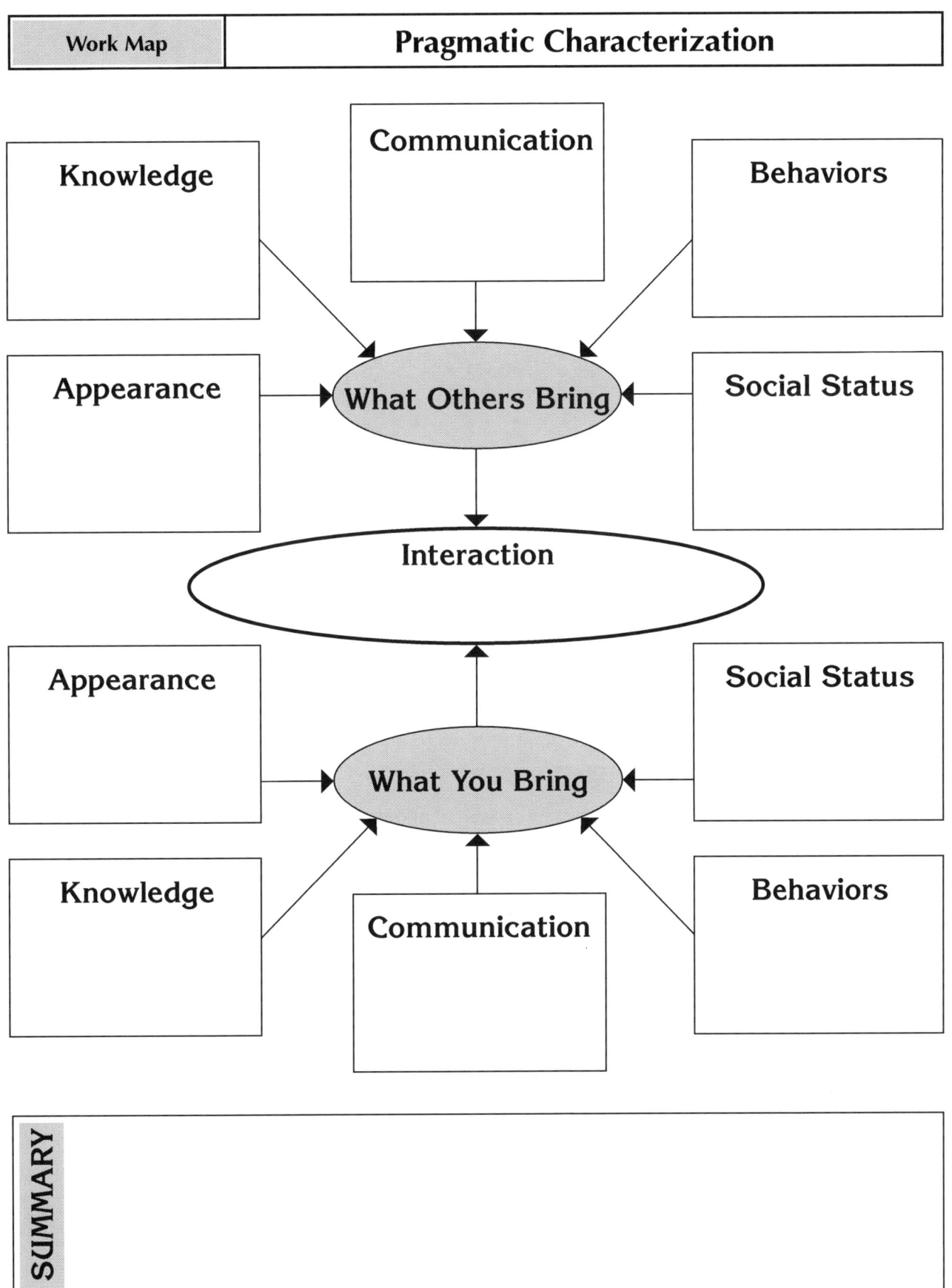

SUMMARY

© 2001 by E.H. Wiig and C.C. Wilson
Duplication permitted for educational use only.

Map It Out

Unit 33: Perspective Taking

Educational Levels

Upper elementary through secondary

Objectives

(1) Identify important dimensions and features of self-awareness; (2) analyze and discuss the level of awareness of others; and (3) integrate these elements for dynamic perspective taking in true-life situations.

Completed Map

For this map, students in Grade 5 were preparing to welcome a classmate back after she suffered an injury. The teacher guided the students in identifying some of the important features to consider in order to take their classmate's perspective. The teacher began by telling students to be sensitive to their classmate's needs and not overwhelm her with attention or questions. They then discussed what to be aware of and how to behave in a considerate way.

Show the Completed Map to students and say, for example:

This map shows an example of how some students analyzed their awareness of themselves and a classmate. Let's talk about the students' awareness and how that might influence the way they welcomed their classmate back.

You may want to follow up by asking, for example:

How could you analyze your self-awareness and needs in order to be more sensitive to the needs of a friend?

Work Map

Show the Work Map to students and say, for example:

This map is empty. Let's talk about an interaction or relationship in your life that requires sensitivity. First analyze the awareness you have of yourself. Second analyze the awareness you have of your friend. After you complete your analyses, we will discuss what is good about your awareness of self and others and what you may need to think about and do to become more sensitive to others.

Extended Activities

1. Select a story or novel that is part of the curriculum and in which one or more of the characters show sensitivity to the needs of other characters (e.g., *Charlotte's Web* by E.B. White). Read one or more excerpts that exemplify a character's sensitivity and perspective taking. Guide students in identifying what made a character sensitive to others in his or her environment.

2. Identify a character in a story, novel, or play who is insensitive to others (e.g., Ebenezer Scrooge in Dickens's *A Christmas Carol*). Read excerpts that illustrate the character's lack of sensitivity. Then ask students to identify what seems to be lacking in the character's ability to take another person's point of view.

3. Identify a topic or theme that is part of the curriculum and find students with special interests or experiences related to the topic (e.g., deserts or coin collecting). Ask these students to prepare a short oral presentation about the topic. Guide the students by eliciting evidence of what the other students know or do not know about the topic. Then ask the students to look inward and identify feelings, reactions, and memories associated with the topic.

4. Select an episode from a current TV series that shows characters who have a high degree of sensitivity to others and characters who lack sensitivity. Show the episode, and have each student analyze the characteristics of a sensitive and an insensitive character. Then ask students to share their findings and compare and contrast the characters.

5. Have each student think of either a positive or negative relationship he or she has with another person. Have each student identify how sensitive or insensitive he or she is to the needs of the other person. Then discuss how his or her sensitivity to the other person can be increased (e.g., by spending time together or asking questions).

Map It Out

| Master Map | Perspective Taking |

Self
- Reactions
- Feelings
- Changes in feelings

Memory
- Reactions at given points in time
- Facts about others
- Prior interactions
- Knowledge gained from being self-aware

Awareness of Self

Perspective Taking

Communication
- Meanings of words and expressions
- Implied meanings
- Style
- Body language

Knowledge
- Past experiences
- Prior knowledge
- Information about a theme or topic
- Level of attention

Awareness of Others

SUMMARY — Plan for perspective taking

220

© 2001 by E.H. Wiig and C.C. Wilson
Duplication permitted for educational use only.

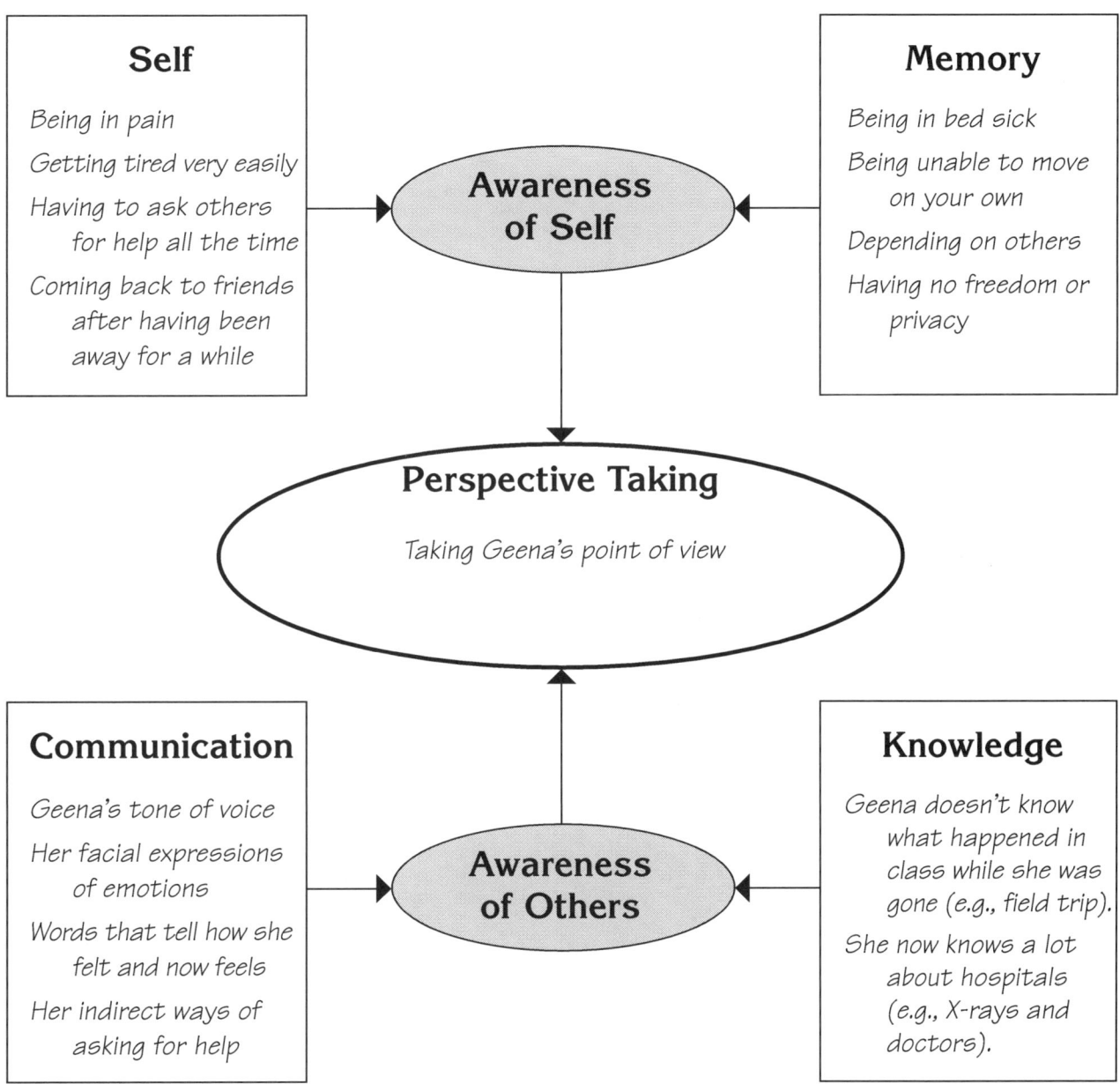

Map It Out

| Work Map | Perspective Taking |

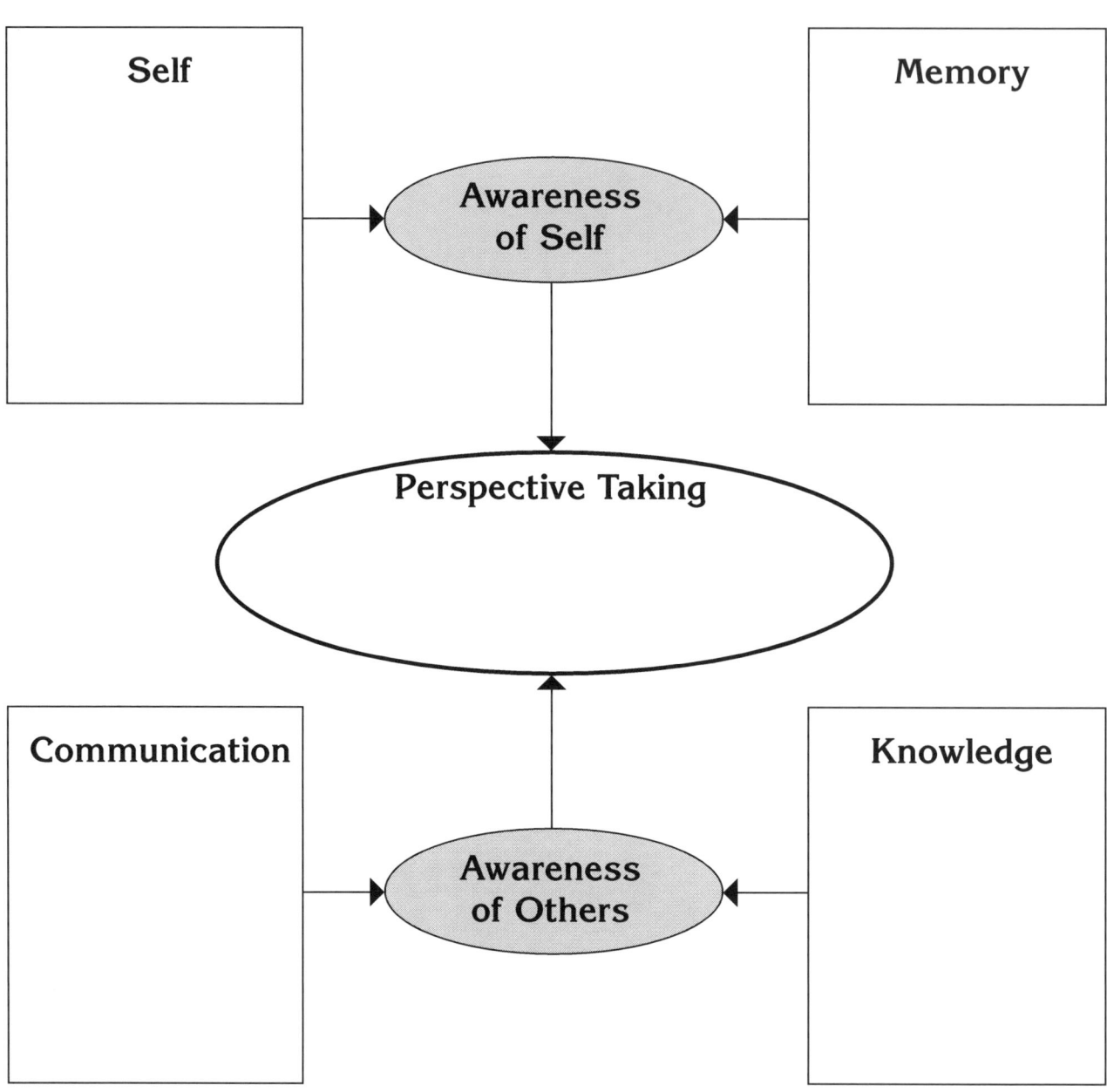

SUMMARY

222

© 2001 by E.H. Wiig and C.C. Wilson
Duplication permitted for educational use only.

Context (Pragmatics)

Unit 34: Sharing, Borrowing, and Exchanging

> ## Educational Levels
>
> Elementary through secondary
>
> ## Objectives
>
> (1) Identify the needs of self and others; (2) analyze and discuss mutual benefits of sharing, borrowing, or exchanging items; and (3) integrate this knowledge to negotiate sharing, borrowing, or exchanging items with others

Completed Map

This map shows how students in Grade 4 prepared for a field trip. The teacher told the students that they wanted to bring as few food and drink supplies as possible. This required that the students share foods, drinks, and equipment. Each student specified what he or she wanted to bring. The students then worked together in small groups and discussed what each of them wanted to bring. They came up with a compromise list of the foods, drinks, and equipment that would benefit and be liked by the majority of the students in the class.

Show the Completed Map to students and say, for example:

> *This map shows an example of how some students managed to bring as few supplies as possible on a field trip by sharing, borrowing, and exchanging necessities. Let's talk about how the students analyzed the situation, their needs, and the mutual benefits.*

You may want to follow up by asking, for example:

> *How would you analyze and plan for sharing something with a friend during a day at a community pool or in a park?*

Map It Out

Work Map

Show the Work Map to students and say, for example:

> *This map is empty. Let's talk about a situation in your daily life where you have to share, borrow, or exchange something. We'll analyze your needs and the needs of other people involved. Then we'll identify possible mutual benefits of sharing and plan how to negotiate the deal.*

Extended Activities

1. Set up a simulated activity for creating a collage with a minimum of tools. Give students only one object for each task involved (e.g., one pair of scissors, one tube of glue, and one picture source). Tell students that they will have to share and exchange tools. Prepare them by reviewing how they might ask to borrow or exchange an object. Then engage them in the activity. Listen for and record examples of what they say to negotiate. Review the examples with the students after the activity.

2. Randomly give each student in a small group a magazine (e.g., fashion or technical) or book (e.g., fiction or nonfiction). Tell students to prepare themselves for negotiating exchanges of the magazines or books. Remind them to take another person's perspective before they begin to negotiate as this will increase their chances of success. You may want to prepare the students by reviewing perspective taking and verbal scripts for negotiating exchanges.

3. Set up a simulated activity in which the students have been shopping and come home with some items they did not want or need. You may want to make up a realistic shopping list for the students that details what they bought. Then ask each student to identify an item she or he does not want and prepare to return or exchange the item at the store. Have students role-play some interactions at a fictitious customer-service desk and to get feedback from peers.

4. Have each student write a note to ask permission to borrow something from someone (e.g., a helmet for biking or a lawn mower for a yard job). Prepare students by guiding them to consider the lender's needs and points of view on the matter. Share and discuss the request notes.

Context (Pragmatics)

| Master Map | **Sharing, Borrowing, and Exchanging** |

Situation

What I Want

Objects/Entities
Tasks/Situations
Goals
Benefits
Desired Outcomes

What They Want

Objects/Entities
Tasks/Situations
Goals
Benefits
Desired Outcomes

Mutual Benefits

Negotiate to Share, Borrow, or Exchange

SUMMARY: Highlight of the process and its outcomes

Map It Out

| Completed Map | Sharing, Borrowing, and Exchanging |

Situation
Negotiating supplies for a field trip

What I Want

Sandwich—white bread, mayo, mustard, ketchup, cold cuts, and cheese
Snack—cupcakes and candy
Drinks—canned sodas
Emergency—meat and potatoes

What They Want

Sandwich—whole wheat bread, cold cuts, lettuce, tomatoes, and mayo
Snack—fruits, cereals, snack bars, dried fruits, and nut mix
Drinks—fruit juices
Emergency—chocolate-flavored energy bars and distilled water

Mutual Benefits

Limit the types and increase the amounts of lunch foods
Select snacks that are compact, won't spoil, and give energy (e.g., granola bars and apples)
Bring emergency foods that give protein, grains, and carbohydrates (e.g., instant soups with beans and rice or energy bars), and bring distilled water

Negotiate to Share, Borrow, or Exchange

SUMMARY

We were planning a field trip. Our teacher said to limit what we brought along and share everything. The problem was that everyone wanted to bring something different. We first listed our individual preferences. Then we worked in teams to compare our lists and compromise.

Context (Pragmatics)

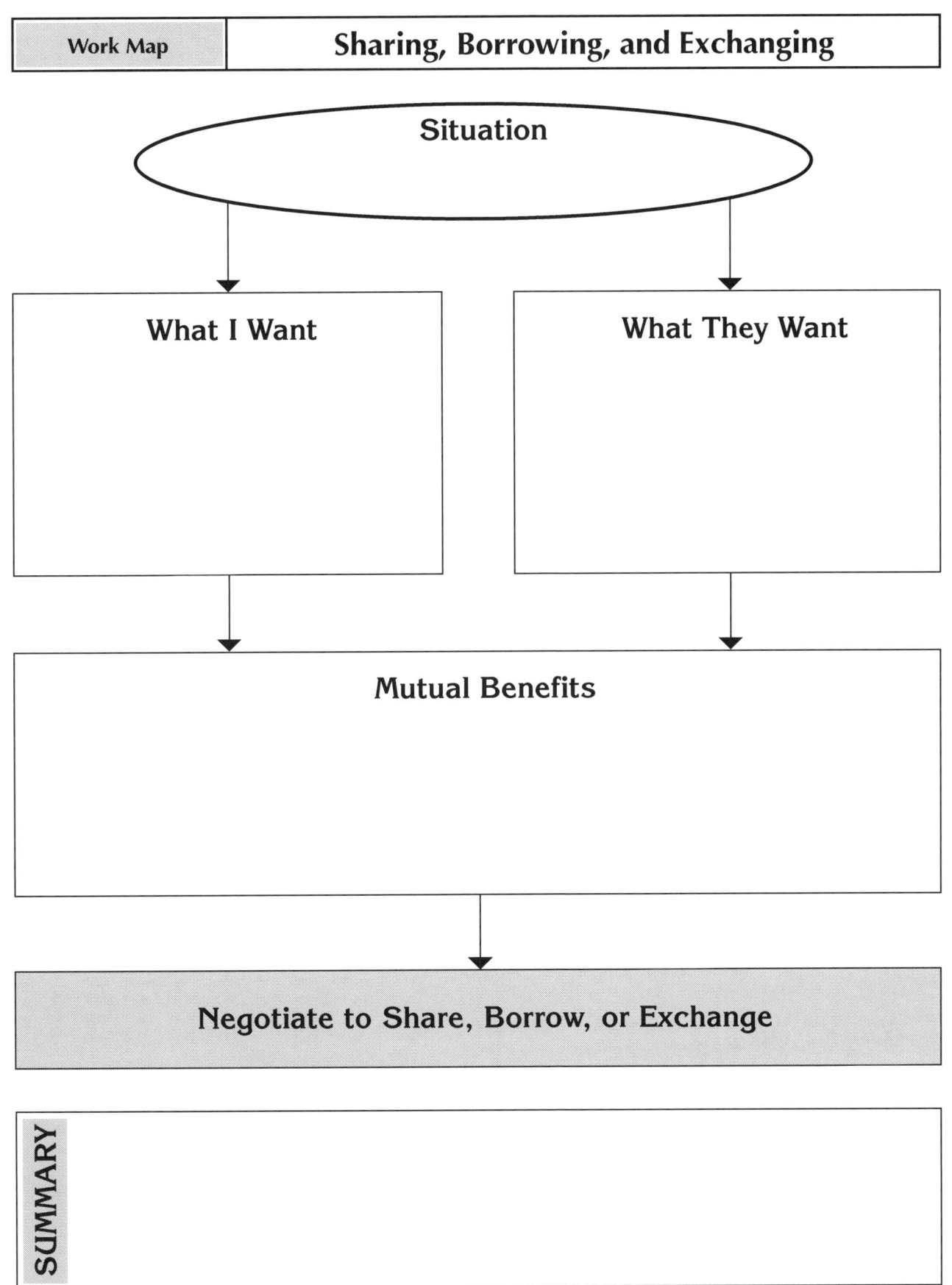

Map It Out

Unit 35: Negotiating Terms

Educational Levels

Upper elementary through secondary

Objectives

(1) Identify similarities and differences in goals, interests, and personal perspectives; (2) analyze and discuss points and counterpoints; and (3) integrate this knowledge to negotiate win-win solutions

Completed Map

This map shows how a student in Grade 9 negotiated terms for a day trip with a friend. The friend wanted to go downhill skiing all day. The student, however, did not like downhill skiing. He preferred cross-country skiing and loved to hike. The student analyzed the two points of view and came up with a negotiation of the terms for the trip.

Show the Completed Map to students and say, for example:

This map shows an example of how a student dealt with opposing ideas about what to do on a day trip. To begin, let's talk about the different views or perspectives the two students had. Then we'll look at the points and counterpoints.

You may want to follow up by asking one or both of the following questions:

What side would you have taken on this issue? What would you consider to be a win-win agreement or contract?

Work Map

Show the Work Map to students and say, for example:

This map is empty. Let's identify a situation where there could be different points of view. Then we'll identify some possible points and counterpoints.

Extended Activities

1. Have each student identify a situation in his or her family that might call for negotiating terms (e.g., chores or bedtime) and arriving at a better solution for both parties. Have each student analyze the situation. Share and role-play how several of the students would approach the task of negotiating.

2. Identify some current terms for student work, activities, or classroom chores you want changed. Record your points on a map, and share the map with the class to elicit their points of view on the issues. Afterward negotiate a change in terms.

3. Have each student identify a job he or she is being paid to do and what he or she would like changed about the job. Then have students role-play negotiating for some of the new terms.

4. Identify a community issue that is in the news (e.g., building a new road). Then ask students to take sides on the issue and prepare to negotiate with the opposite side. Have students role-play a negotiation on the issue.

5. Identify a broad social issue with opposing views (e.g., gun control). Then ask the students to take sides on the issue and team up to prepare for a discussion and negotiation for a compromise.

Map It Out

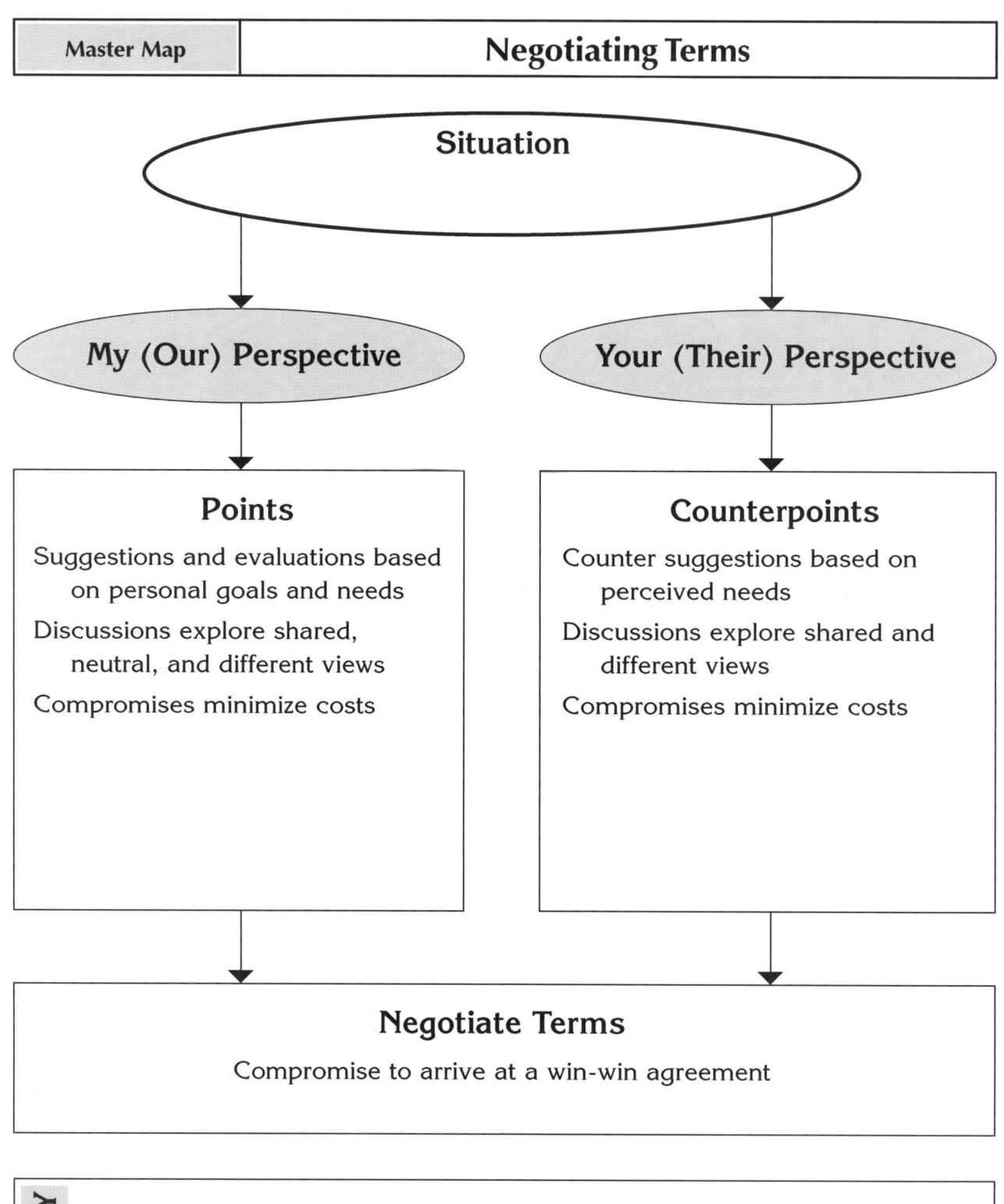

230

Context (Pragmatics)

| Completed Map | **Negotiating Terms** |

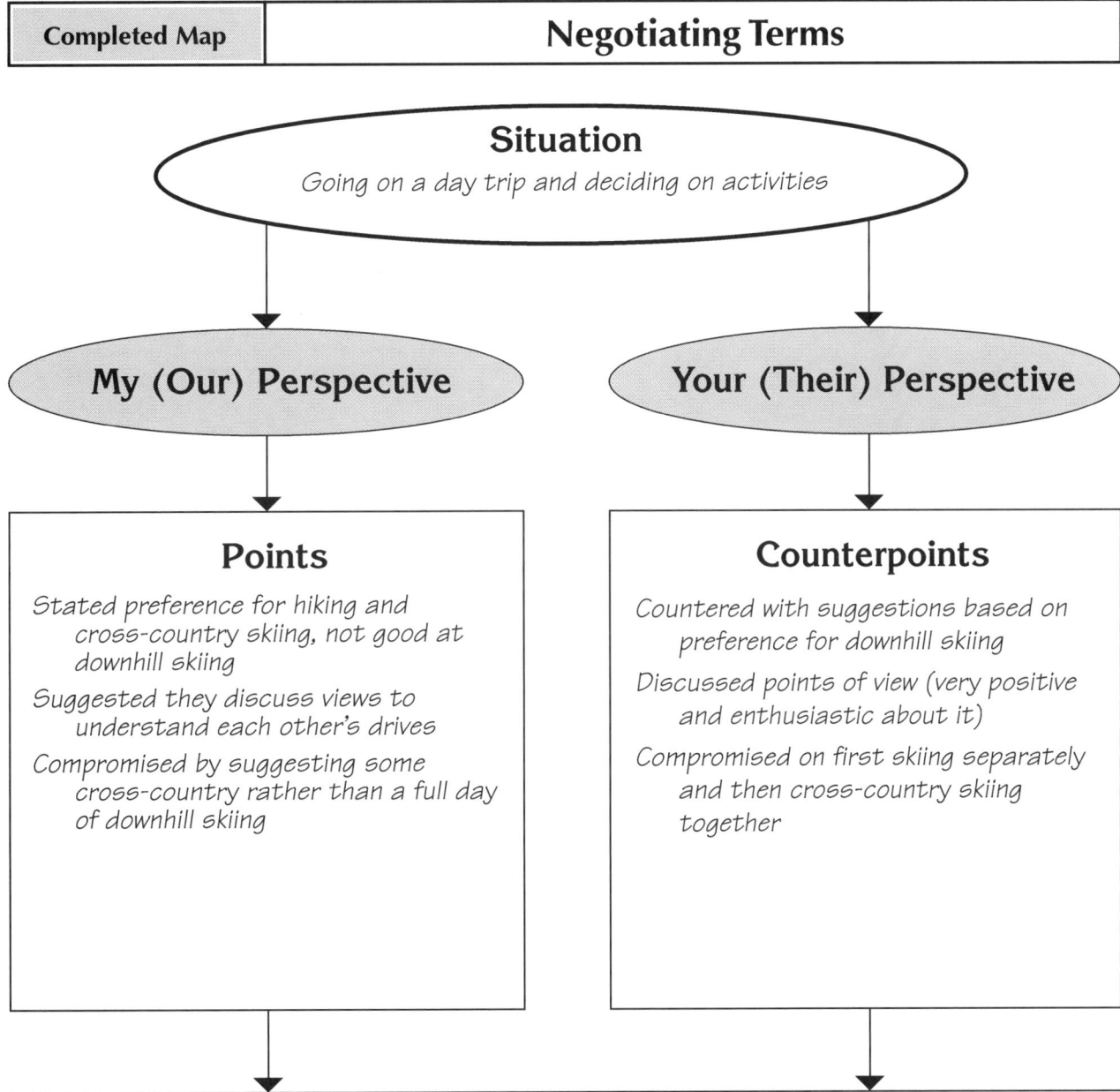

Situation
Going on a day trip and deciding on activities

My (Our) Perspective

Points

Stated preference for hiking and cross-country skiing, not good at downhill skiing

Suggested they discuss views to understand each other's drives

Compromised by suggesting some cross-country rather than a full day of downhill skiing

Your (Their) Perspective

Counterpoints

Countered with suggestions based on preference for downhill skiing

Discussed points of view (very positive and enthusiastic about it)

Compromised on first skiing separately and then cross-country skiing together

Negotiate Terms

A win-win agreement resulted based in positive attitudes, cooperation, collaboration.

A win-win agreement required willingness to understand, accept, and cooperate.

SUMMARY

When we started out, I didn't want to go skiing. My friend wanted to ski downhill all day. We discussed how we could negotiate to make the day fun for both of us. It helped to share why I didn't want to ski downhill. My friend understood. I suggested that we could cross-country ski together either in the morning or afternoon and that my friend could ski downhill while I went hiking. My friend accepted these terms.

© 2001 by E.H. Wiig and C.C. Wilson
Duplication permitted for educational use only.

Map It Out

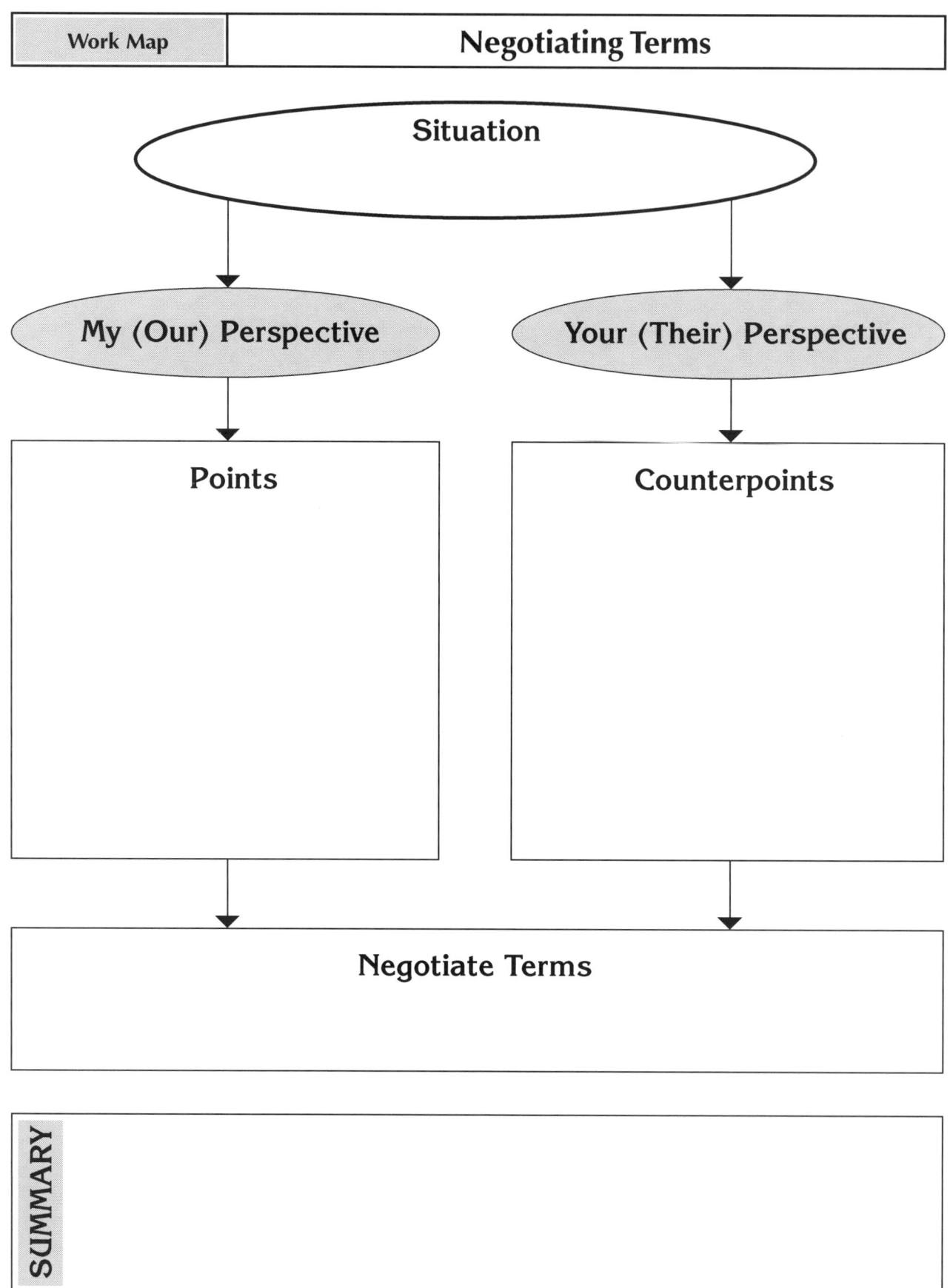

232

Context (Pragmatics)

Unit 36: Establishing Better Relationships

> **Educational Levels**
>
> Elementary through secondary
>
> **Objectives**
>
> (1) Identify and analyze verbal and nonverbal behaviors, needs, attitudes, and perspective-taking abilities in self and others; (2) determine which of these features could contribute to a positive and which to a negative relationship; and (3) integrate this understanding to control the dynamics of personal relationships

Completed Map

For this map, students in Grade 7 analyzed the relationship between two classmates who could not get along. The teacher guided a discussion about the quality of the relationship and possible causes for the problem. Afterward students analyzed features of the relationship.

Show the Completed Map to students and say, for example:

> *This map shows an example of how some students analyzed two classmates who were involved in a negative relationship. Let's talk about the verbal and nonverbal communication traits and behaviors the students in the relationship had.*

You may want to follow up by asking, for example:

> *How could you analyze the relationship between you and a friend or enemy? Let's figure out the reasons for positive or negative qualities in the relationship.*

Work Map

Show the Work Map to students and say, for example:

> *This map is empty. Let's talk about a relationship in your life that you would like to maintain or improve. Analyze your verbal and nonverbal communication traits and behaviors in the relationship.*

Map It Out

Extended Activities

1. Have each student identify a relationship in his or her life that went from bad to good. Have each student analyze the relationship when it was negative and after it became positive. Ask students to share and compare their findings.

2. Ask students to think about a collaborative relationship (e.g., working on a project with a classmate) and analyze what features supported the collaboration.

3. Have each student think about a competitive relationship in his or her life and analyze the features that might be causing the competition.

4. Identify a TV series in which there are positive and negative relationships among characters. Have each student view one or more episodes in the series and identify a relationship for analysis. Ask students to share and compare their findings.

5. Select or develop skits that show positive and negative relationships between people or groups. Guide students in preparing for and presenting a skit. Afterward ask students to analyze the contributing features to and dynamics of the interactions between characters.

Context (Pragmatics)

| Master Map | **Establishing Better Relationships** |

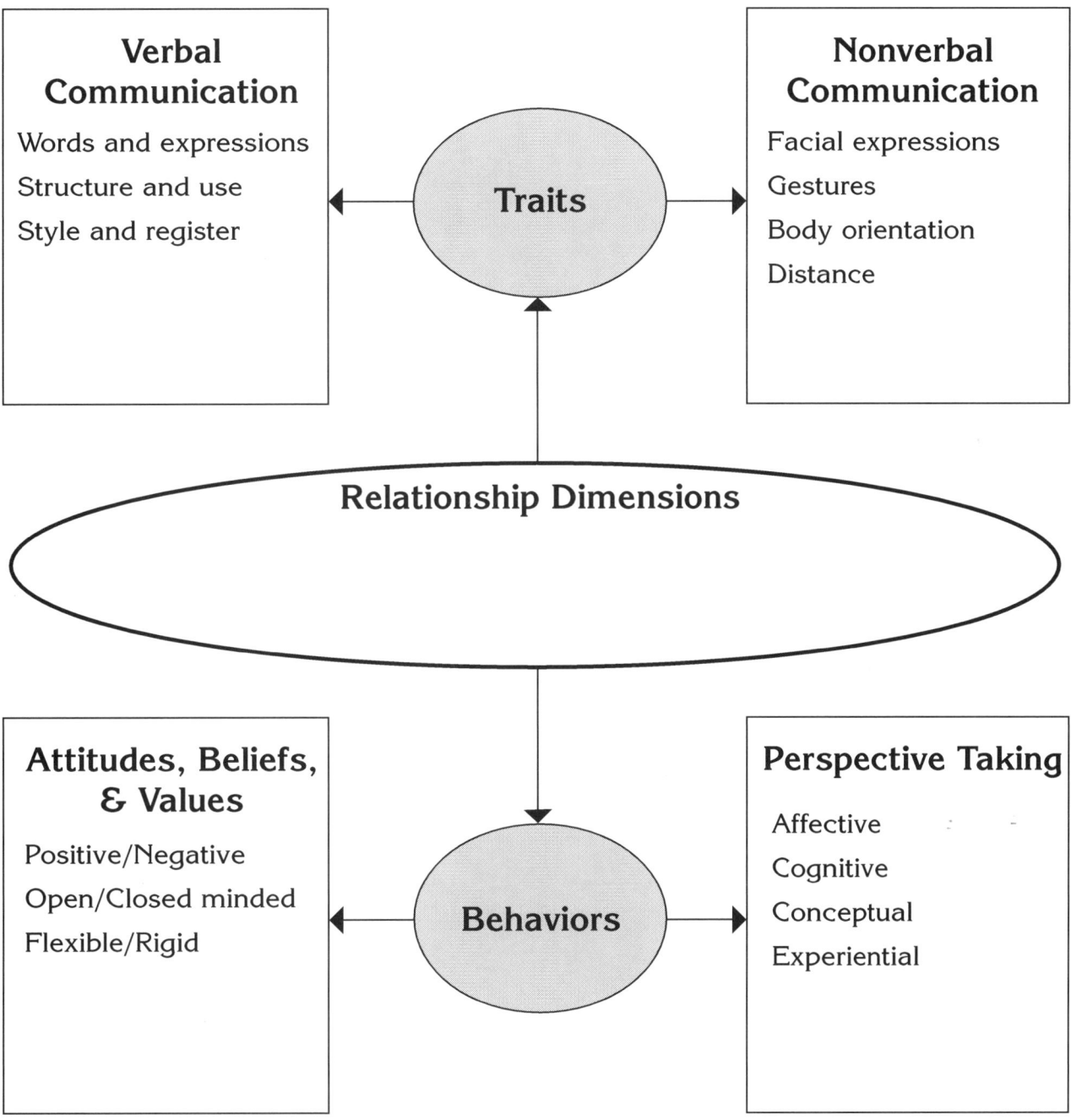

Verbal Communication
Words and expressions
Structure and use
Style and register

Nonverbal Communication
Facial expressions
Gestures
Body orientation
Distance

Attitudes, Beliefs, & Values
Positive/Negative
Open/Closed minded
Flexible/Rigid

Perspective Taking
Affective
Cognitive
Conceptual
Experiential

SUMMARY: Summary of competition, cooperation, or collaboration (i.e., the overall nature of the relationship)

© 2001 by E.H. Wiig and C.C. Wilson
Duplication permitted for educational use only.

Map It Out

| Completed Map | **Establishing Better Relationships** |

Verbal Communication

First teen—name calls and swears, blames other for what happens

Second teen—responds to name calling, blaming, and other negative statements with anger and/or aggression

Nonverbal Communication

First teen—shows no emotion in face or voice, crowds others

Second teen—depends on body talk to understand attitudes, feels rejected when others don't show positive emotions

Traits

Relationship Dimensions

Two teens who cannot get along

Attitudes, Beliefs, & Values

First teen—negative in attitudes and reactions, closed to opposite views, rigid or ritualistic

Second teen—positive, open to opposite views, flexible

Perspective Taking

First teen—insensitive to feelings in others, unaware of what others know

Second teen—sensitive to feelings of others, often unaware of what others know or think

Behaviors

SUMMARY

Our teacher helped us analyze the behaviors and reactions of two teens who can never get along in school and often abuse each other. We first discussed and listed everything we knew about the first teen. Then we did the same for the second teen. Then we talked about what could be done to help each of the teens change a little to make the relationship better or at least tolerable.

Context (Pragmatics)

| Work Map | **Establishing Better Relationships** |

Establishing Better Relationships

Verbal Communication

Nonverbal Communication

Traits

Relationship Dimensions

Attitudes, Beliefs, & Values

Perspective Taking

Behaviors

SUMMARY

© 2001 by E.H. Wiig and C.C. Wilson
Duplication permitted for educational use only.

Map It Out

Unit 37: Developing Trust

Educational Levels

Upper elementary through secondary

Objectives

(1) Identify verbal and nonverbal communication characteristics and personal values; (2) take another's point of view or perspective; and (3) integrate this knowledge to understand the dynamics of trust and the means and potentials for developing or regaining a relationship of trust

Completed Map

This map shows the results of an analysis of a relationship of trust in *Of Mice and Men* by John Steinbeck. Students in Grade 9 were asked to analyze the relationship between Lenny and George and examine the trust George had in Lenny. They identified Lenny's characteristics that inspired trust or distrust.

Show the Completed Map to students and say, for example:

> *This map shows an example of analyzing two characters in the novel* Of Mice and Men. *The focus was on analyzing which of Lenny's characteristics helped George to trust him. Let's talk about Lenny's verbal and nonverbal communication, personal values, and perspective-taking abilities.*

You may want to follow up by asking, for example:

> *How could you analyze a relationship of trust between you and a friend, sibling, or relative?*

Work Map

Show the Work Map to students and say, for example:

> *This map is empty. Let's talk about a trusting or a nontrusting relationship in your life. Then we'll describe the aspects of the relationship.*

Extended Activities

1. Ask the students to describe a collaborative effort (e.g., teamwork in sports). Then guide students in analyzing and identifying the role that trust plays in maintaining a positive and collaborative relationship.

2. Have each student identify a person who trusts him or her and who he or she trusts too. Then have each student analyze, from his or her perspective, which characteristics might have contributed to the mutual trust.

3. Have each student analyze if he or she is the type of person others would place their trust in. If a student finds that he or she does not have the qualities that lead to trust, spend one-to-one time to discuss wanted or needed changes in communication behavior.

4. Identify a story, novel, or play in which the characters first trust each other and then lose that trust (e.g., Brutus and Mark Anthony in Shakespeare's *Julius Caesar*). Ask students to identify segments that describe the relationship of trust and segments that reflect the loss of trust. Then guide an analysis of the features and dynamics that contributed to the loss of trust.

5. Select or develop a skit for role-playing a relationship between two characters who do not trust each other. Prepare students for role-playing by discussing how the characters might behave and what they might say to each other. Then give students cue cards to role-play the skit. Afterward guide students in a discussion of the relationship and how it might be changed or improved.

Map It Out

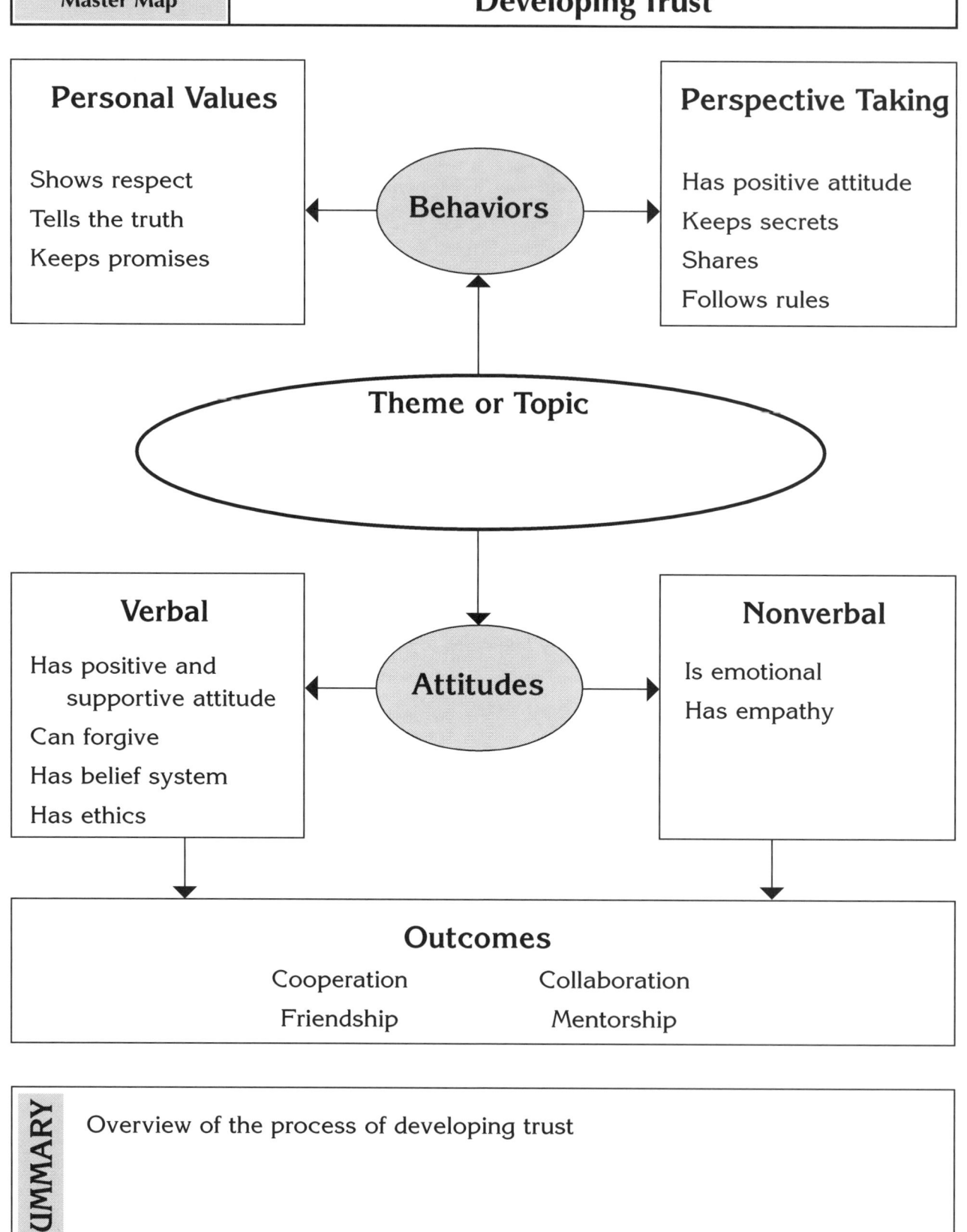

Context (Pragmatics)

Completed Map — **Developing Trust**

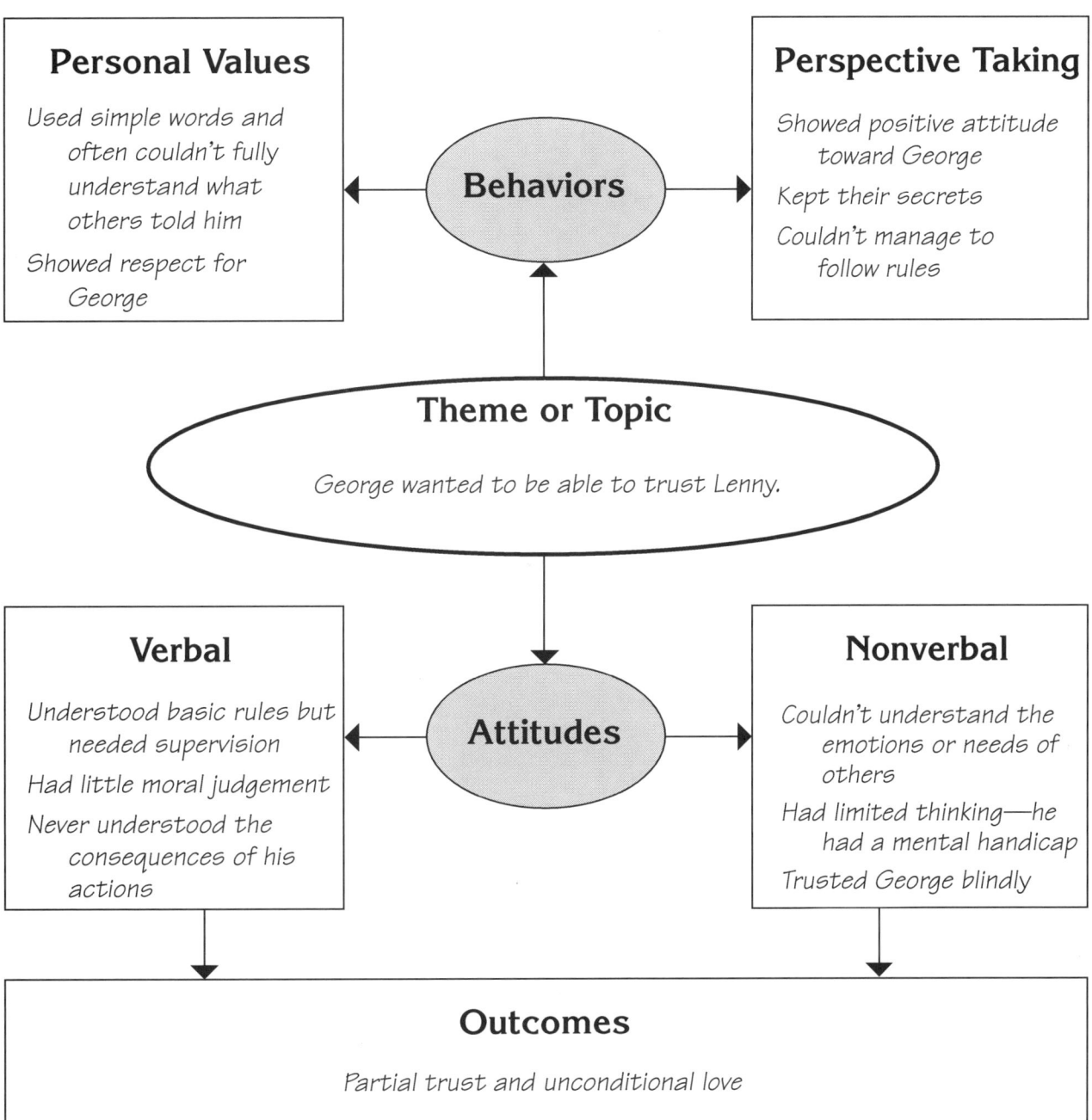

Personal Values
- Used simple words and often couldn't fully understand what others told him
- Showed respect for George

Perspective Taking
- Showed positive attitude toward George
- Kept their secrets
- Couldn't manage to follow rules

Behaviors

Theme or Topic
George wanted to be able to trust Lenny.

Attitudes

Verbal
- Understood basic rules but needed supervision
- Had little moral judgement
- Never understood the consequences of his actions

Nonverbal
- Couldn't understand the emotions or needs of others
- Had limited thinking—he had a mental handicap
- Trusted George blindly

Outcomes
Partial trust and unconditional love

SUMMARY
George wanted to but could never trust Lenny completely, because of his impulsive actions and limited ability to judge what was right and wrong. Still, Lenny showed respect for George and kept their secrets. George recognized Lenny's limitations and trusted him when they were together.

© 2001 by E.H. Wiig and C.C. Wilson
Duplication permitted for educational use only.

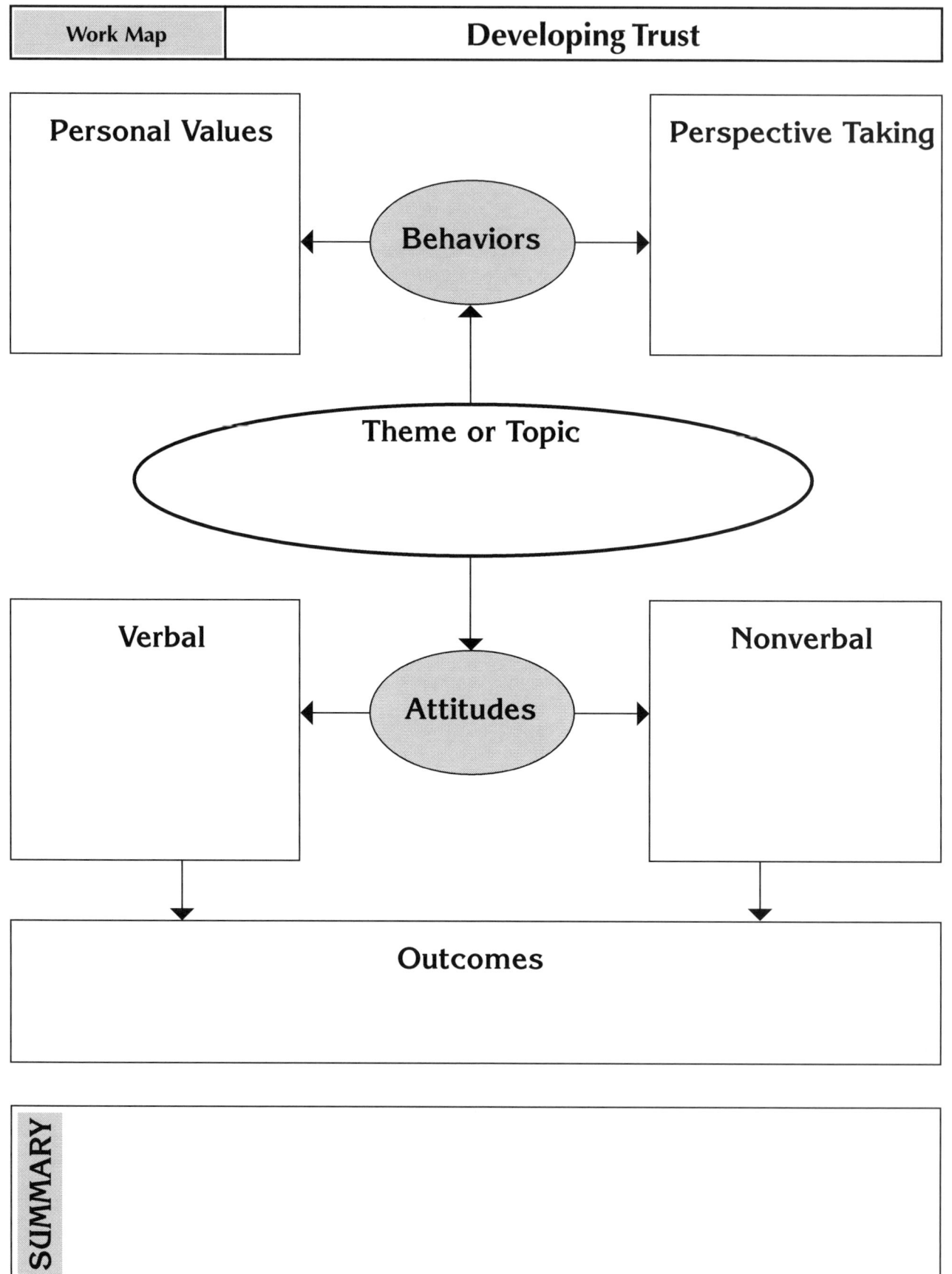

Context (Pragmatics)

Unit 38: Causes for Conflict or Disagreement

Educational Levels

Upper elementary through secondary

Objectives

(1) Analyze verbal and nonverbal behaviors that can cause conflicts or disagreements at school, in the home, and in the community; (2) identify reactions and responses to situations of conflict or disagreement; and (3) prepare to avoid or control conflict-provoking behaviors and reactions

Completed Map

This map shows an example of how students in Grade 5 analyzed a recent conflict between two players on a school team. They were asked to identify the conflict situation and discuss the verbal and nonverbal behaviors of the person that caused it (i.e., the team captain). Then they were asked to analyze and discuss reactions and responses that might have fueled the conflict or disagreement (i.e., causes).

Show the Completed Map to students and say, for example:

> *This map shows an example of verbal and nonverbal behaviors and responses that created a conflict between players on a team. Let's talk about the team captain's verbal and nonverbal behaviors. Then let's consider how the rejected player responded.*

You may want to follow up by asking, for example:

> *How could you analyze a disagreement or conflict between you and another person?*

243

Map It Out

Work Map

Show the Work Map to students and say, for example:

> *This map is empty. Let's talk about an important disagreement or conflict you have experienced. To begin, we'll describe behaviors that could have caused the conflict. Then we'll describe responses to those behaviors.*

Extended Activities

1. Have each student identify a recent disagreement or conflict in his or her immediate environment. Then have each student analyze the verbal and nonverbal behaviors that started the conflict and the reactions and responses to the conflict.

2. Ask students to identify a current TV series that deals with disagreements or conflicts between people. Assign an episode for students to view at home or show a videotape of an episode in class. Ask students to analyze one of the featured conflict situations to identify verbal and nonverbal behaviors that led to and intensified the conflict.

3. Select or develop a skit in which a disagreement or conflict develops or an ongoing conflict is intensified. Ask students to analyze and record verbal and nonverbal behaviors that led to or fueled the conflict. Then identify and discuss reactions and responses to the causes and how these might accelerate the conflicts. Emphasize the circular interactions and accelerations that occur in unresolved conflicts.

4. Guide students in rewriting a skit or piece of dialogue from a story or play that shows a conflict. Ask the students to go through the text and identify behaviors and reactions in the conflict situation. Then guide them in rewriting the dialogue to avoid or lessen the conflict situation.

5. Identify an ongoing conflict that is in the news involving two or more individuals, groups, or countries. Ask students to view a TV news report on the conflict. Ask them to identify and write down verbal and nonverbal behaviors by individuals or groups that could maintain or intensify the already existing conflict.

6. Review one of the conflict situations the students analyzed earlier. Then guide them in a discussion of which aspects—behaviors or reactions—might contribute the most to creating the dynamics of the conflict or disagreement.

Context (Pragmatics)

| Master Map | Causes for Conflict or Disagreement |

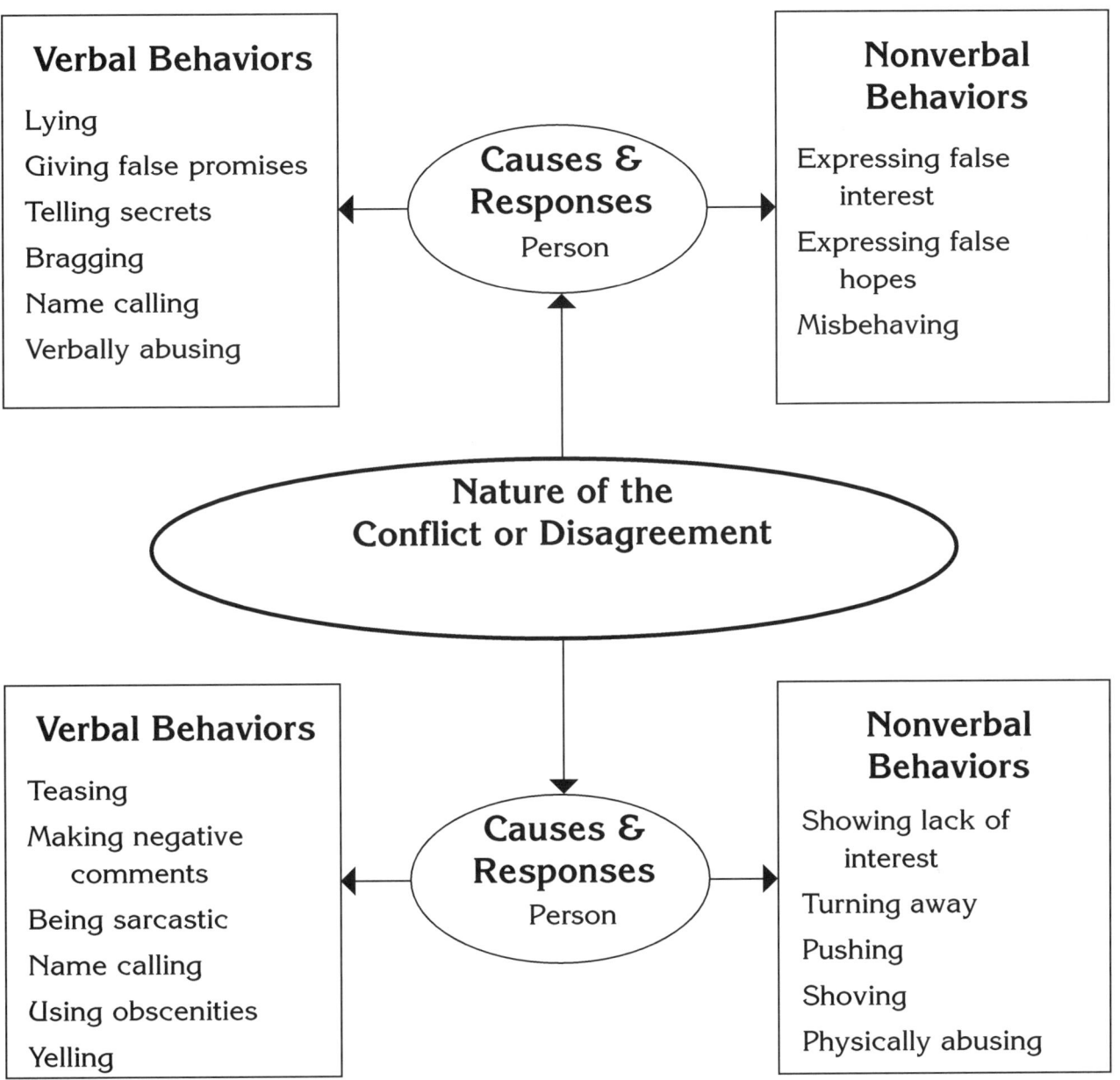

Verbal Behaviors
- Lying
- Giving false promises
- Telling secrets
- Bragging
- Name calling
- Verbally abusing

Causes & Responses — Person

Nonverbal Behaviors
- Expressing false interest
- Expressing false hopes
- Misbehaving

Nature of the Conflict or Disagreement

Verbal Behaviors
- Teasing
- Making negative comments
- Being sarcastic
- Name calling
- Using obscenities
- Yelling

Causes & Responses — Person

Nonverbal Behaviors
- Showing lack of interest
- Turning away
- Pushing
- Shoving
- Physically abusing

SUMMARY: Description of the conflict and suggestions for how it could have been avoided

© 2001 by E.H. Wiig and C.C. Wilson
Duplication permitted for educational use only.

Map It Out

| Completed Map | Causes for Conflict or Disagreement |

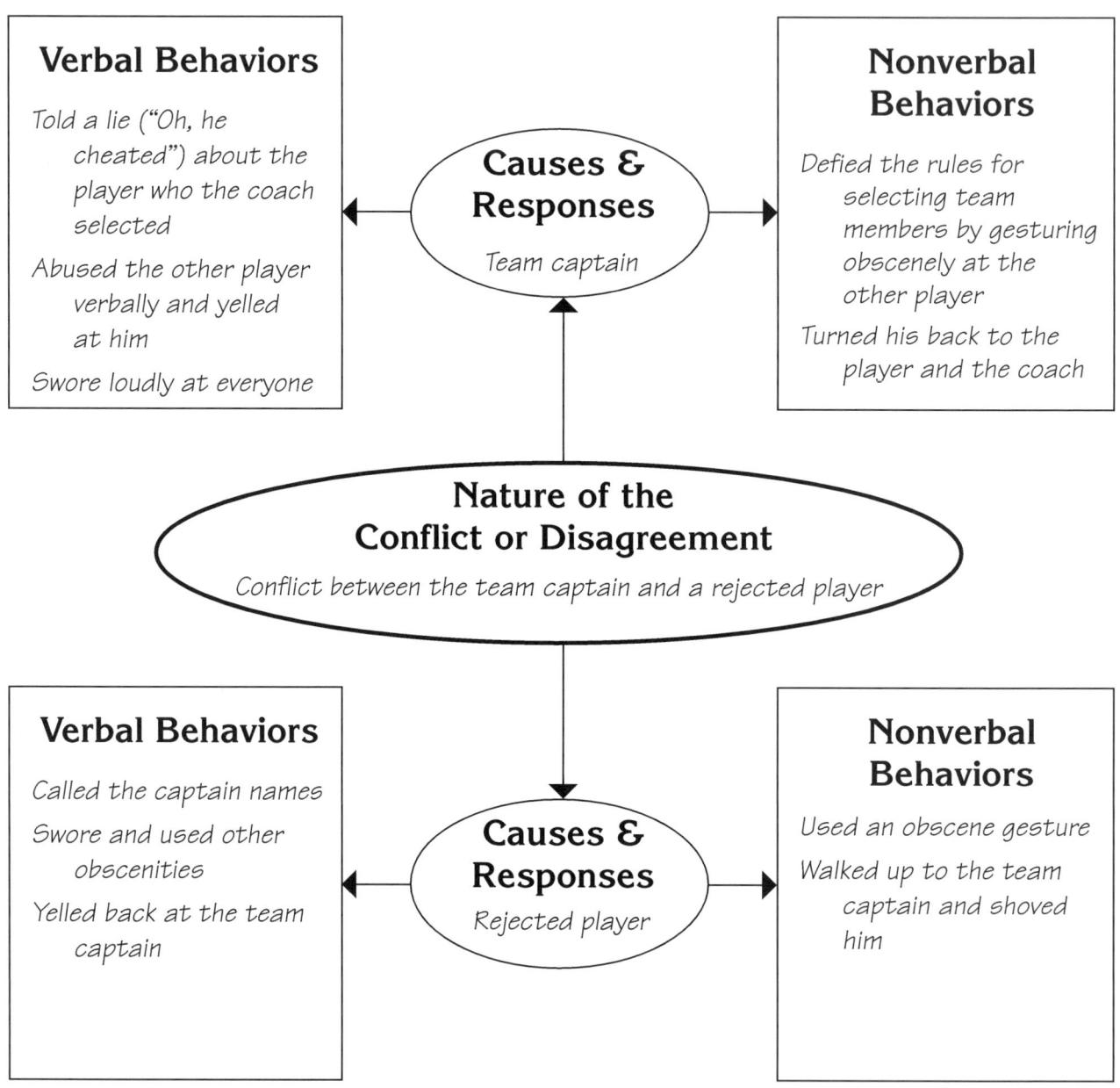

Verbal Behaviors
Told a lie ("Oh, he cheated") about the player who the coach selected
Abused the other player verbally and yelled at him
Swore loudly at everyone

Nonverbal Behaviors
Defied the rules for selecting team members by gesturing obscenely at the other player
Turned his back to the player and the coach

Causes & Responses
Team captain

Nature of the Conflict or Disagreement
Conflict between the team captain and a rejected player

Causes & Responses
Rejected player

Verbal Behaviors
Called the captain names
Swore and used other obscenities
Yelled back at the team captain

Nonverbal Behaviors
Used an obscene gesture
Walked up to the team captain and shoved him

SUMMARY
There was a nasty incidence on the playing field today. The team captain rejected a player the coach selected for the team. The team captain violated all rules for behavior and was taken off the team for four weeks. The rejected player also used obscenities and yelled at the team captain. If the team captain and rejected player had expressed their feelings in an appropriate way, the conflict could have been avoided.

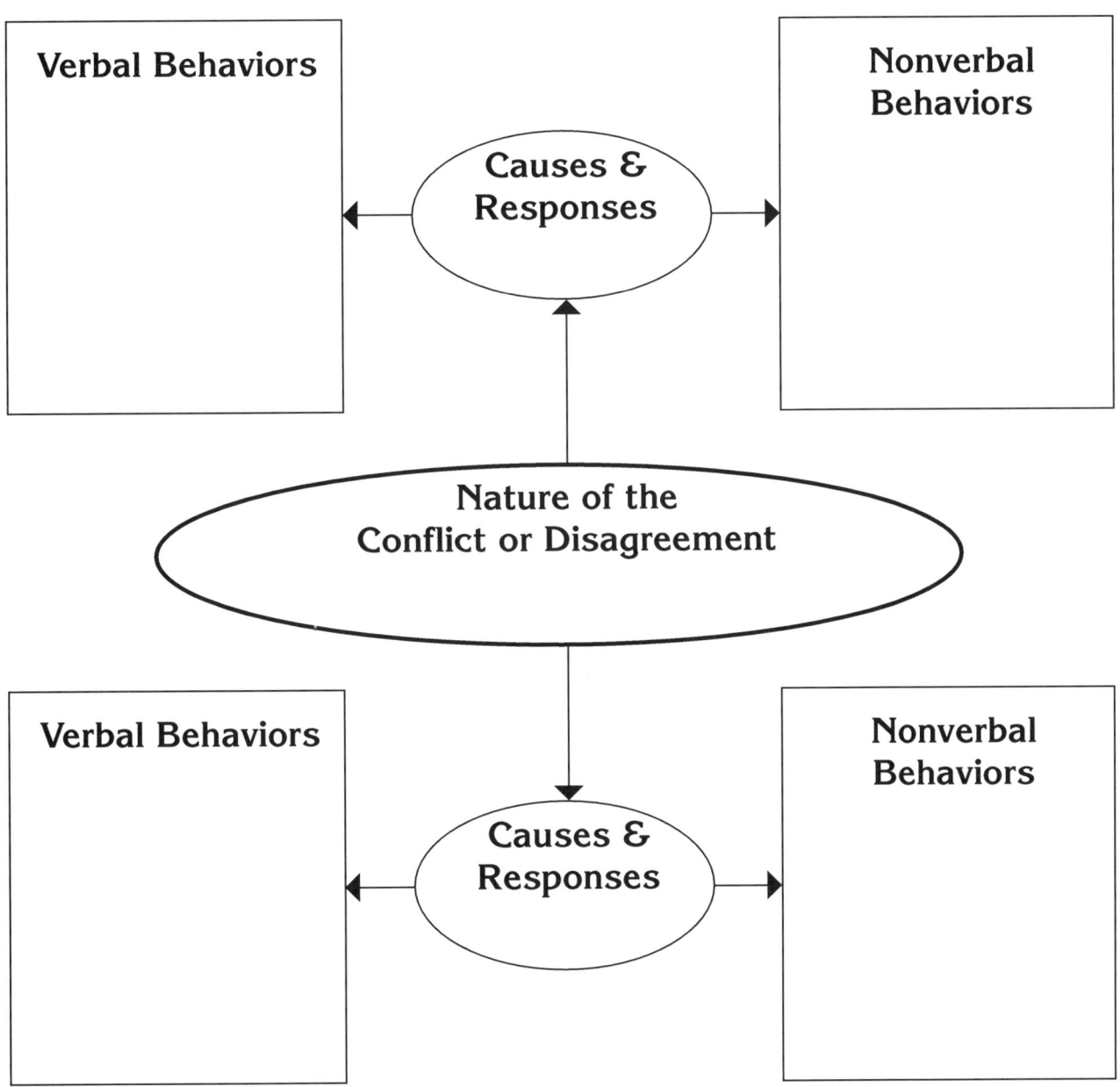

Map It Out

Unit 39: Ongoing Conflict Resolution

Educational Levels

Upper elementary through secondary

Objectives

(1) Analyze actions, underlying causes, reactions, and consequences of conflicts in the home, among friends, at school, or at work; and (2) provide and implement suggestions for solving conflicts

Completed Map

For this map, students in Grade 6 were asked to identify a conflict situation in their lives that needed to be resolved. Each student identified and delineated aspects of an ongoing conflict. The students shared their analyses and discussed options for reaching solutions to the conflicts. The student whose map serves as the example made a contractual agreement with the group to initiate and contribute positively to a process of resolving the conflict in her family. The teacher guided the students to become aware of which aspects contributed to the conflict and suggested how the conflict might be solved.

Show the Completed Map to students and say, for example:

> *This map shows an example of behaviors and responses that created a conflict between a student and her family. Let's talk about the student's actions and reactions. Then let's consider how the family members responded to the student. Finally we'll look at the suggestions that were given for resolving the family conflict.*

You may want to extend the activity by asking, for example:

> *How could you analyze an ongoing disagreement or conflict between yourself and another person?*

Work Map

Show the Work Map to students and say, for example:

> *This map is empty. Let's talk about an important disagreement or conflict you have experienced. To begin, describe behaviors that could have caused the conflict. Then describe how you or others responded to the behaviors. Finally we'll discuss what might be done to resolve the conflict.*

Extended Activities

1. Have each student identify a recent conflict situation in his or her immediate environment. Have each student analyze the causes, actions, and reactions that started the conflict and the consequences in the relationship between the contributors. Elicit suggestions for some immediate actions by students and others that might help to resolve the conflict. Share and discuss the analyses, and prepare students to implement some of the suggestions.

2. Ask students to identify a current TV series that deals with disagreements or conflicts between people. Assign an episode for students to view, or show a videotape of an episode in class. Ask students to analyze the conflict situation and suggest immediate actions that might help resolve it. You may want to use the Completed Map from Unit 38: Causes for Conflicts or Disagreements (see page 246) to get students started.

3. Select or develop a skit in which a disagreement or conflict develops or an ongoing conflict is intensified. Ask students to analyze and record the factors that either led to or fueled the conflict. Then identify and discuss possible actions that might lead to an immediate and long-term resolution.

4. Help students write a skit or select a piece of dialogue from a story or play that shows a conflict. Ask students to analyze the conflict and give suggestions for immediate and long-term actions that might resolve it.

5. Identify an ongoing conflict that is in the news and involves two or more individuals, groups, or countries. Ask students to view a TV news report of the conflict. Ask them to analyze the situation, discuss factors that might have led to the conflict, and consider how the conflict might be managed in the short-term by immediate action. Then ask students to come up with some suggestions for a long-term resolution of the conflict.

6. Review a conflict situation that students analyzed earlier. Guide them in a discussion of which actions or aspects might contribute the most to resolving the conflict. Ask students to rank their suggestions for conflict resolution in two ways: from most to least important and from immediate to long-term actions and implementations.

Map It Out

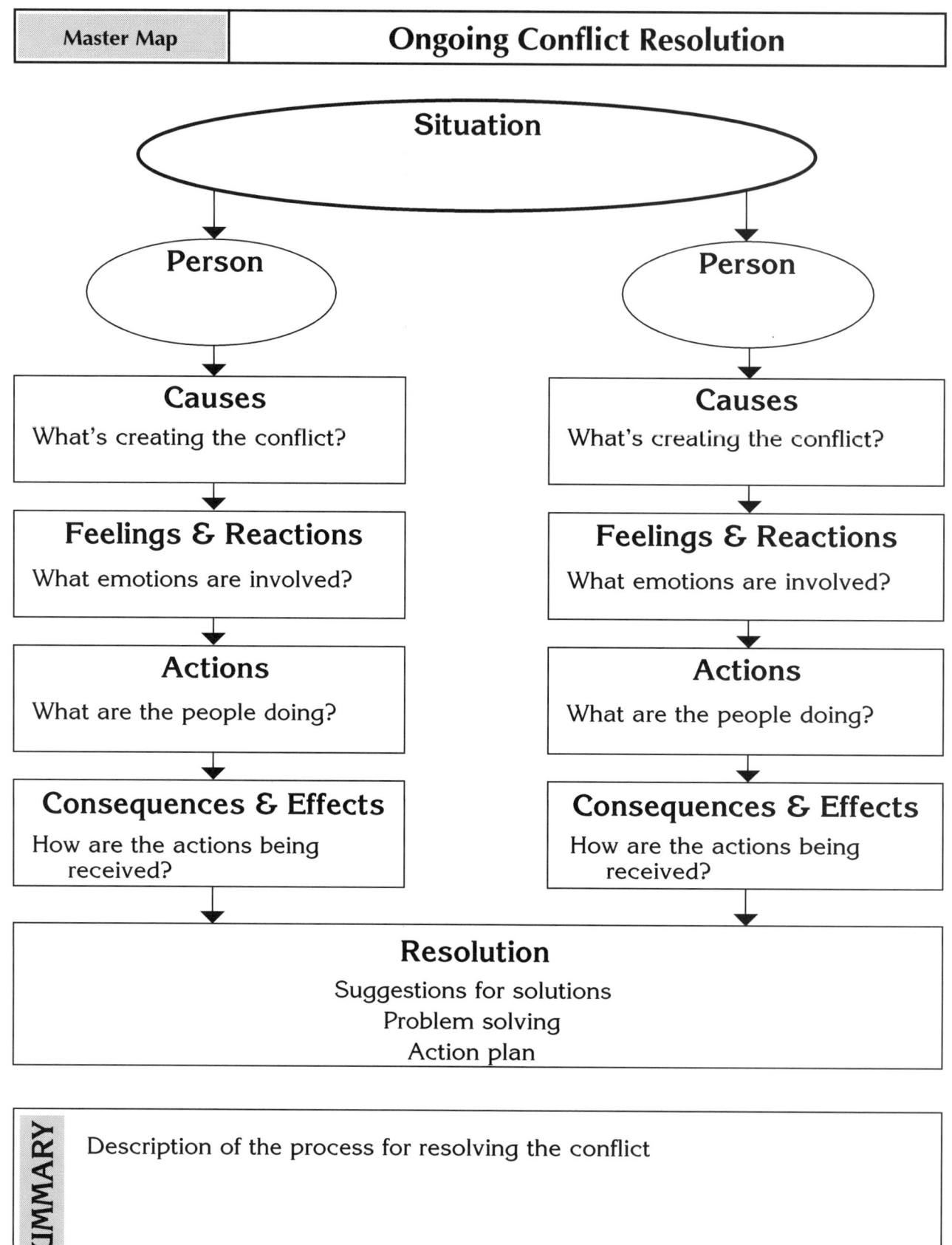

250

Context (Pragmatics)

| Completed Map | **Ongoing Conflict Resolution** |

Situation
Teenager and family get into daily verbal fights

Person
Teenager

Person
Parents and brother

Causes
Picked on for being a perfectionist

Causes
Teenager doesn't study enough/not doing well in school

Feelings & Reactions
Wanted to be popular, wanted revenge for being picked on

Feelings & Reactions
Parents—upset
Brother—felt superior

Actions
Became lazy, blamed others for her failures

Actions
Parents—lectured and grounded her
Brother—teased her constantly

Consequences & Effects
Felt pressure from family, became defensive, created conflict

Consequences & Effects
Frustrated that teenager hasn't changed her behavior

Resolution
Teenager—will study daily, listen and ask questions, and spend less time with friends
Parents—will stop daily lectures and meet with school counselor
Brother—will stop teasing and give his sister space

SUMMARY
The family realized everyone had to change some of their actions to reduce the conflict. Each of them committed to acting differently on a day-to-day basis.

Map It Out

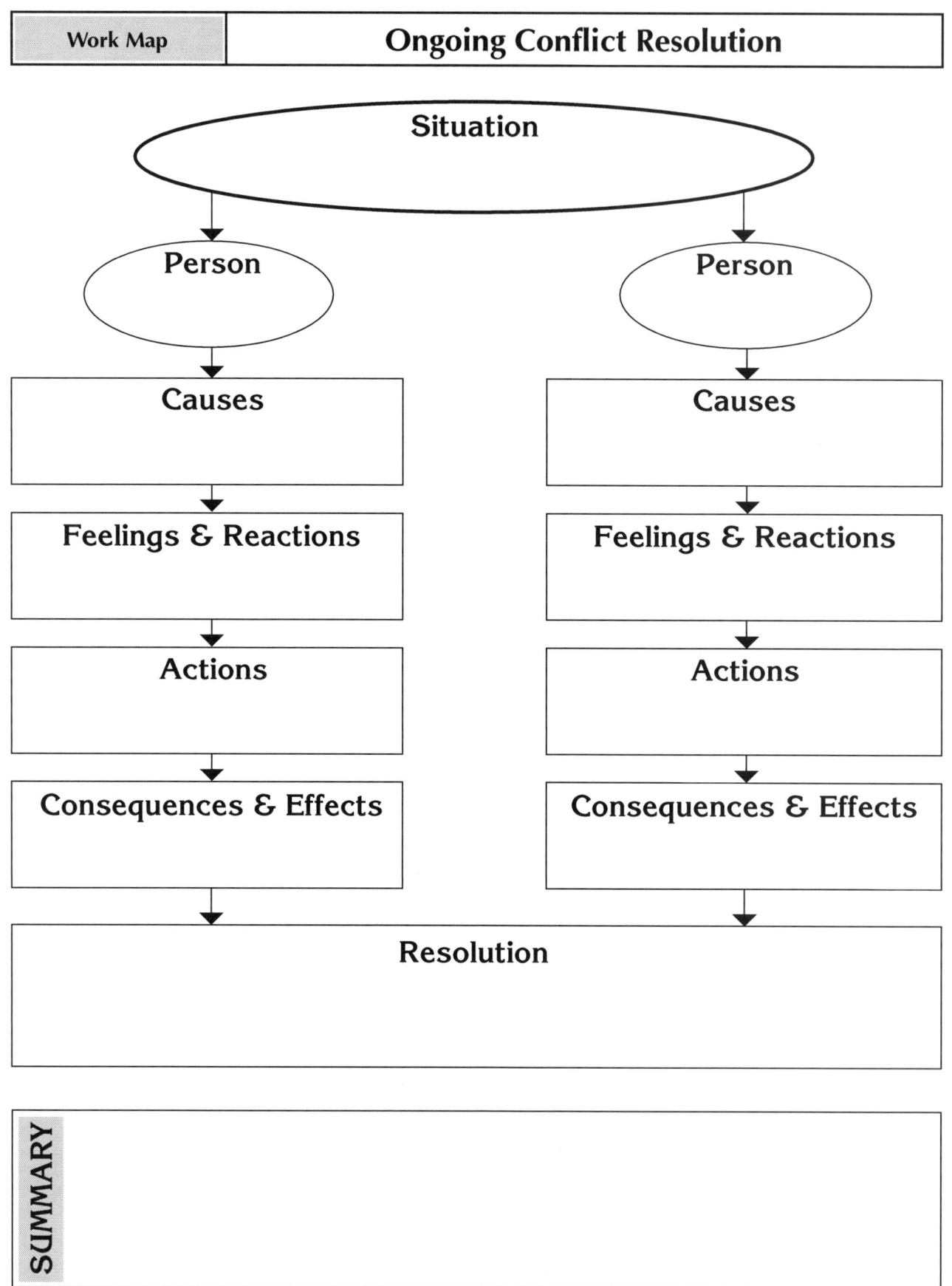

Unit 40: Understanding Relationship Changes

> **Educational Levels**
>
> Upper elementary through secondary
>
> **Objectives**
>
> (1) Analyze contributing factors, driving forces, and conditions and outcomes before and after changes in the quality of a personal relationship; and (2) use this knowledge to change or control relationships

Completed Map

For this map, students in Grade 10 formed small groups to identify relationships in their lives that had changed from positive to negative or negative to positive. Each student took a turn identifying a turning point or time period of change in the relationship; describing the relationship before the change; and delineating causes, conditions, and driving forces. As a follow up, students shared their maps with the class; discussed their experiences, feelings, and reactions; and made suggestions for how they might handle the relationships in the future.

Show the Completed Map to students and say, for example:

> *This map shows an example of how a student analyzed changes in her relationship with her best friend. Let's talk about the relationship before and after the turning point. Then we'll look at the causes for the changes and existing conditions and analyze how they are related.*

You may want to follow up by asking, for example:

> *How could you analyze an important relationship in your life that changed from good to bad or bad to good according to causes and effects? What were some of the driving forces in changing the relationship? What was the turning point and when did it happen?*

Map It Out

Work Map

Show the Work Map to students and say, for example:

> *This map is empty. Let's talk about a relationship in your life. Then we'll analyze and evaluate important changes in your relationship and factors that caused the changes.*

Extended Activities

1. Ask if any of the students have a long-term friendship that changed due to a move or other separation. Guide students in analyzing and recording what the relationship was like before the move when the friends were always together. Then guide them in analyzing how the friendship changed after the move and how the two friends keep in contact.

2. Ask students to identify a TV series that portrays a friendship or relationship that changed for some reason (e.g., a move or divorce). Ask students to view one or more episodes in the series. Then guide them in analyzing the cause of the change and the quality of the relationship before and after the change.

3. Ask students to analyze changes they have observed in relationships between others (e.g., friends or family members). Ask them to analyze and record features of the relationship before and after the change occurred. Then ask them to identify and record a turning point or time period of change in the relationship. Discuss the types of events that can change a relationship from negative to positive or vice versa.

4. Identify a relationship in literature that is part of the curriculum (e.g., *Ethan Frome* by Edith Wharton or *Gone With the Wind* by Margaret Mitchell). After students have read a part or all of the text, ask them to sketch out the relationship over time and discuss how and why the relationship changed.

5. Have each student analyze a dating relationship or male-female friendship he or she has experienced. Tell students that they need not share the details with others. Then have each student sketch out the relationship over time and analyze how the relationship changed. Then have each student identify how, when, and why the greatest relationship changes occurred and how to deal with the changes in the future.

6. Have each student identify a work relationship (e.g., collaborative, competitive, or neutral) in his or her life. Have each student analyze the relationship over time to determine if it has been stable or changed. If the relationship has changed, ask the student involved to identify what caused the changes. If the relationship has not changed, ask the student what kinds of changes she or he would like to see in the relationship and how they might be achieved.

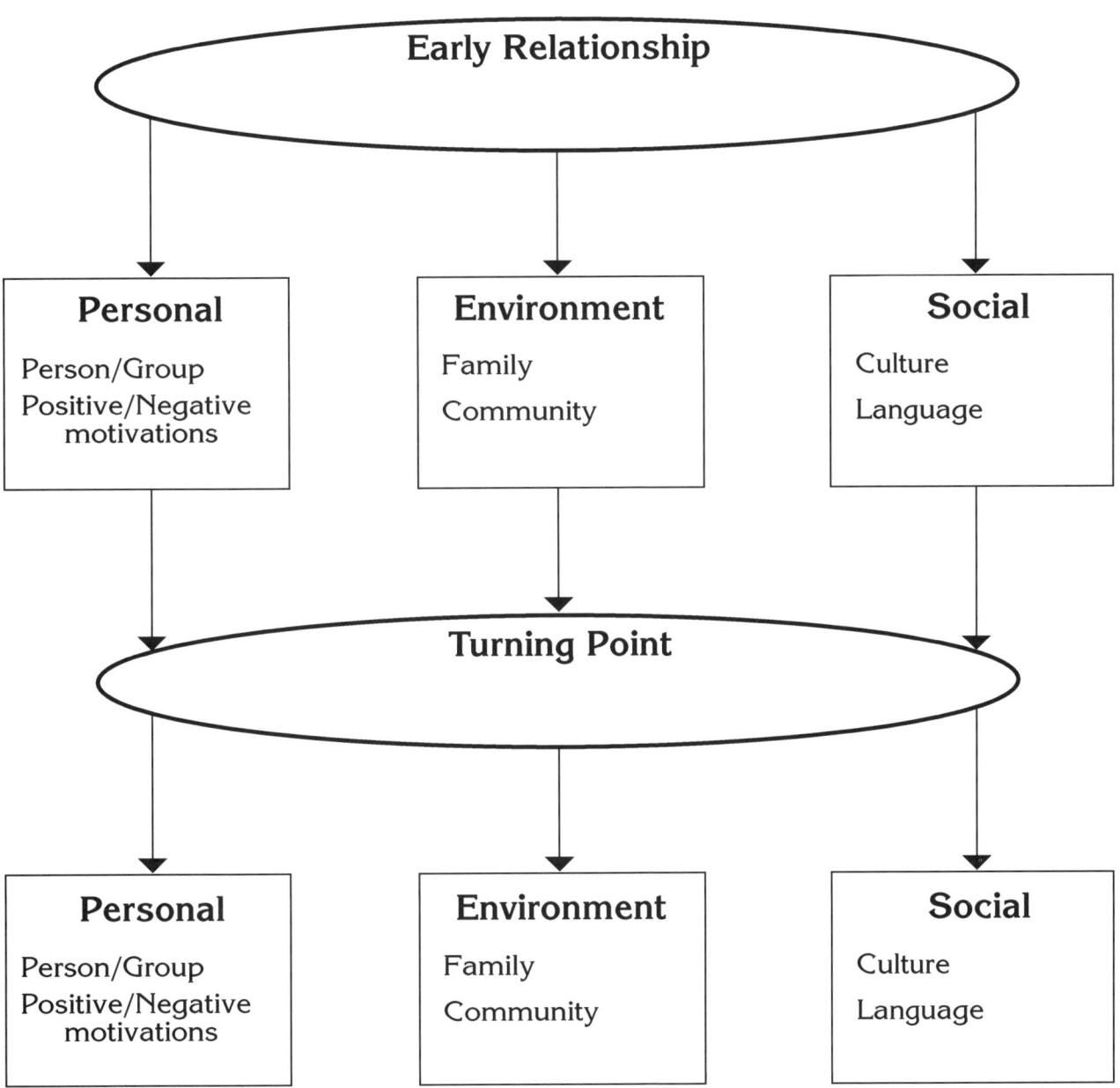

Map It Out

| Completed Map | **Understanding Relationship Changes** |

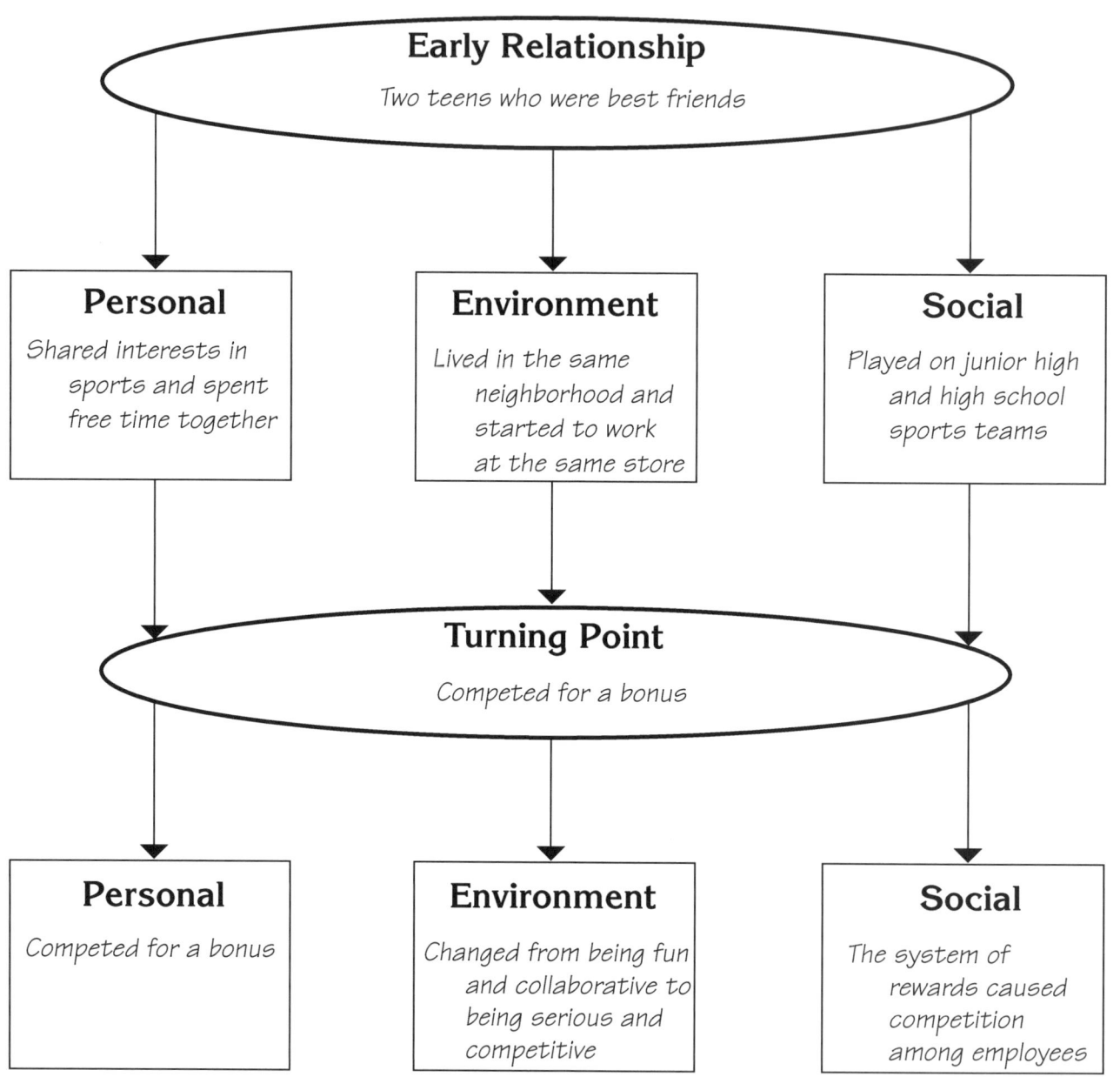

SUMMARY: The two girls were best friends that trusted each other and had fun together. Once they got employed, the relationship changed from being collaborative to being competitive. In the store, they competed for a bonus. That competition ruined their friendship and stopped their shared activities.

256

© 2001 by E.H. Wiig and C.C. Wilson
Duplication permitted for educational use only.

Context (Pragmatics)

| Work Map | **Understanding Relationship Changes** |

Early Relationship

- Personal
- Environment
- Social

Turning Point

- Personal
- Environment
- Social

SUMMARY

© 2001 by E.H. Wiig and C.C. Wilson
Duplication permitted for educational use only.

257

Map It Out

Unit 41: Preparing for Role-Playing

> ## Educational Levels
>
> Elementary through secondary
>
> ## Objectives
>
> (1) Analyze and identify major traits in characters; (2) determine which features of communication will best portray a given character; (3) analyze and discuss how to communicate the traits through role-playing; and (4) present the character effectively through role-playing

Completed Map

This map shows how students in Grade 6 analyzed the major characters in a social-interaction skit, "Letting the Cat Out of the Bag" by Elisabeth Wiig and J. McCracken. Small groups of students were asked to analyze a specific character and write down how they would use verbal and nonverbal communication dimensions to portray the character's essential traits. The map shows an analysis of the bully who "let the cat out of the bag." After completing their maps, students discussed how the traits of one character would play off against those of another (e.g., a wimp and an authority figure). One student from each team then assumed the role the team had analyzed and presented the skit to the class.

Show the Completed Map to students and say, for example:

> *This map shows an example of how a team of students analyzed the major character in a skit called "Letting the Cat Out of the Bag." Let's talk about the personality and behavior traits the students saw in the character. Then we'll look at the character's verbal and nonverbal communication.*

You may want to follow up by asking, for example:

> *How could you portray a considerate and polite teenager through your communication while role-playing a skit? How would you talk? How would your body talk? How would you use space?*

Work Map

Show the Work Map to students and say, for example:

> *This map is empty. Let's talk about a character role you are going to play in a skit. We'll analyze the character you are going to play. Then we'll discuss how you can portray that character through your way of communicating.*

There are suggestions for role-playing activities throughout this section (Section 3). The Work Map in this unit can be used to prepare for role-playing.

Extended Activities

1. Select a short story with dialogue (e.g., *The Outsiders* by S.E. Hinton), and assign a reading to each student. Have each student prepare for reading the text by analyzing actions, characteristics, and verbal and nonverbal communication features. Then allow each student to present his or her reading to the class.

2. Select an act from a play that is part of the assigned curriculum (e.g., *Romeo and Juliet* by William Shakespeare). Ask students to analyze the major character traits for each role and identify how to communicate the traits in words, tone of voice, and body talk. Rehearse a role-playing or reading session, and then ask students to present it to others (e.g., another class).

3. Have each student identify a favorite actor or actress in a popular TV series. Direct each student to view one or more episodes and identify what the performer does to show the personality traits of his or her character. Ask students to share their observations in class.

4. Ask students to analyze the verbal and nonverbal communication characteristics of a current political figure based on the role he or she plays for the public. Show students a news segment that profiles the figure. Then ask them to make inferences about the figure's character traits based on the behaviors and reactions shown to the public.

5. Ask students to analyze, compare, and contrast the verbal and nonverbal communication characteristics of two people who are in the public eye. Have students compare and contrast expressions by the two people and make inferences about the personalities each wants to portray to the public. Then ask students to describe and show how they would imitate one or both of the people.

Map It Out

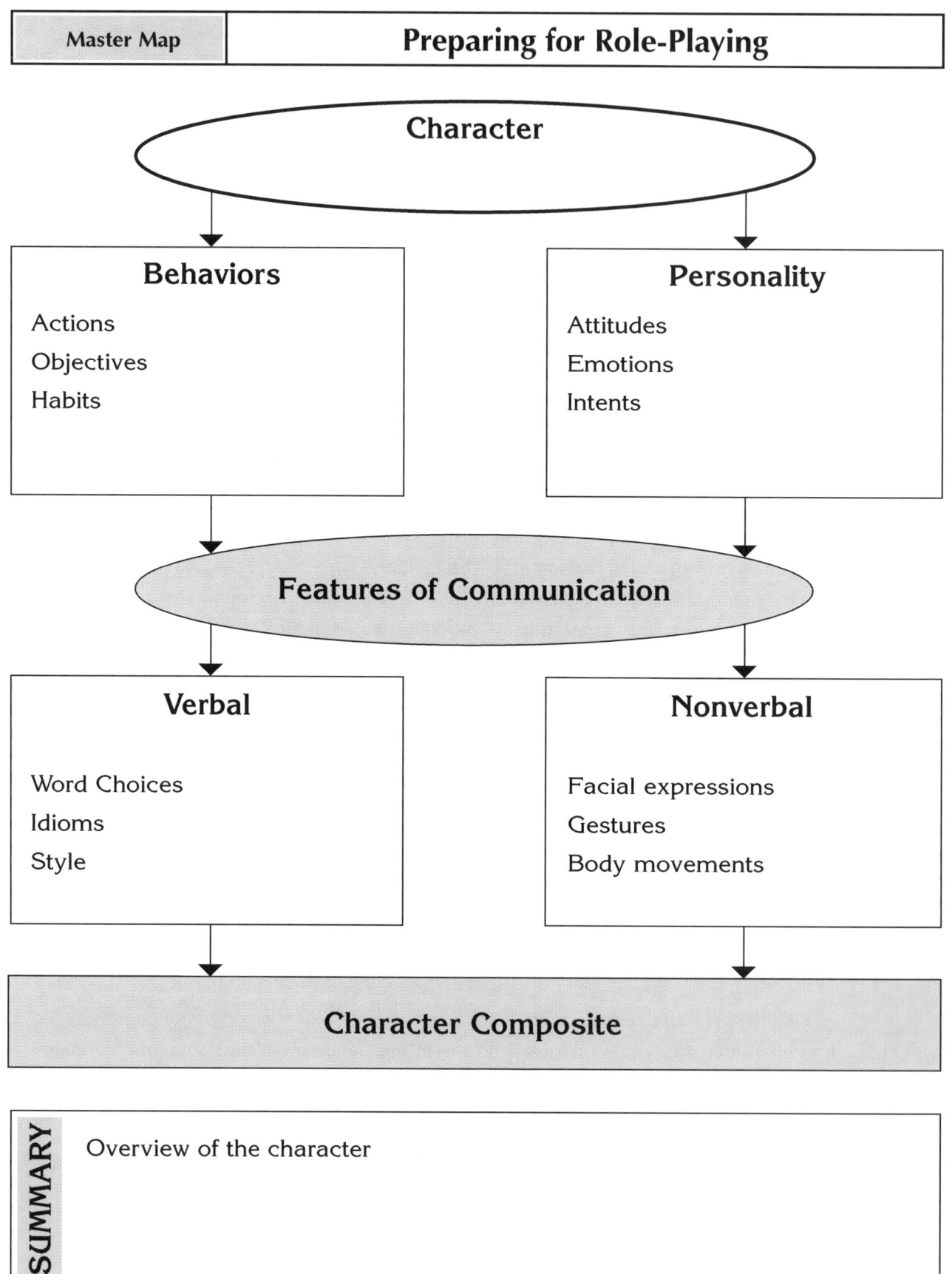

Context (Pragmatics)

| Completed Map | **Preparing for Role-Playing** |

Character
The bully

Behaviors
- Was aggressive but not violent
- Bullied others
- Told secrets he should have kept
- Was direct and offensive

Personality
- Was negative toward others
- Was impulsive
- Was angry
- Was jealous
- Defied authority

Features of Communication

Verbal
- Used slang
- Didn't apologize
- Was abrupt and direct
- Didn't understand subtle hints
- Didn't understand rules of friendship

Nonverbal
- Pushed his way
- Frowned a lot
- Sounded negative and angry
- Couldn't read or understand body talk

Character Composite

SUMMARY

The boy I have to play is not likable. He is a big bully with a loud voice and rude actions to go with it. He is negative and impatient. What is worse, however, is that he doesn't understand how much he hurts a friend and classmate by telling a very personal secret that he was trusted with.

© 2001 by E.H. Wiig and C.C. Wilson
Duplication permitted for educational use only.

Map It Out

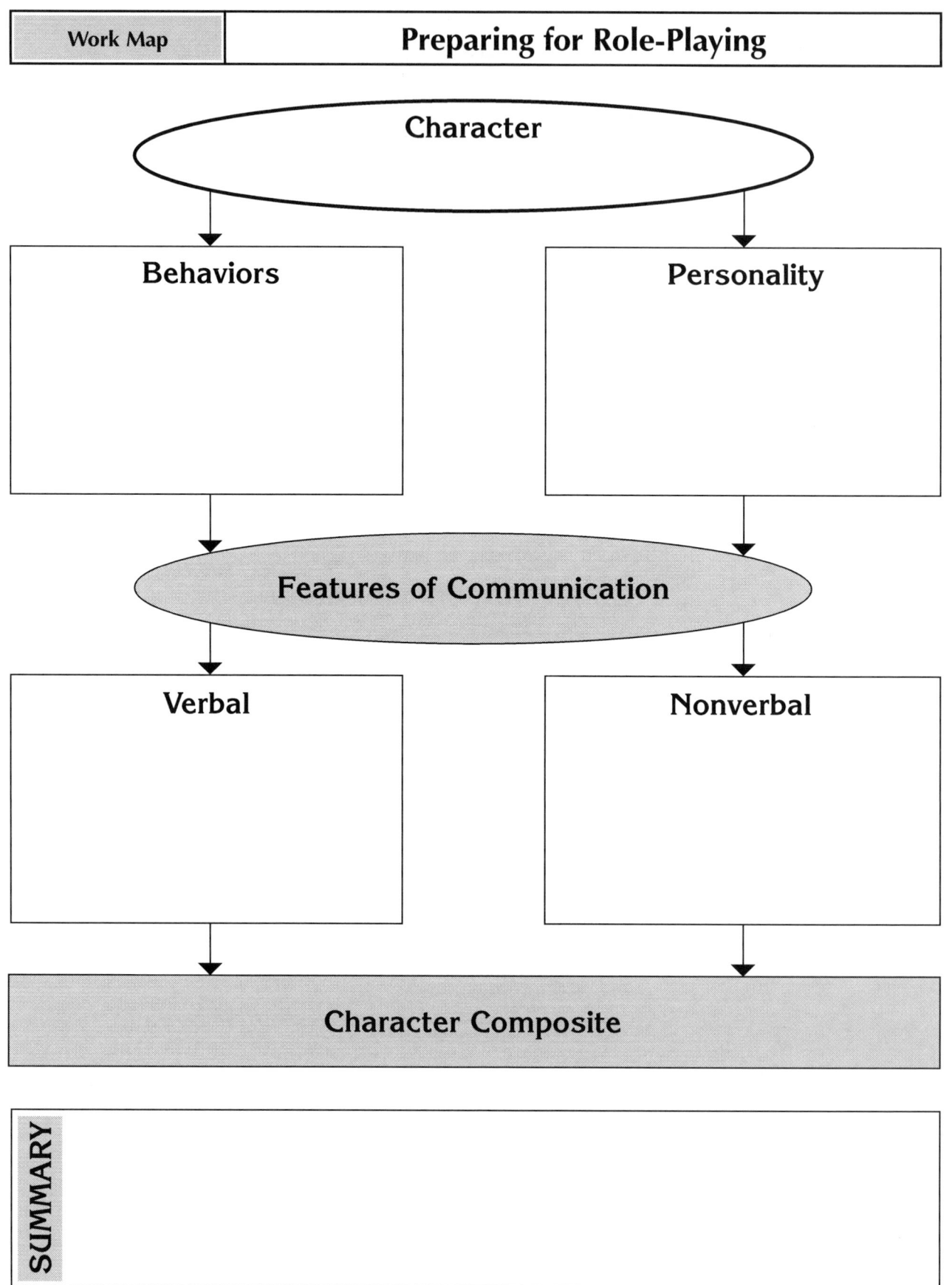

Section 4
School Knowledge/Study Skills

Unit 42: Remembering Events 265

Unit 43: Remembering Messages 270

Unit 44: Remembering Directions to Locations 275

Unit 45: Remembering Teacher Instructions 280

Unit 46: Understanding Rules and Regulations 285

Unit 47: Social Hierarchies and Communication 290

Unit 48: School (Organizational) Culture...295

Unit 49: Understanding Cultural Diversity...300

Unit 50: Decision-Making Process for Options 305

School Knowledge/Study Skills

Unit 42: Remembering Events

> ## Educational Levels
> Upper elementary through secondary
>
> ## Objectives
> (1) Analyze, store, and recall actions, reactions, and outcomes of positive or negative events at home, at school, and in life; and (2) integrate actions, reactions, and outcomes into an understanding of the dynamics of the situation

Completed Map

For this map, students in Grade 11 were asked to identify and analyze a recent event that left a long-term impression on them. The student whose map serves as an example analyzed and recorded what she perceived through the senses and how she acted and reacted during and immediately after an auto accident. She shared the map with the class. The students discussed the event; analyzed her memories, actions, and reactions; and evaluated her ability to stay cool and take the perspective of the other driver.

Show the Completed Map to students and say, for example:

> *This map shows how a student analyzed and remembered a traumatic event in her life. Let's talk about the event, an auto accident, and what the student saw, heard, felt, and did. Then we'll look at the student's positive and negative reactions.*

You may want to follow up by asking, for example:

> *Can you think of a memorable event in your life? What can you remember about it? What did you or another person do that was either good or bad in response to the event?*

Map It Out

Work Map

Show the Work Map to students and say, for example:

> *This map is empty. Let's talk about some events you have been involved in recently. Then we'll pick a memorable event and analyze what you remember and what your reactions were.*

Extended Activities

1. Have each student analyze a recent, positive event at home, in school, or in the community (e.g., a birthday party) based on his or her memory of it. Then ask students to share their memories and discuss what they no longer remember (e.g., visual or auditory stimuli).

2. Have each student analyze a school event (e.g., a concert or science fair). Ask students to pay attention to what they experience through their senses and how they act and react in response to the stimuli. Students may record aspects of the event as it happens or immediately after.

3. Select a popular TV series in which each episode features a different event. Assign an episode for students to watch. Have each student analyze the event featured in the episode. Tell students that they can make inferences about feelings and reactions based on the actions they observe. Share the analyses in class, and discuss any differences in observations.

4. Select a short story or play that is part of the curriculum. Ask students to read a segment that describes a pivotal event. Have students analyze aspects of the event, either in small teams or individually. Then share and discuss the students' observations and inferences.

5. Select a skit or segment of a play for role-playing. Assign roles to some students and have them role-play the interactions. Have other students observe. After the presentation, have each student analyze the events in the segment or skit. Compare the analyses completed by the students involved in role-playing to the analyses completed by those who observed. Point out similarities and differences in their observations, and discuss what might have caused the different perceptions (e.g., involvement in one's own role to the exclusion of observing others).

School Knowledge/Study Skills

| Master Map | **Remembering Events** |

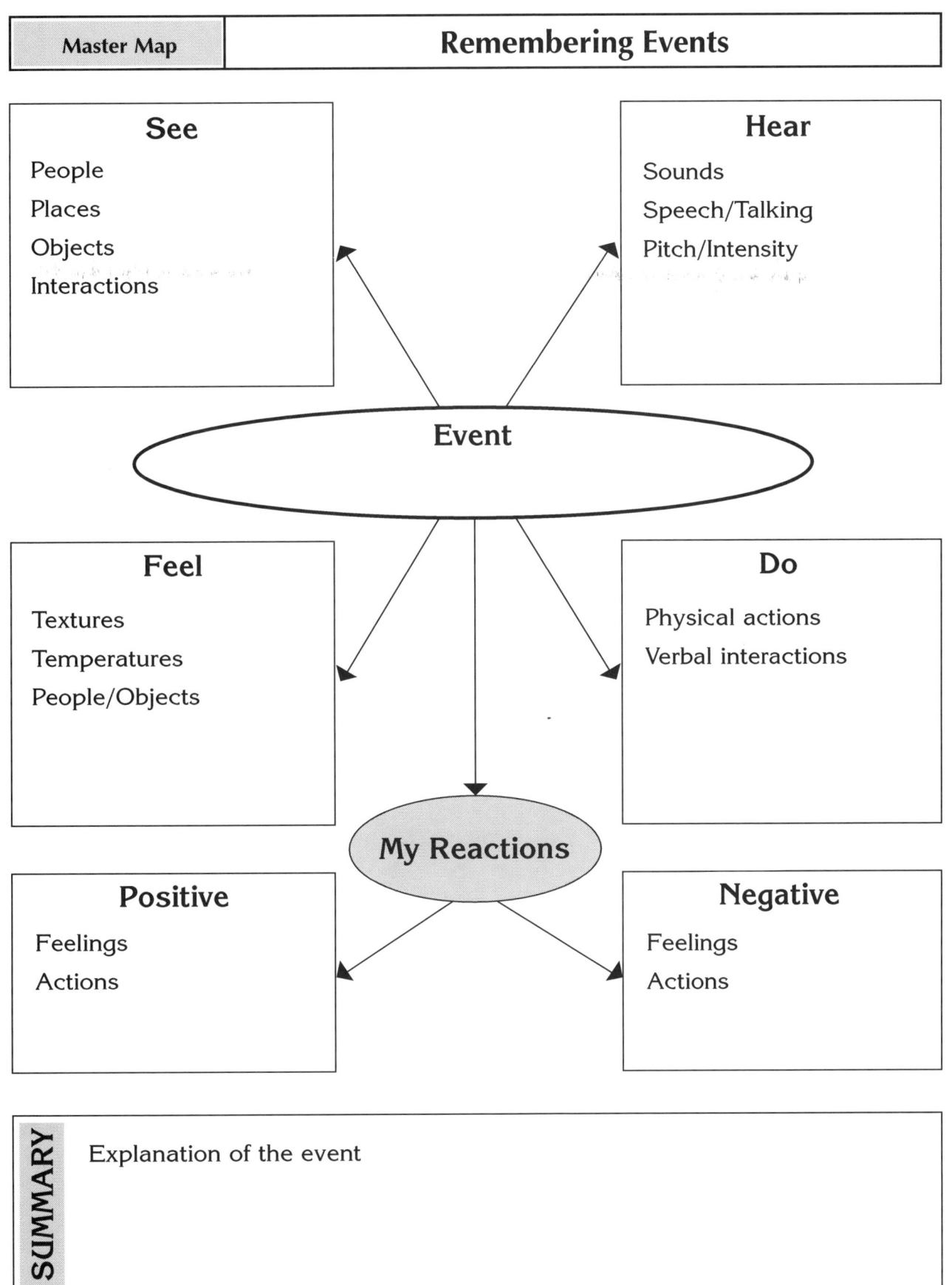

See
People
Places
Objects
Interactions

Hear
Sounds
Speech/Talking
Pitch/Intensity

Event

Feel
Textures
Temperatures
People/Objects

Do
Physical actions
Verbal interactions

My Reactions

Positive
Feelings
Actions

Negative
Feelings
Actions

SUMMARY — Explanation of the event

© 2001 by E.H. Wiig and C.C. Wilson
Duplication permitted for educational use only.

Map It Out

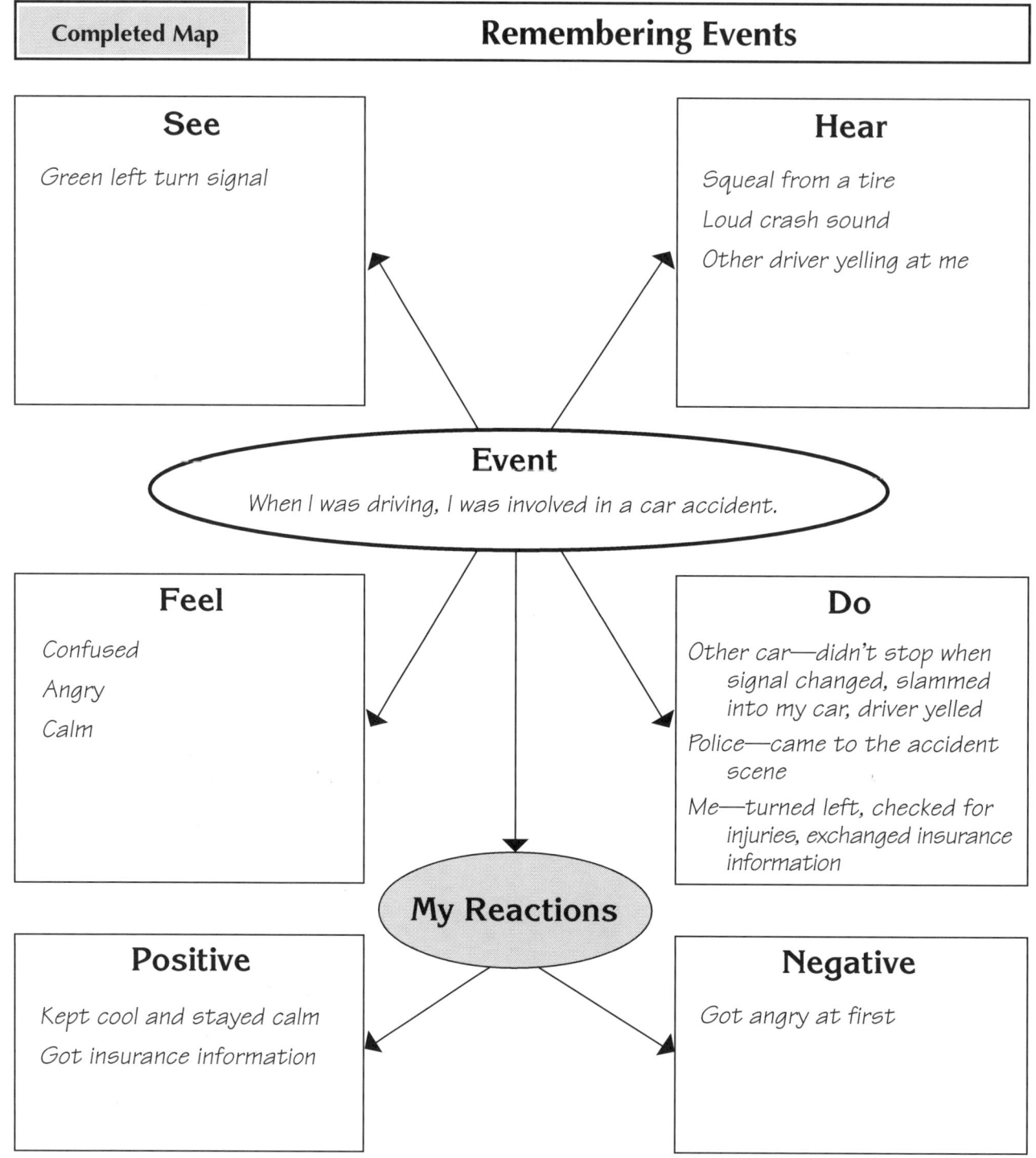

School Knowledge/Study Skills

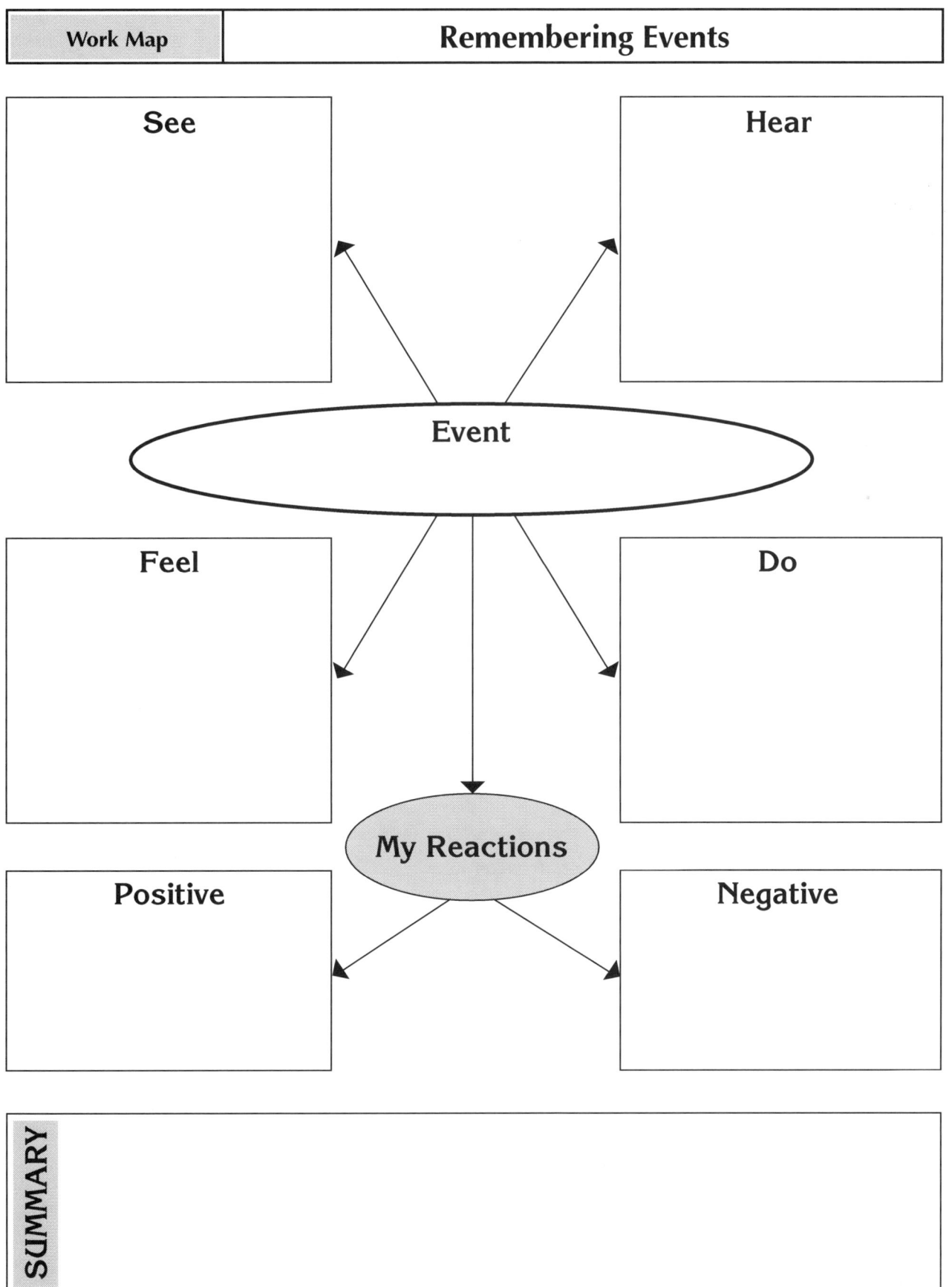

Map It Out

Unit 43: Remembering Messages

> **Educational Levels**
>
> Upper elementary through secondary
>
> **Objectives**
>
> (1) Identify important or key information in spoken messages; and (2) reconstruct the content of spoken messages in a paraphrase form that is easy to remember and transmit to the intended recipient

Completed Map

This map shows how a student in Grade 6 analyzed a telephone message that was part of a role-playing activity. The student first watched a skit that was presented by classmates. Then he wrote down the essentials of the telephone message given in the skit. The student shared his written record and discussed what he had remembered easily and what he had left out.

Show the Completed Map to students and say, for example:

> *This map shows how a student analyzed a telephone message that was part of a skit. Let's talk about the essential elements of the message and how the student recorded them.*

You may want to follow up by asking, for example:

> *Can you remember a message you were asked to give to another person? What can you remember about it? Can you analyze the message by using the process shown on this map?*

Work Map

Show the Work Map to students and say, for example:

> *This map is empty. I will give you a message. Listen to my message and record the essential information.*

Discuss and illustrate various strategies for remembering spoken information, such as chunking, imaging, and relating to prior knowledge.

Extended Activities

1. Have each student make up a true-life example of a message for someone else in the class. Then assign some students to record and others to transmit each message. Emphasize the importance of abstracting; recording only the essential content; and avoiding the tendency to repeat, rehearse, or record messages verbatim.

2. Prepare a series of messages for students to present to someone outside the classroom face to face. Tell the messages to students, and ask them to record and paraphrase each message. Then assign each student a message and recipient (e.g., a school secretary or librarian).

3. Prepare a series of messages for one group of students to record on a telephone-answering device. Ask another group of students to listen to the messages, analyze them, and deliver them to the students who recorded the messages. Ask students to compare how the telephone messages were recorded to how they were presented face to face.

4. Design a series of messages for students to listen to and analyze in class. Tell students that they are practicing for taking notes on presentations. Ask students to share and discuss their note-taking experiences.

5. Select examples of messages from home, school, or work settings. Use a round robin format in which the teacher whispers a message to one student, who then records, reconstructs, and whispers it to another student. Compare the final message with the original. Expand the activity to note taking for school or work.

Map It Out

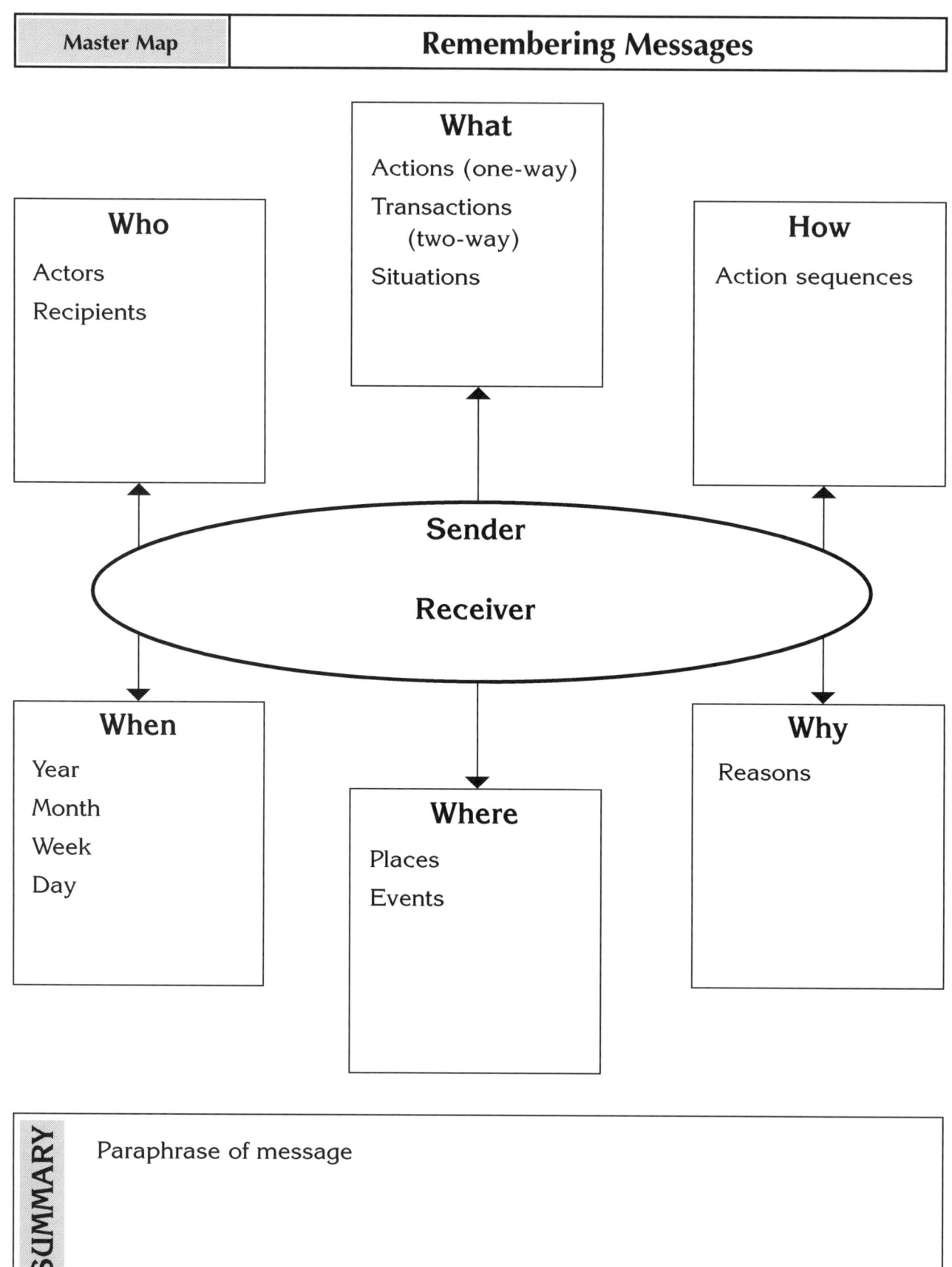

School Knowledge/Study Skills

| **Completed Map** | **Remembering Messages** |

What
Open door
Hand out registration cards
Lead meeting

Who
Mom
Club members

How
Order doesn't matter

Sender
Mrs. Jones
Receiver
Mom

When
Tonight
Get there early

Where
The club

Why
Mrs. Jones is sick.

SUMMARY — Mom, Mrs. Jones called. She wants you to lead the club meeting tonight. She asked that you get there early, open the door, hand out registration cards, and lead the meeting. She is sick and won't be there.

Map It Out

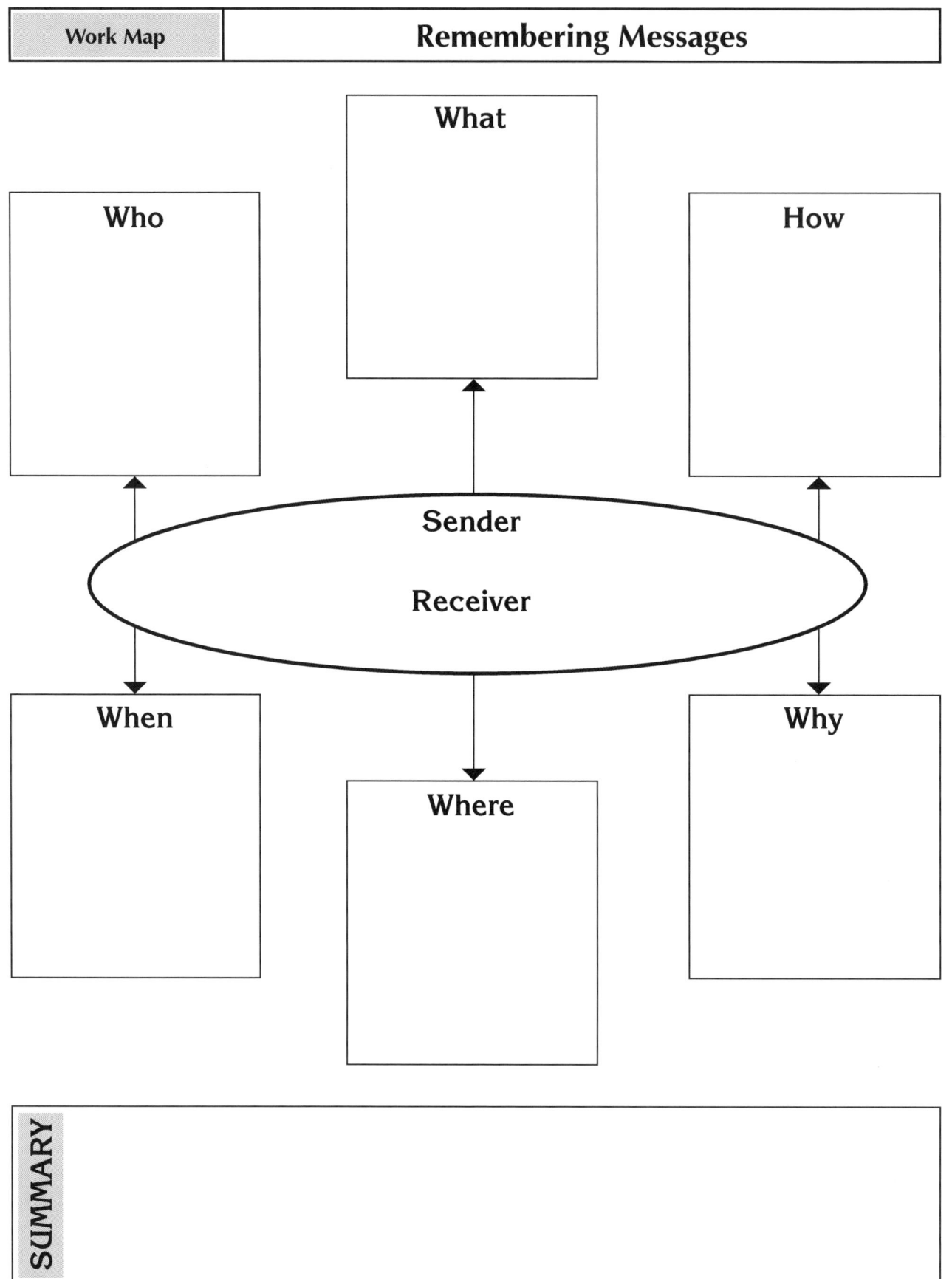

274

© 2001 by E.H. Wiig and C.C. Wilson
Duplication permitted for educational use only.

School Knowledge/Study Skills

Unit 44: Remembering Directions to Locations

> ## Educational Levels
> Upper elementary through secondary
>
> ## Objectives
> (1) Identify important information in directions to locations; (2) recode and record directions to locations in short form; and (3) recall or reconstruct spatial directions in a telegraphic, easy-to-remember format

Completed Map

This map shows how students in Grade 7 analyzed spoken directions to locations in their community. Students listened to the teacher giving a direction from one location to another. They recorded the important elements of each direction.

Show the Completed Map to students and say, for example:

> *This map shows how students recorded directions to a location given by a teacher. Let's talk about the sequence of and essential elements in directions to locations. Then we'll look at how the students recorded the directions.*

You may want to follow up by asking, for example:

> *What do you find easy and hard to remember when you listen to spoken directions to an unfamiliar place? Can you think of directions to a location you have given to another person? What can you remember about giving the directions?*

Work Map

Show the Work Map to students and say, for example:

> *This map is empty. I will give you directions to a location. Listen to my spoken directions. Record the essential information and circle any directional terms—like north or left—contained in the direction.*

Map It Out

Discuss and illustrate memory strategies students can use. Explain how they can use the column at the right to circle the critical directional terms (i.e., right, left, north, south, east, and west).

Extended Activities

1. Have each student prepare spoken directions from the classroom or school to a familiar place. Ask some students to read their directions to the class. Guide the other students in a shared activity of recording important details and paraphrasing each spoken direction. Identify the sequence in the directions, and record actions and spatial terms to help students recall the directions. Emphasize the importance of keeping the sequence accurate; recording only essential actions and directional terms; and avoiding the tendency to repeat, rehearse, or record spoken directions verbatim.

2. Give students a map of their community. Assign a final destination to each student. Have each student prepare a set of directions from the school to the assigned location. Then have each student read his or her directions while the other students follow along on the map. Discuss and clarify any difficulties the students experience while following directions.

3. Use spoken directions to locations in the community in a round robin game. Read a direction to the first student who then repeats the direction to the next and so on. Ask the last student to repeat the directions in their final form and compare them to the directions in the original version.

4. Role-play telephone calls with spontaneous, unprepared spoken directions to locations in the school or community. Ask the listeners to record each telephone message. Then ask the listeners to request clarification if they feel a direction is unclear or incomplete.

5. Play the informal game Guess My Destination. The game can focus on listening to directions and identifying destinations within the classroom, school, or immediate neighborhood without using maps or within the larger community by using maps.

School Knowledge/Study Skills

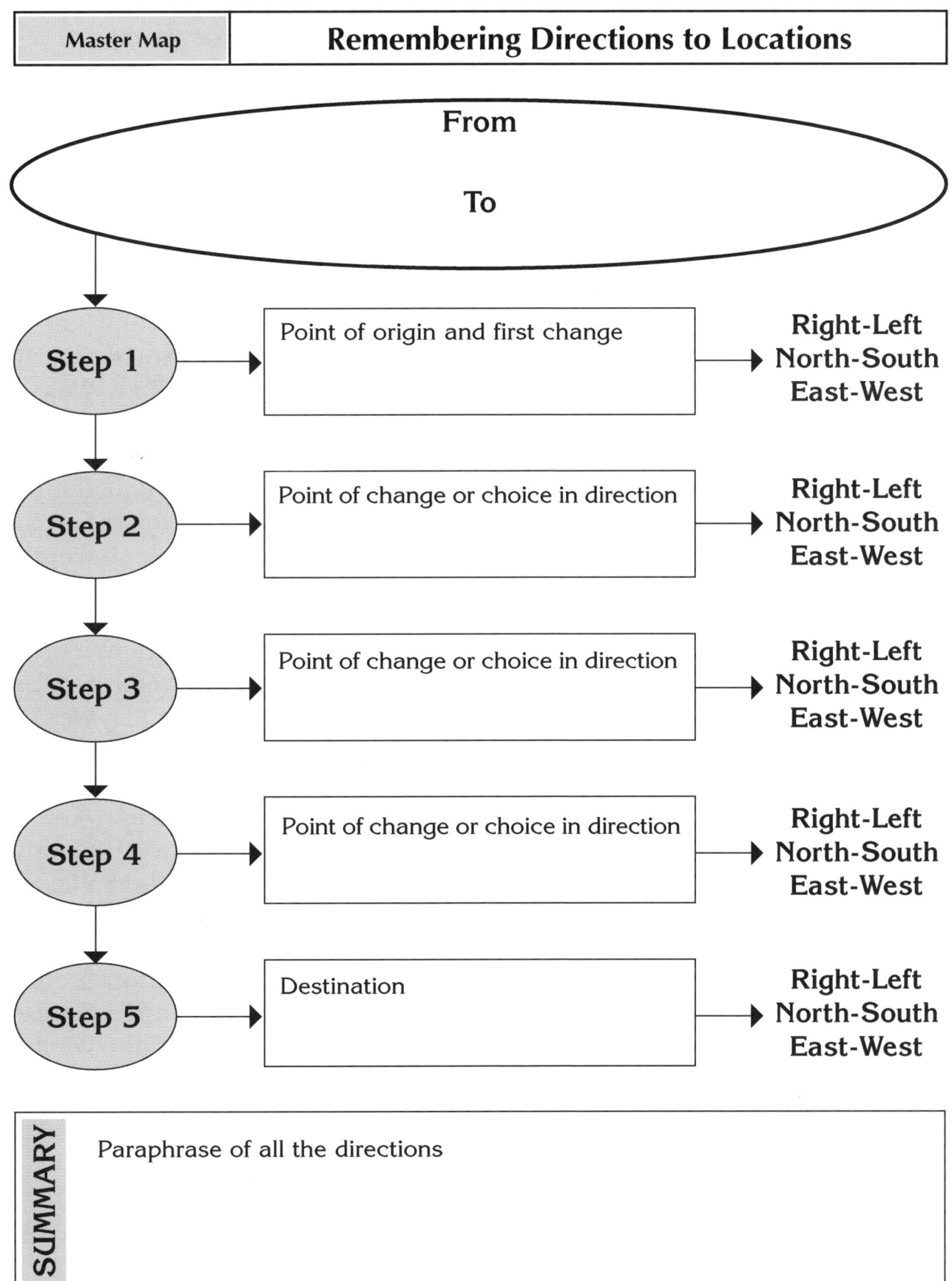

Map It Out

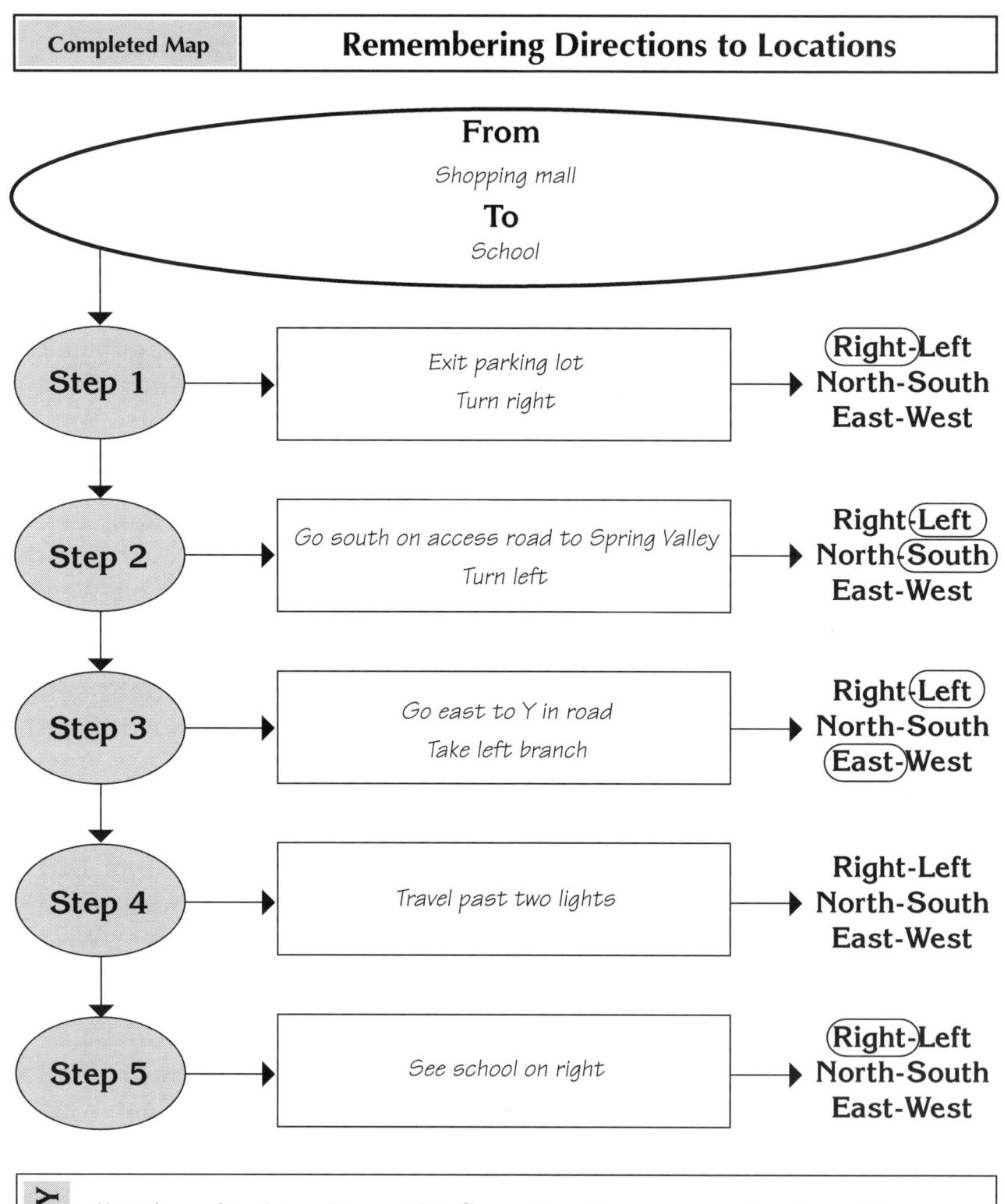

278

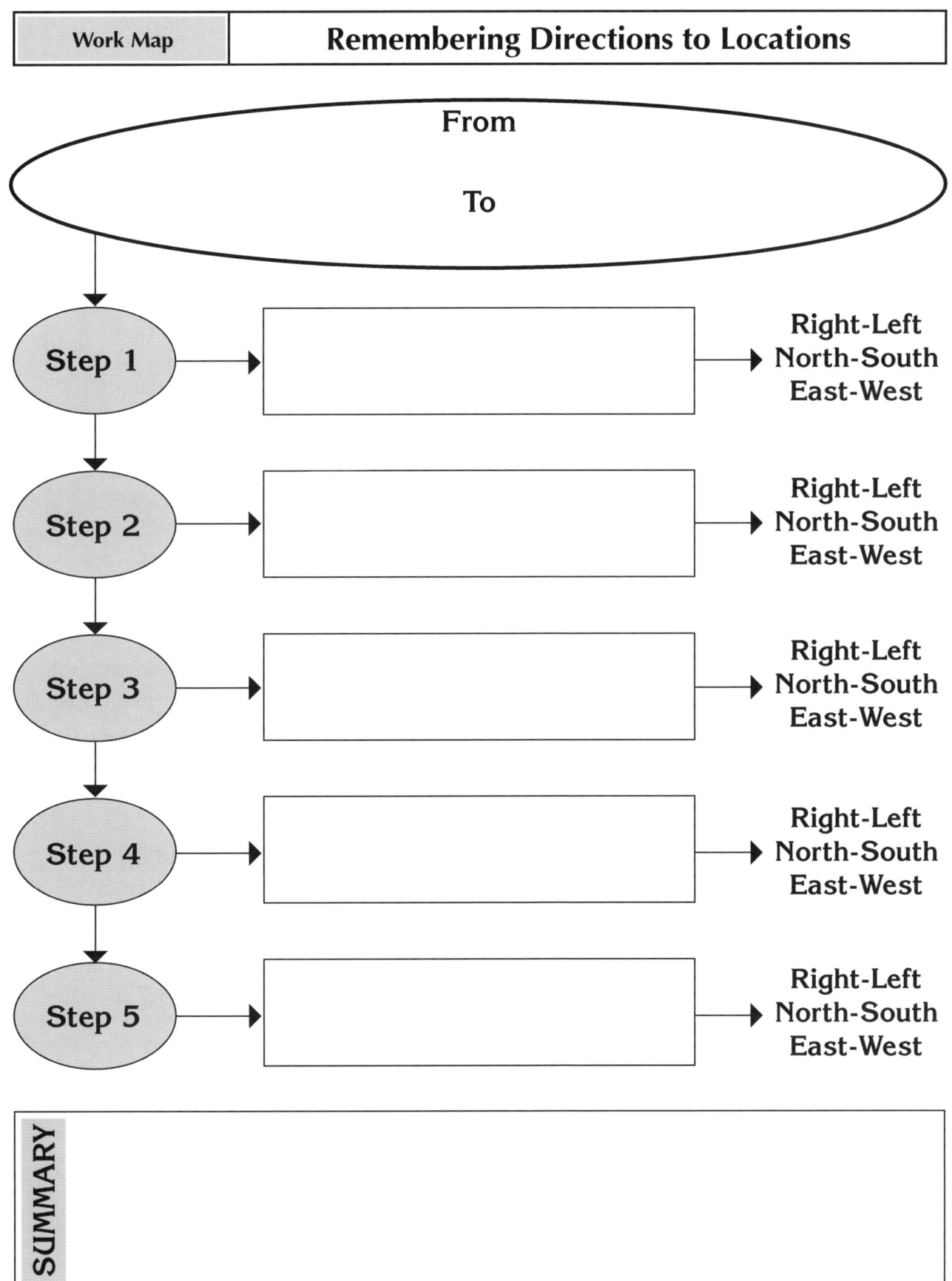

Map It Out

Unit 45: Remembering Teacher Instructions

> **Educational Levels**
>
> Upper elementary through secondary
>
> **Objectives**
>
> (1) Identify important information in spoken instructions; (2) record information in short form (i.e., take notes); and (3) follow instructions to complete a task

Completed Map

This map shows how students in Grade 6 responded to instructions. Students were told that they were going to research a country of their choice. The teacher gave instructions for the research project after asking the students to take notes on the instructions. Then the students formed teams to plan for and implement the details of the assignment.

Show the Completed Map to students and say, for example:

> *This map shows how a team of students recorded a teacher's instructions for a team project in geography. Let's talk about the essential elements in the instructions.*

Emphasize the importance of recording only essential information; making logical inferences; and avoiding the tendency to repeat, rehearse, or record instructions verbatim. Emphasize the underlying plans (e.g., scripts or schema) for instructions teachers use regularly to tell about the expected action sequences in a given subject area (e.g., mathematics or arts).

You may want to follow up by asking, for example:

> *Can you remember an instruction a teacher recently gave you? What can you remember about it? Can you analyze the instruction using the process shown on this map?*

Work Map

Show the Work Map to students and say, for example:

> *This map is empty. I will give you instructions for a task. Listen to my instructions, and write the essential information on the map. Then we'll talk about the essential elements of instructions.*

Discuss and illustrate various memory strategies, such as chunking, imaging, and relating to prior knowledge.

Extended Activities

1. Ask students to come up with some examples of how teachers in other classes give instructions for a task. Guide the students in taking notes on the instructions by recording only the essential details. Then ask students to share notes and paraphrase each instruction.

2. Play the informal game Guess What I Teach. Prepare somewhat long instructions that follow the underlying plan that is commonly used in a subject area. Read the instructions to students at a faster than normal rate. Ask students to listen to the structure and important details and then guess the subject area.

3. Have each student write an instruction for a classroom task and read the instruction to the class. While students listen to instructions, have them take notes. If any instruction was not clear, tell the listeners to identify what was missing. Select some of the instructions that were read, and ask students to paraphrase them in easy-to-remember terms.

4. Record on audiotape some classroom instructions spoken by several teachers. Select some of the instructions, and play them to the class. Have each student take notes and then retell each instruction in his or her own words.

5. Play a round robin instruction game using a simple classroom task (e.g., preparing for reading). Tell the instructions to the first student in line. At the end of the game, ask the last student to perform the instructions as she or he heard them. Afterward compare the final instructions to the original instructions.

6. Form small teams, and prepare each team to play a barrier game. Set up a barrier between two halves of each team. Then give each team the same materials to work with (e.g., construction paper, glue, and scissors). Select one student on each team to be the "instructor." Give the instructors a map that has only the details of the instructions filled in (i.e., the map has been filled in backwards with the details but without the instructions) and requires the materials to be handed out. Ask the instructors to make up spoken instructions for their teammates using full sentences and their own words.

Map It Out

| Master Map | **Remembering Teacher Instructions** |

What (Actions)
Actions (one-way)
Transactions (two-way)

What (Materials)
Texts
Projects
Parts
Pages
Equipment
Software

Where
General areas
Specific places
Virtual places

From

To

Why
Reasons
Expectations

How
Action sequences
Follow ups

When
Immediate/Delayed actions
Due dates

SUMMARY: Paraphrase of the instructions and a plan for implementation

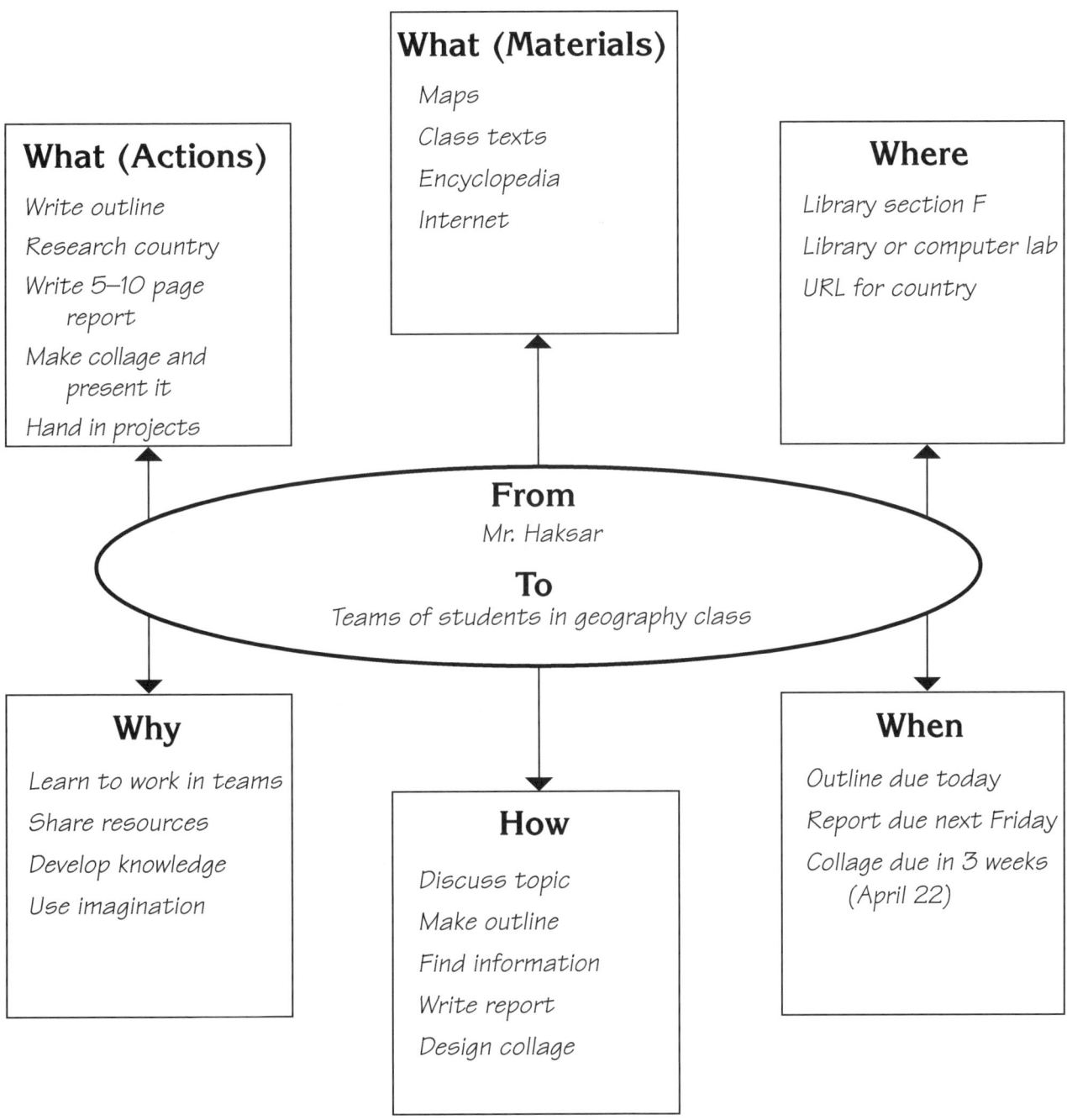

Map It Out

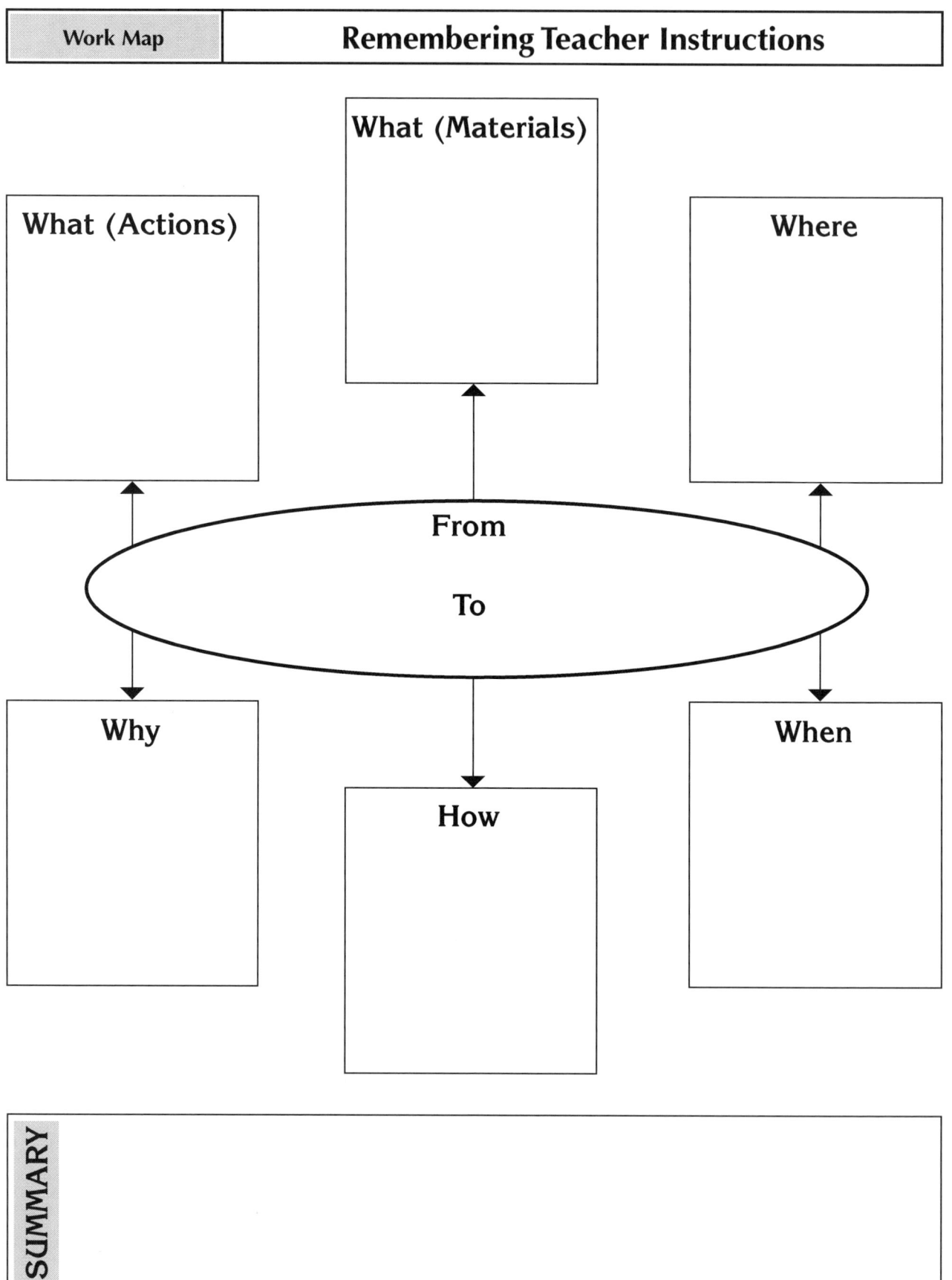

School Knowledge/Study Skills

Unit 46: Understanding Rules and Regulations

Educational Levels

Upper elementary through secondary

Objectives

(1) Analyze existing school or community rules and regulations that are stated in short forms; (2) understand intentions behind rules and implications of violating rules; and (3) interpret and create new examples of rules and regulations

Completed Map

This map shows how students in Grade 7 interpreted a new school rule, "Zero Tolerance for Violence." The teacher asked students to analyze each important word or concept for its meaning and write down words that were similar in meaning and could cause confusion.

Show the Completed Map to students and say, for example:

This map shows an example of a new school rule that everyone needed to understand. Let's look at the important words and concepts in the rule and discuss how a group of students interpreted them.

You may want to follow up by showing students examples of signs around the school that state a rule without using words (e.g., no smoking or no guns).

Work Map

Show the Work Map to students and say, for example:

This map is empty. Let's think of a school or community rule. We'll look at each important word and interpret its meanings.

Map It Out

Extended Activities

1. Select an existing school rule, regulation, or slogan that is stated in short form in words or images (e.g., no smoking or no guns). Ask students to identify important words and concepts; analyze them for interpretation; and discuss the meaning of the concept, intent of the creator, and possible benefits of the rule. Then ask students to discuss the possible implications of violating the rule.

2. Have each student identify and select abbreviated expressions of rules, regulations, or slogans from his or her memory or from a curriculum text. Have each student analyze the meaning and intent of the rules.

3. Have each student search the community for signs that tell about rules and regulations (e.g., traffic signs). Then have them draw or write some of the rule statements. Ask students to share their findings. Guide an analysis of what each rule means and how to act according to the rule. Then ask students to suggest how the rule might be violated and what the punishments might be.

4. Ask students to listen to TV ads or look at magazines to identify slogans or short expressions that are supposed to "tell it all" and sell a product. Have each student analyze one or more of the examples and present his or her findings to the class. Guide a class discussion of the example and the results of the student's analysis. You may want to ask questions, such as, "What did you like most about the ad?" "How did you react to the ad?" or "Would you buy the product? Why? Why not?"

5. Have each student identify a setting he or she is familiar with or visits regularly that has posted rules for behavior (e.g., a library or community pool). Have each student identify and record the posted rules. Then have each student show one or more of the rules in their original forms, interpret each rule for classmates, and discuss possible violations and probable punishments for violations.

6. Select slogans or short quotes from famous people's speeches (e.g., "Read my lips"). Organize students in small teams, and have each team analyze one or more of the slogans or quotes. Then ask each team to present its analysis to the class.

School Knowledge/Study Skills

| Master Map | Understanding Rules and Regulations |

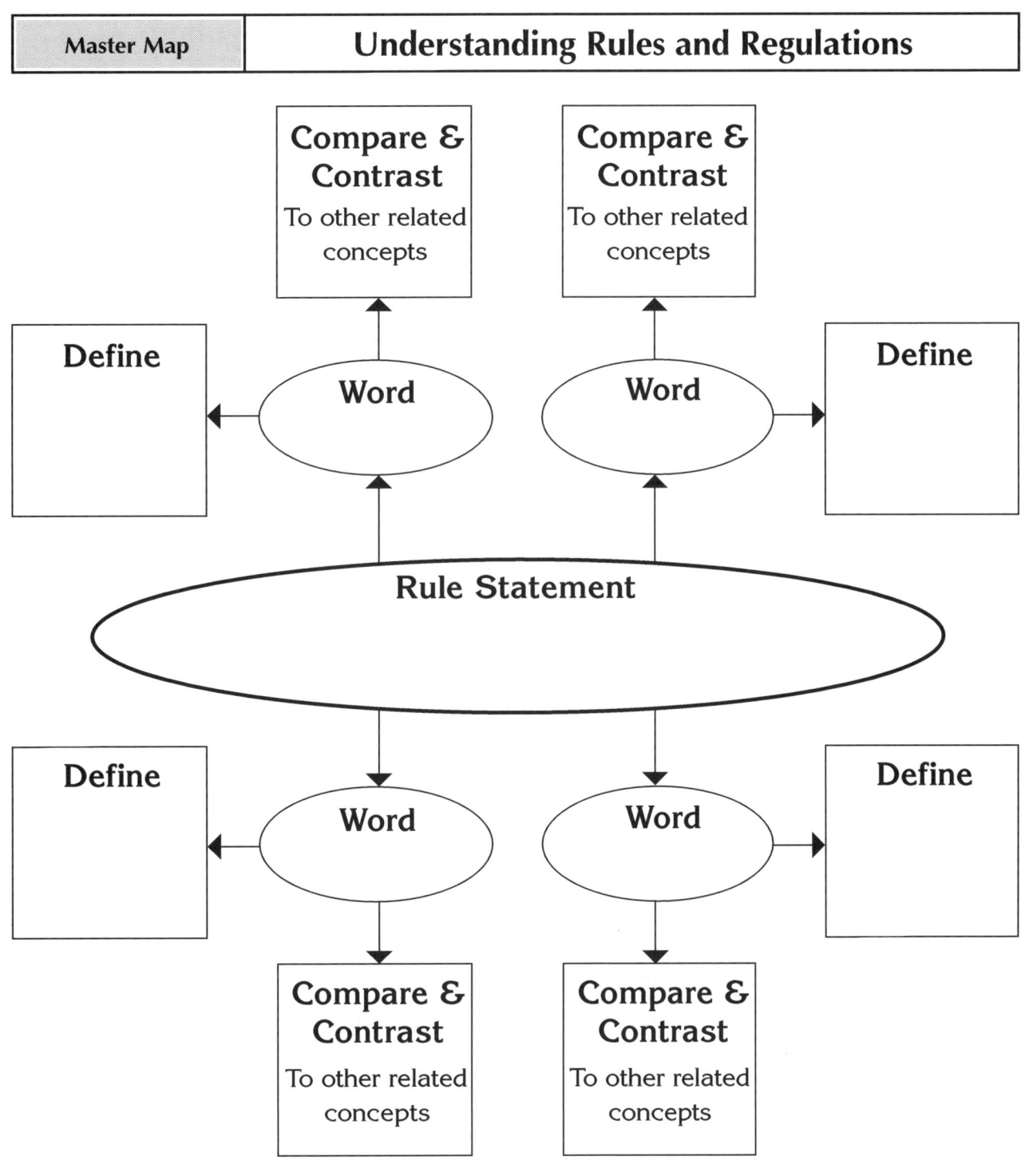

SUMMARY: Paraphrase of the rule or regulation and discussion of its associated intentions, implications, and consequences

Map It Out

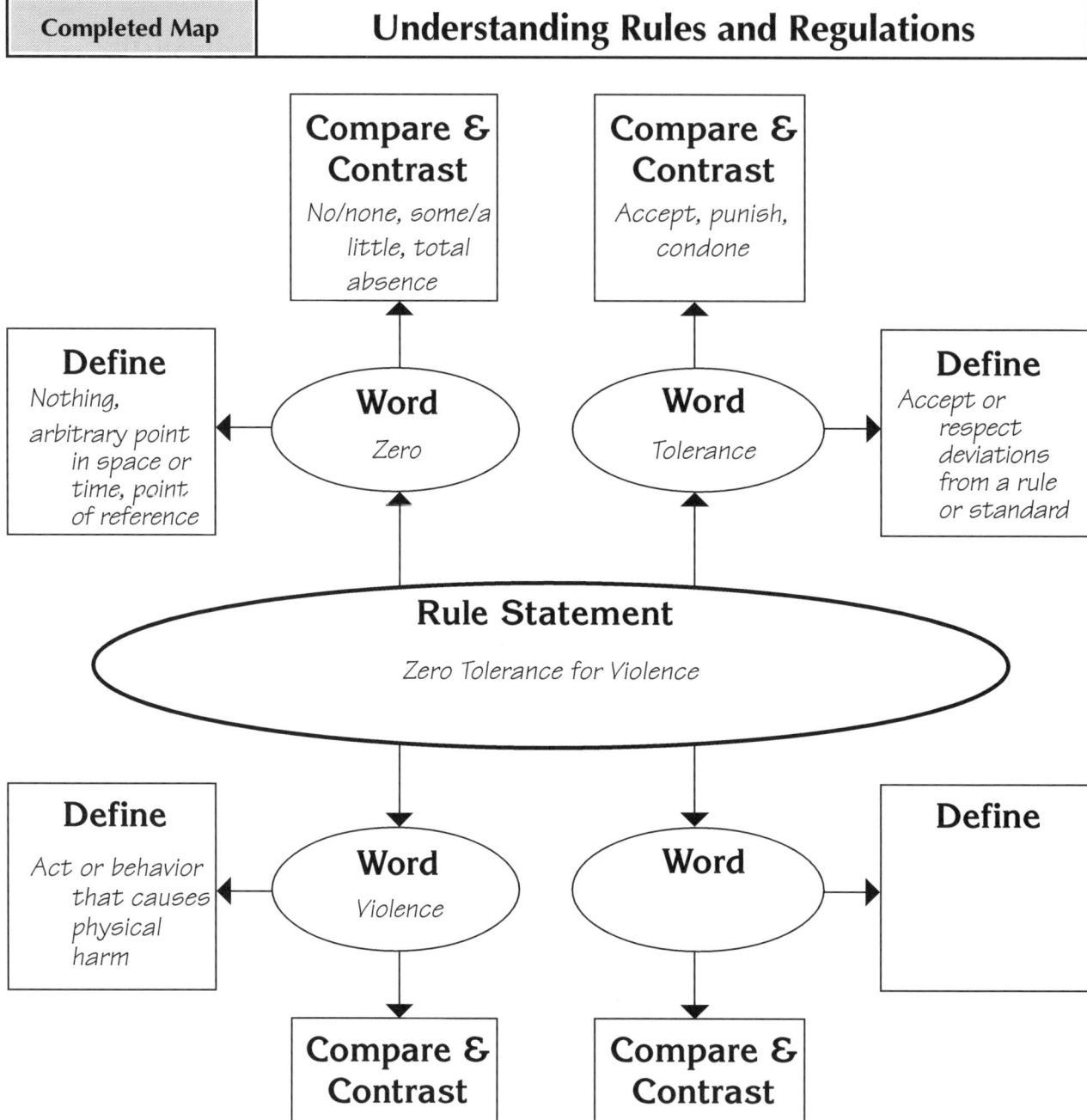

288

School Knowledge/Study Skills

| Work Map | Understanding Rules and Regulations |

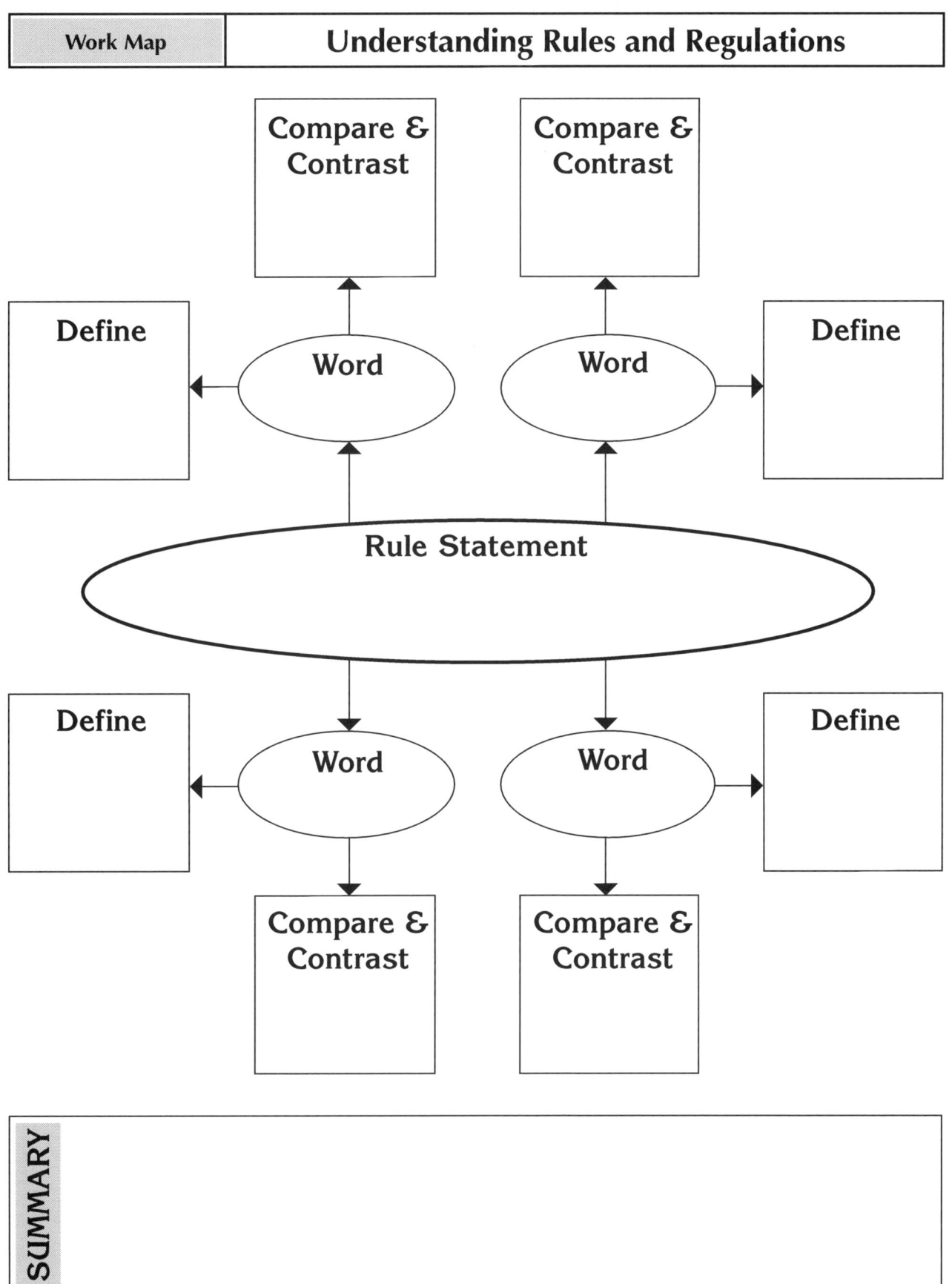

SUMMARY

289

Map It Out

Unit 47: Social Hierarchies and Communication

> **Educational Levels**
>
> Elementary through secondary
>
> **Objectives**
>
> (1) Analyze levels within cultural or social hierarchies; (2) identify features that indicate level and control in social interactions; (3) identify features and characteristics of behavior and communication within a social hierarchy to understand interactions and communications within it better; and (4) apply the process to communicating and responding within social hierarchies in academic, vocational, and social settings

Completed Map

This map shows how students in Grade 9 analyzed behaviors and communication as they prepared to interview for summer jobs. The class discussed examples and characteristics of levels within a social hierarchy in the working community. The teacher elicited features the students should be aware of and discussed behaviors they might want to control when they went for interviews. The class then identified and discussed some differences in behavior and communication between two levels within a social hierarchy.

Show the Completed Map to students and say, for example:

> *This map shows how a group of students analyzed features of behavior and communication to be aware of when they interviewed for summer jobs. Let's talk about the social levels and expectations within the social hierarchy of work. Then we'll look at the specific features to consider when interviewing for a job.*

Emphasize that social hierarchies are part of any organization and that they are determined by all members.

You may want to follow up by asking, for example:

> *How is the social hierarchy in the world of work like the hierarchy in schools? How is it different? What is the social hierarchy in this class?*

School Knowledge/Study Skills

Work Map

Show the Work Map to students and say, for example:

> *This map is empty. Let's think of a social structure and hierarchy you know about. It could be in your family, a club you belong to, or a public institution. Then we'll analyze the features of the social hierarchy you select.*

Extended Activities

1. Have each student analyze and compare social hierarchies within the class and the school at large. Ask students to share their findings and come up with examples of how to start or respond to a conversation with participants in each setting (e.g., with friends in the schoolyard or with the principal in a school office).

2. Have each student take a close look at his or her family and how the members communicate with each other. Ask them to analyze how children talk parents, how parents talk to children, and how siblings communicate with each other. Then have each student relate his or her findings to the levels on the social-hierarchies map.

3. Find a TV series with a distinct social hierarchy among the characters. TV series with legal or medical settings and interactions (e.g., between client and attorney or doctor and patient) are especially good for this type of analysis. Guide an analysis of the social hierarchies in the series and how social level or status influences behavior and nonverbal and verbal communication.

4. Select a story, novel, or play that is part of the required literature (e.g., *The Outsiders* by S.E. Hinton or *Julius Caesar* by William Shakespeare). Ask students to read all or a segment of the selection. Then ask them to form small teams to analyze levels in the social hierarchies and how the participants from different levels communicated with each other.

5. Ask students to identify hierarchies in the city, state, and federal government. Ask them to identify the levels and participants at each level. Then have them select a role and an objective to communicate to an official in the hierarchy (e.g., present an opinion to the school board). Ask students to role-play this interaction. Then guide a discussion of the style and possible effectiveness of the interaction.

6. Ask students to identify a situation where they take the role of middle- or top-level supervisor (e.g., captain of a sports team or baby sitter). Ask them to consider and analyze how they would interact with individuals at other levels. Discuss the results of the analysis.

Map It Out

| Master Map | Social Hierarchies and Communication |

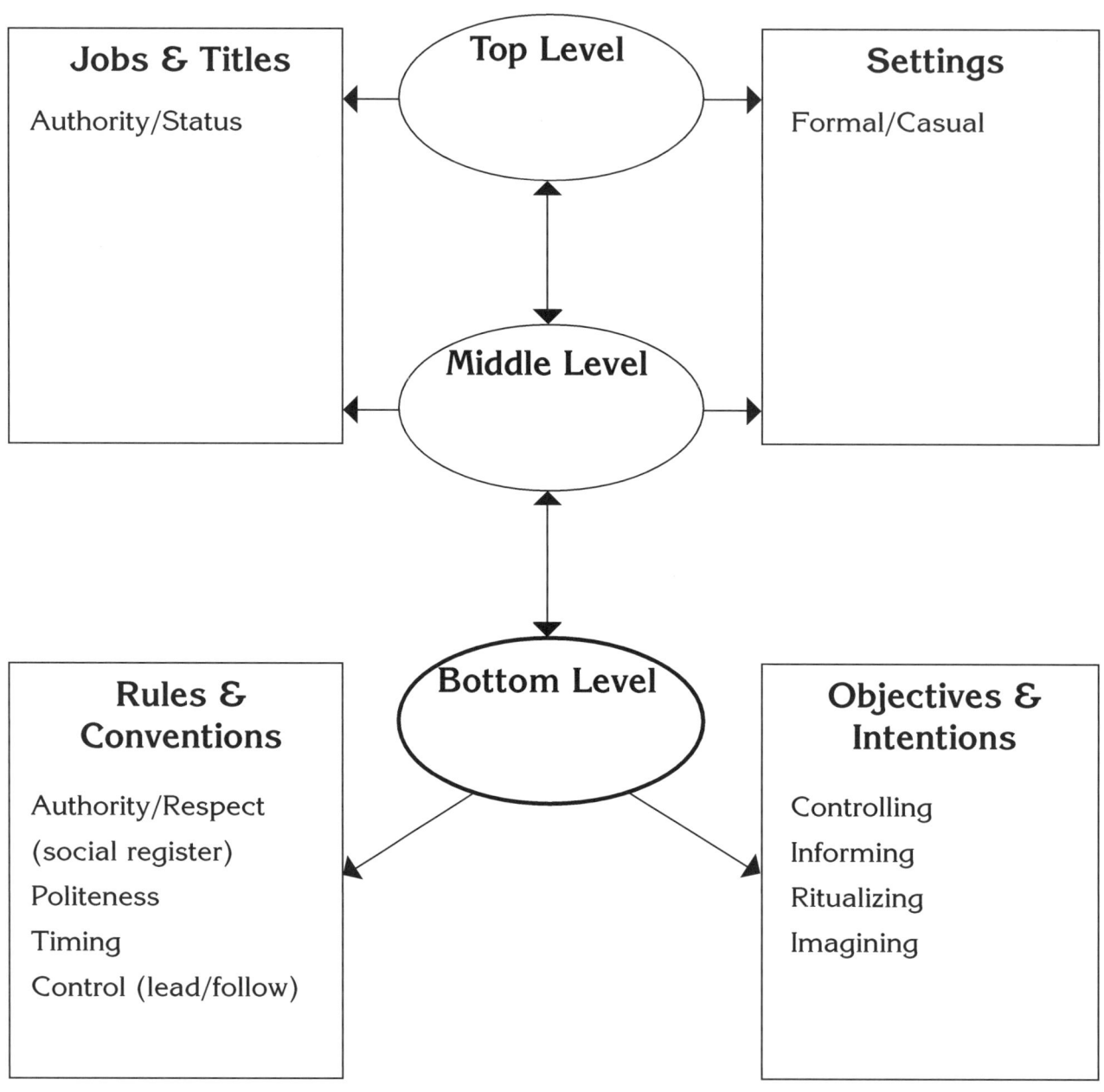

SUMMARY: Observations about the social hierarchy and communication styles

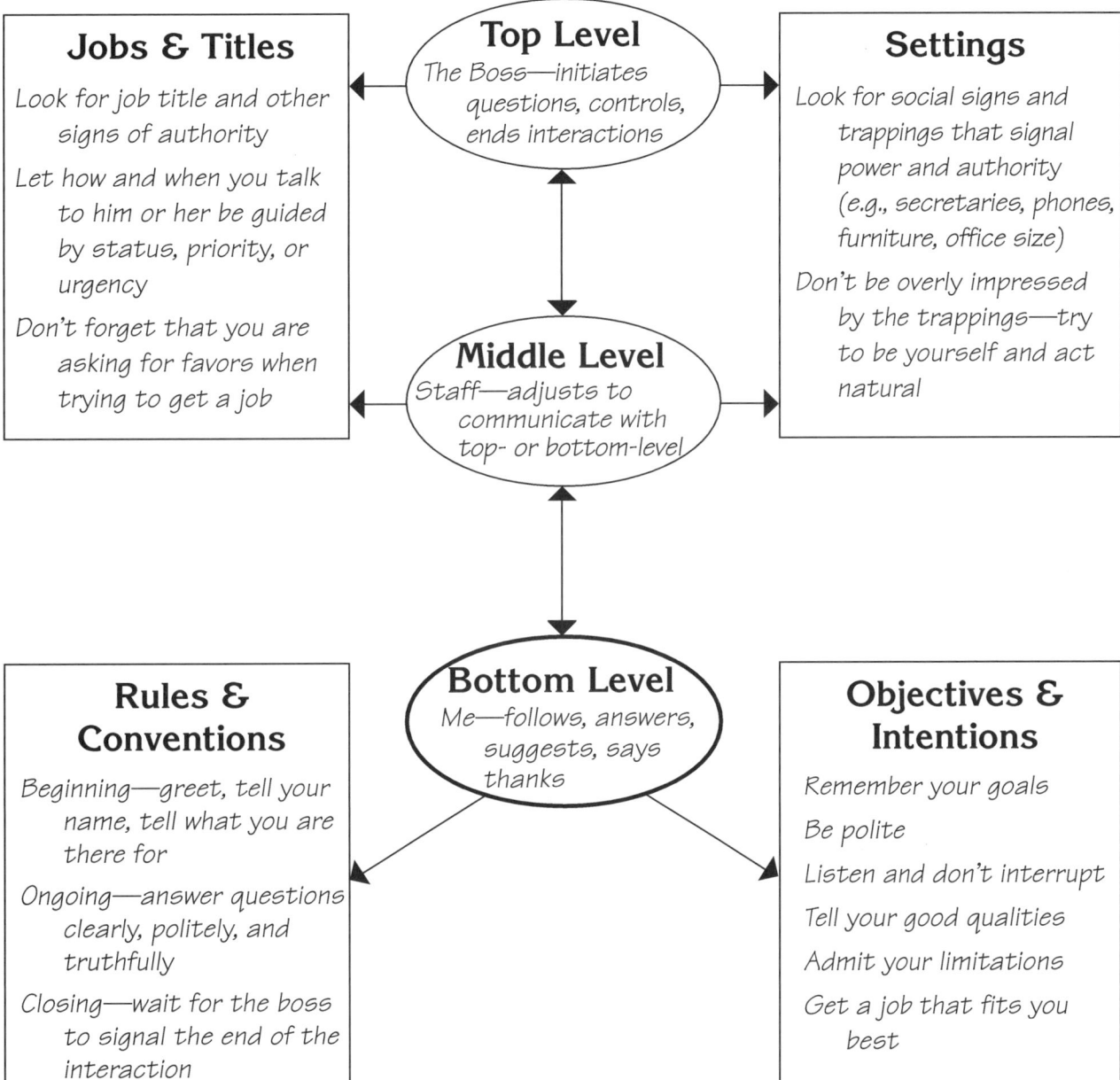

Map It Out

Work Map | **Social Hierarchies and Communication**

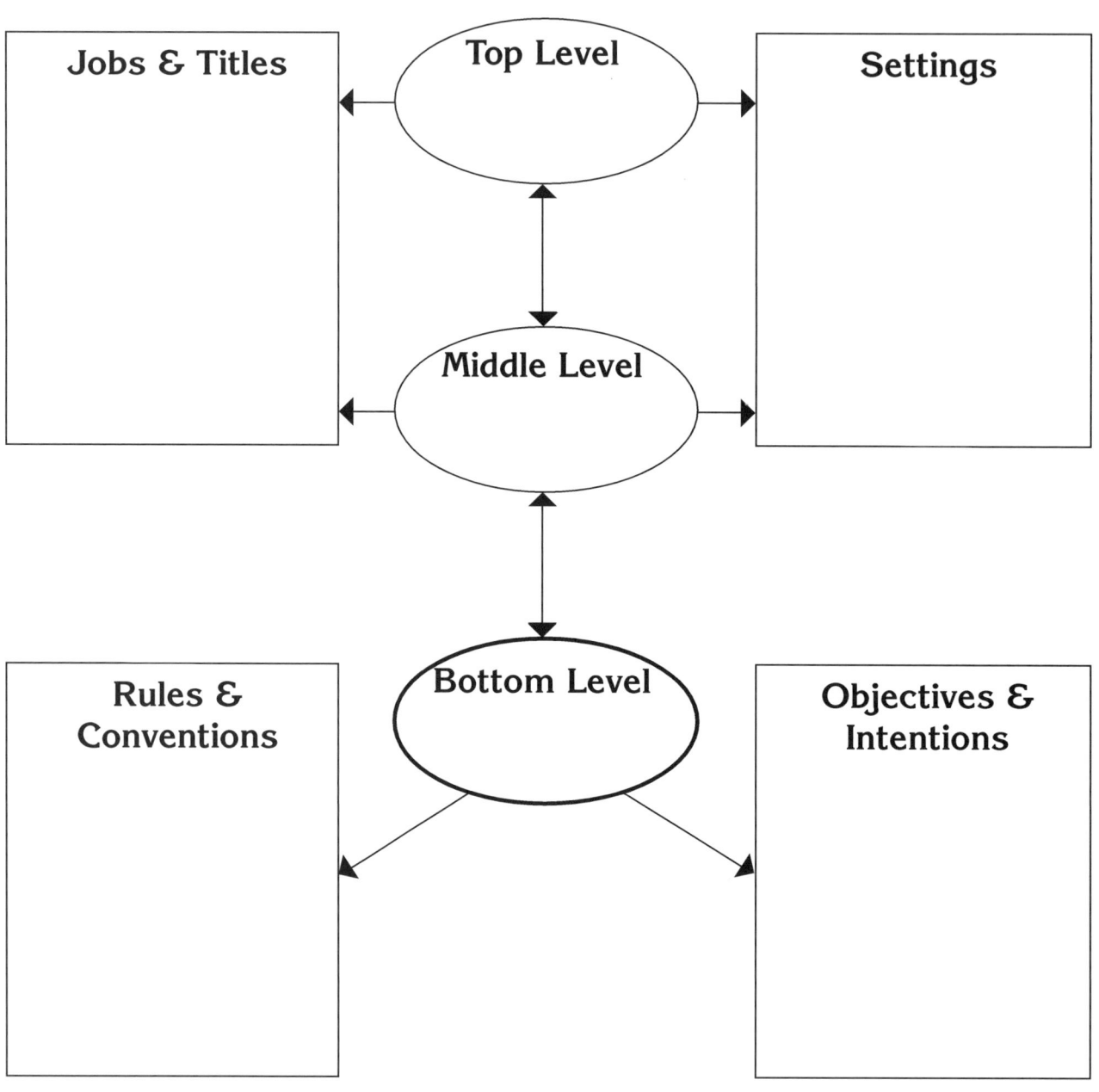

294

© 2001 by E.H. Wiig and C.C. Wilson
Duplication permitted for educational use only.

Unit 48: School (Organizational) Culture

> **Educational Levels**
>
> Upper elementary through secondary
>
> **Objectives**
>
> (1) Analyze dimensions and features of the culture of groups, organizations, and societies; (2) compare and contrast organizations to arrive at a better understanding of what creates an organizational culture and how it influences its members; and (3) understand how these elements contribute to a cultural identity

Completed Map

This map shows how a group of students in Grade 6 analyzed the organizational culture of their school. Students were asked to pretend that they were going to tell a new student about their school. Small teams identified important features (e.g., external factors) and described their perceptions of philosophies and dominant values in the school. The teams reported their findings to the class and discussed differences in their perceptions of the school culture. Afterward the students role-played how to introduce a new student to the culture.

Show the Completed Map to students and say, for example:

> *This map shows how a group of students analyzed the culture of their school so that they could give a new student advice about how to behave. Let's talk about the rules, standards, and behaviors expected from students in that school. Then let's look at the unspoken attitudes in the school, such as how students feel, what they value, and what drives teaching and learning.*

Discuss features that are observable, unspoken, or unique to the school culture. Emphasize that the culture of an organization, such as a class or school, is created and maintained by all members.

You may want to follow up by asking, for example:

> *How is the culture of that school like ours? How is it different? What would you like to see changed in our school's culture?*

Map It Out

Work Map

Show the Work Map to students and say, for example:

> *This map is empty. Let's think of an organization with a culture you know about. It could be your family, a group of close friends, or a club you belong to. Then we'll analyze features of the culture you select.*

Extended Activities

1. Ask students to think of the various classrooms they attend as representatives of different educational cultures. Have each student select a favorite classroom (e.g., a physics classroom or computer lab) and analyze the culture of that classroom. Afterward ask students to share and compare classroom cultures.

2. Have each student analyze the culture that exists within his or her family or immediate environment. Ask students to share and compare their analyses.

3. Ask students to compare the cultures of two different grade-level schools (e.g., elementary and junior high or high school and college). Guide students in an analysis and comparison of the organizational cultures at different levels of education. Ask them to discuss reasons for the differences and evaluate what they liked or disliked in each setting.

4. Ask students to explore different types of stores or fast-food restaurants. Ask them to look at each store as representing its own organizational culture. Have them look for uniforms and other evidence of status hierarchies. Tell them to look for slogans, ads, and other sources that tell about the culture of the organization. Have each student analyze a store and report his or her findings to the class.

5. Analyze the organizational culture of the students' immediate community. Ask them to work together to describe characteristics of the neighborhood or community culture. You may want to get brochures about the community from local realtors or the business bureau. Have students follow up by making collages to illustrate the organizational culture of their community.

School Knowledge/Study Skills

| Master Map | **School (Organizational) Culture** |

Behaviors
- Rules and norms
- Ceremonies
- Language use
- Deference and demeanor

Rules
- Attendance
- Compliance
- Use of resources

Norms & Standards
- Attention
- Behavior
- Performance

Observable (Explicit) Factors

School or Organization

Unspoken (Tacit) Factors

Feelings
- Atmosphere
- Tone of voice
- Attitudes
- Respect

Values
- Set by teachers and administrators
- Shared by students

Philosophies
- Teaching
- Learning

SUMMARY: Explanation of the culture

© 2001 by E.H. Wiig and C.C. Wilson
Duplication permitted for educational use only.

Map It Out

| Completed Map | School (Organizational) Culture |

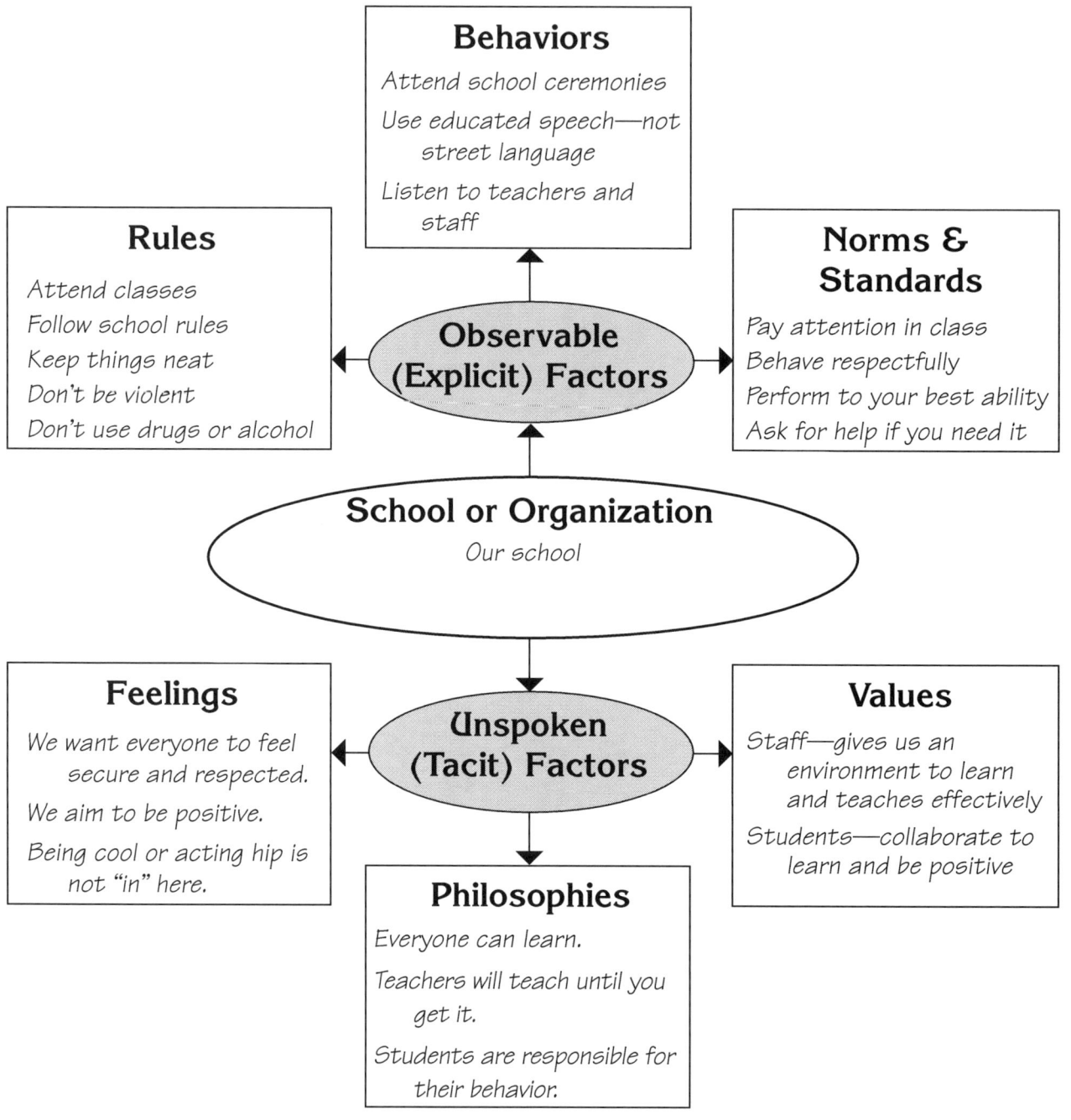

Behaviors
Attend school ceremonies
Use educated speech—not street language
Listen to teachers and staff

Rules
Attend classes
Follow school rules
Keep things neat
Don't be violent
Don't use drugs or alcohol

Norms & Standards
Pay attention in class
Behave respectfully
Perform to your best ability
Ask for help if you need it

Observable (Explicit) Factors

School or Organization
Our school

Unspoken (Tacit) Factors

Feelings
We want everyone to feel secure and respected.
We aim to be positive.
Being cool or acting hip is not "in" here.

Values
Staff—gives us an environment to learn and teaches effectively
Students—collaborate to learn and be positive

Philosophies
Everyone can learn.
Teachers will teach until you get it.
Students are responsible for their behavior.

SUMMARY
When the teachers first started to talk about the culture of our school, we didn't understand what was so important about it. Once we started to discuss the different characteristics of our school's culture, we learned that some students came from schools with very different and often negative cultures. We learned that our school's culture is very positive. We all want to learn and be happy.

School Knowledge/Study Skills

Work Map	School (Organizational) Culture

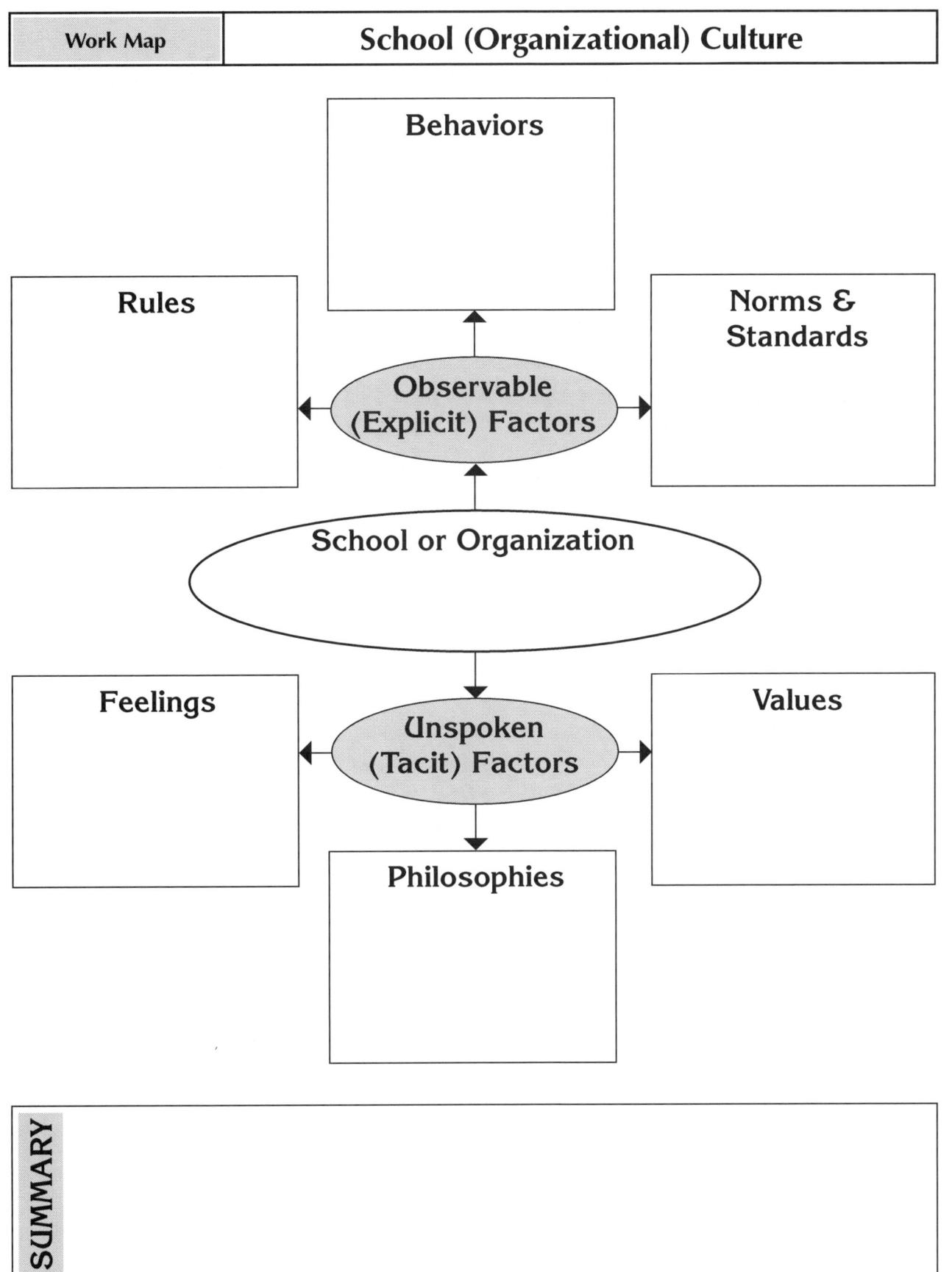

SUMMARY

© 2001 by E.H. Wiig and C.C. Wilson
Duplication permitted for educational use only.

299

Map It Out

Unit 49: Understanding Cultural Diversity

Educational Levels

Elementary through secondary

Objectives

(1) Analyze the dimensions and features of a culture; (2) develop questions to learn more about a culture; (3) apply these skills to unfamiliar cultures; and (4) understand and appreciate cultural diversity

Completed Map

For this map, students in Grade 8 were told that a student from Pakistan would join their class. The teacher wanted to prepare the class to understand and respect the student's cultural and linguistic background. To begin, the teacher elicited prior knowledge about Pakistan. Then she prepared students to talk to and ask questions of the new student so they could learn more about life in Pakistan.

Show the Completed Map to students and say, for example:

> *This map shows how a group of students prepared for a new classmate from Pakistan. Let's talk about what the students already knew about the culture of Pakistan. Then let's look at the questions they developed to ask the new student so that they could get to know more about her background.*

Emphasize the integrity and value of cultural diversity and identity.

You may want to follow up by asking, for example:

> *What do you know about the culture of Pakistan? What surprised you about the culture? How many cultural backgrounds are there in this class? What are they?*

Work Map

Show the Work Map to students and say, for example:

> *This map is empty. Let's select a culture you would like to explore. We'll identify what you already know. Then we'll come up with questions about what you want or need to know.*

Extended Activities

1. Ask students how many different cultural backgrounds there are in the classroom. Remember to count all backgrounds as representatives of cultural diversity. Then have each student analyze some of the important features of his or her cultural background. If there are several students with the same or similar backgrounds, ask them to present their analyses to the class as a team.

2. Guide an analysis and discussion of the characteristics we associate with the mainstream culture of the United States. Elicit commonly accepted features of our shared culture. Expect to find differences in the students' perceptions. The differences may reflect regional, urban, or rural variations in culture. Stress that the mainstream culture of a region is reflected when a diverse group of citizens get together (e.g., at a state fair or community barbecue).

3. Identify cultural groups that are not represented in the classroom or immediate neighborhood. Then discuss some variations in cultural dimensions that exist in the groups. Ask students to research and identify the easily observable (i.e., explicit) as well as unspoken (i.e., tacit) characteristics of the culture.

4. Ask students to analyze a culture. Then ask them to form small groups and make a collage that shows features of that culture.

5. Select literature from the curriculum that introduces readers to new cultures outside of the United States (e.g., *Master Harold and the Boys* by Athol Fugard). Ask students to analyze the culture that is featured in the story.

6. Play a twenty-questions or *wh*-question game for the question, "Where do you think my family comes from?" Have each student analyze his or her family's culture. Then select one student at a time for the game. Tell the other students to ask questions until someone can identify what the student's culture is.

Map It Out

| Master Map | **Understanding Cultural Diversity** |

Government & Social Systems
Levels of development
Infrastructures
Types

Cultural Expressions
Art/Music/Literature
Dress codes
Foods
Holidays
Traditions

Family & Friends
Social units
Professional units
Culture of the units

Country

Values & Beliefs
Attitudes
Customs
Conventions
Taboos
Traditions

Quality of Life
Living conditions
Geographic conditions
Physical/Work conditions
Recreation

Communication
Content/Structure/Use
Nonverbal (facial, gestural)
Conventions
Media and equipment

SUMMARY Description of what needs to be considered to embrace someone from another country or culture

Completed Map | # Understanding Cultural Diversity

Government & Social Systems

They have democracy.

There is education for all children.

Lots of doctors migrate to the United States.

Do you have a House and Senate like here?

Cultural Expressions

Women wear pantsuits made out of colorful silks.

Rice is a staple.

What kind of music do people listen to?

Are there famous painters?

What are sports like?

Family & Friends

The family is central.

How big is your family?

Who came to the United States with you?

What were your friends like?

What was a typical day like in your family?

Country
Pakistan

Values & Beliefs

Most people are Muslim and belong to the Islamic faith.

Are there any Christians or Jews in Pakistan?

Are there any other religions?

What are your holy or special days?

Quality of Life

Karachi is the largest city; it is on the Indian Ocean.

There are great differences between rich and poor.

What did you do for fun?

Communication

The official language is Urdu.

Could you say something to us in Urdu?

What kind of movies do you see?

Do you have telephones and computers?

SUMMARY: A new student from Pakistan will join our class next week. We need to be sensitive to the cultural differences between us. We also need to be able to ask questions so that we can better understand our new classmate and her reactions to all the changes in culture. To help us prepare to talk with the new student, we discussed living conditions in Pakistan and made comparisons with those in the United Sates.

Map It Out

| Work Map | Understanding Cultural Diversity |

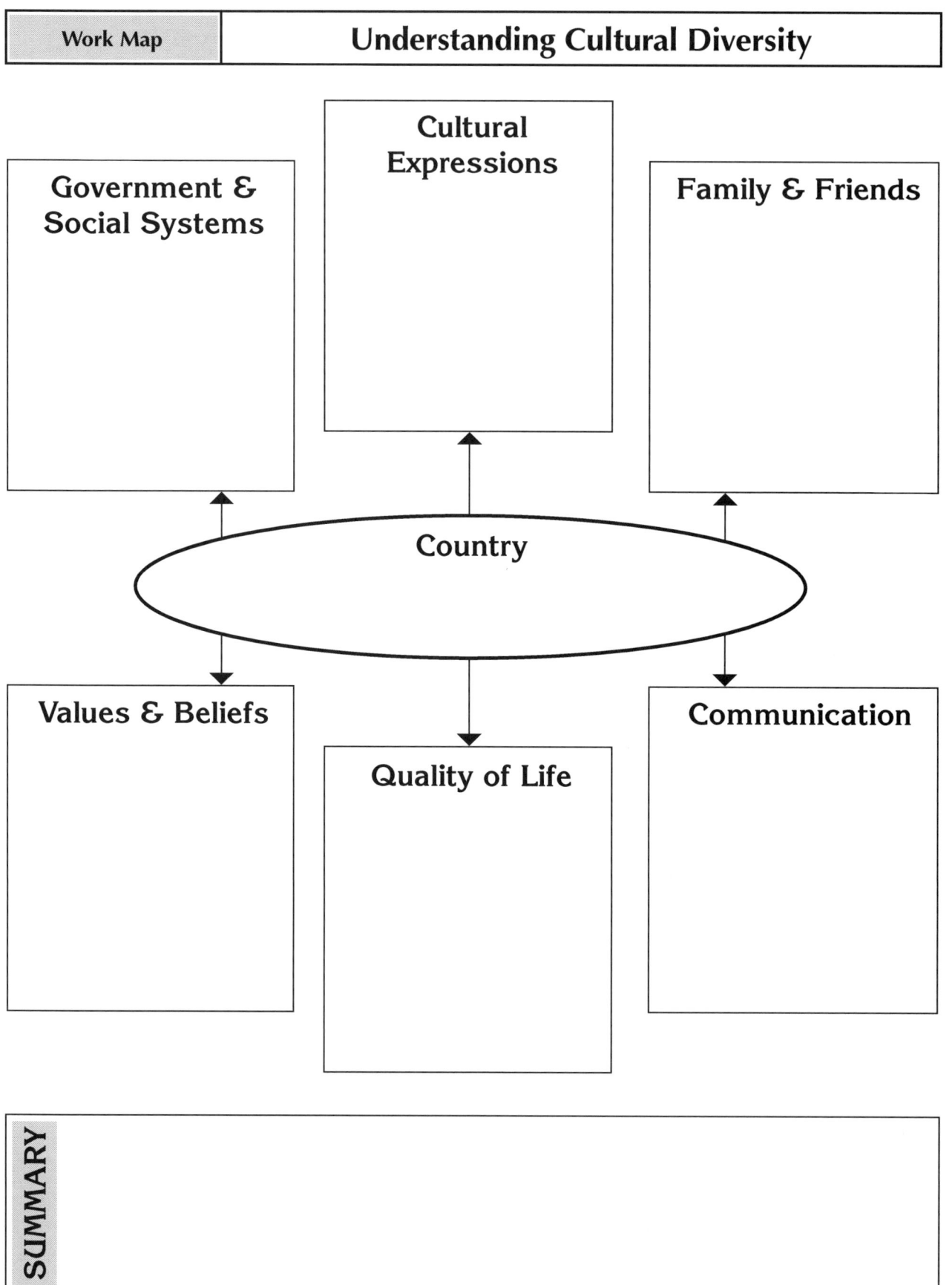

SUMMARY

304

© 2001 by E.H. Wiig and C.C. Wilson
Duplication permitted for educational use only.

School Knowledge/Study Skills

Unit 50: Decision-Making Process for Options

> ### Educational Levels
> Upper elementary through secondary
>
> ### Objectives
> (1) Analyze positive and negative aspects of choices and options; (2) weigh positives against negatives to make decisions about a choice; and (3) apply this process to decision-making in school, work, and personal life

Completed Map

This map shows how students in Grade 8 came up with a fair process for making decisions about how to distribute money to students for an upcoming field trip. The students selected two options for distributing the funds and discussed the positive and negative sides of each option. They then recorded a positive and negative for each point associated with an option. The result was a map with a parallel structure of positives and negatives. The teacher then guided a discussion in which the students weighed the importance of each option against their personal and classroom values and beliefs.

Show the Completed Map to students and say, for example:

> *This map shows how a class decided to distribute money that was set aside for a field trip. Let's look at the two options for giving out the money. Then we'll discuss the positives and negatives given for each option.*

Emphasize that all choices are at best compromises.

Work Map

Show the Work Map to students and say, for example:

> *This map is empty. Let's think of a practical task where you have to make a choice between two options. Then we'll analyze the positives and negatives of both options.*

305

Map It Out

Extended Activities

1. Identify an academic task that requires decision-making among options (e.g., choosing between two theme options for a writing assignment). Ask students to analyze which option would be the best for them (e.g., consider familiarity with the theme, amount of research needed, and other study skills). Guide students in identifying and recording positives and negatives for each option. Then discuss how to weigh the positives and negatives of an option.

2. Ask students to analyze the academic course options for the next term. Have each student analyze the basis for making decisions between two course options. Ask students to share their analyses in small groups.

3. Ask students to pretend that they are going to invite a friend or date to the movies. Ask them to read the reviews of current movie choices. Then have each student identify two movie options and analyze and compare them.

4. Ask students to pretend that they are going to buy a new computer for the class. Have each student research the available options and identify two computers to analyze and compare. Students may use the Internet as a resource or get brochures from computer stores. Have each student share the process he or she went through.

5. Ask students to identify two choices for after-school or social activities (e.g., learning Spanish or taking dance lessons). Have each student analyze the positives and negatives associated with each choice. Compare lists of positives and negatives as a group.

| Master Map | **Decision-Making Process for Options** |

Situation

Option

Option

Positives	Negatives

Positives	Negatives

SUMMARY — Overview of options and analysis of positives and negatives

Map It Out

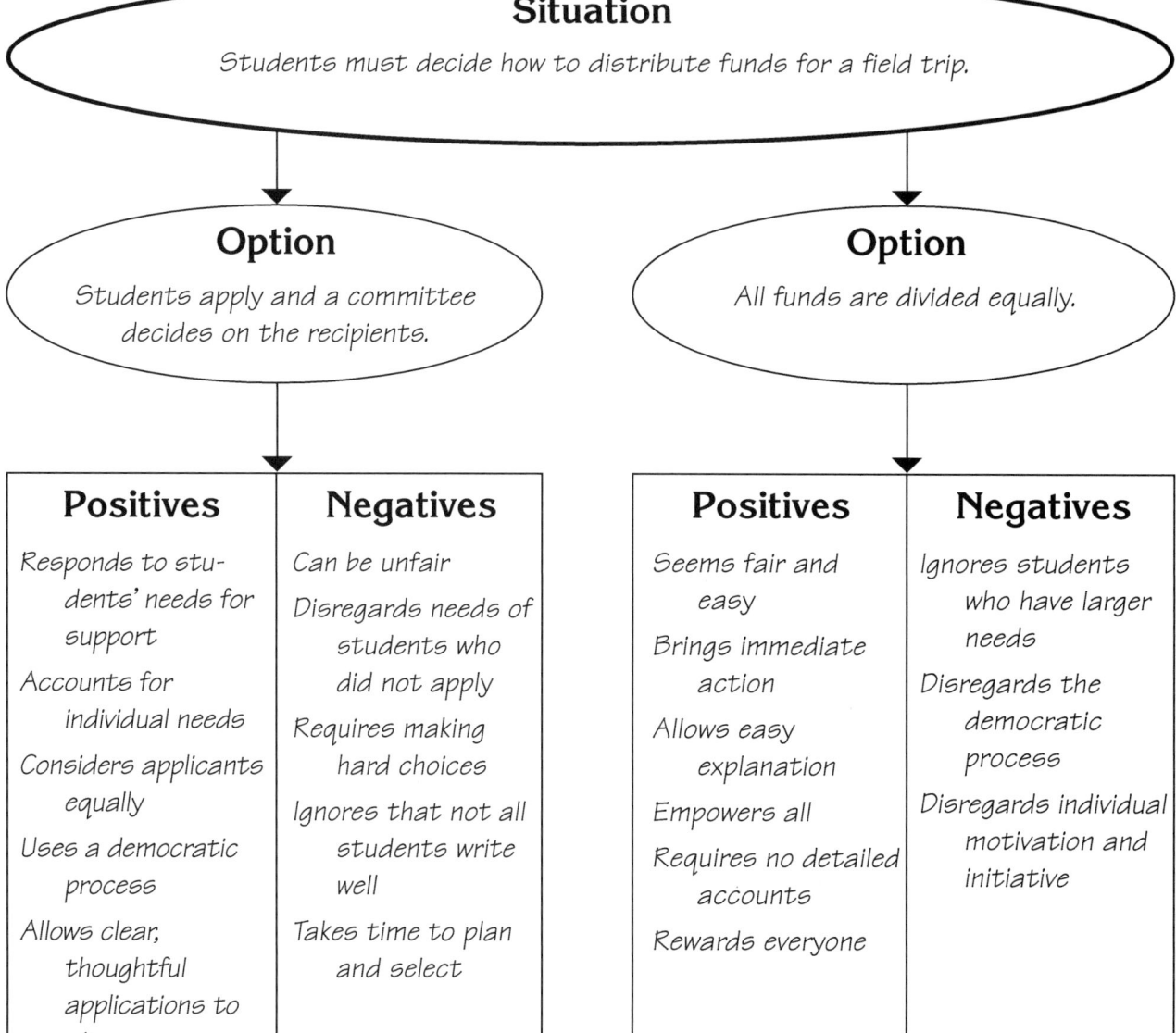

308

School Knowledge/Study Skills

| Work Map | **Decision-Making Process for Options** |

Situation

Option

Option

Positives	Negatives

Positives	Negatives

SUMMARY

Appendices

Appendix A

A Classroom Teaching Example

A teacher field-tested the conceptual mapping approach in an inclusive and culturally diverse classroom. She used Unit 16: Story Pentad (see page 130) with students in Grade 5; the purpose was to review what they had learned from the novel *Homesick* by Jean Fritz. The Master Map was projected on the wall for students to view and discuss. The teacher guided a review of the features and purposes of the map. Students were then asked to fill out the Who and Where and When response boxes on a Work Map in a shared activity. They found this relatively easy to do. Next they were asked to fill out the What, How, and Why question boxes. This task proved more difficult for the class. For the Why question box, the class worked on and reworked answers to the questions "What was the main idea?" and "What was the writer's purpose?" They later said that they thought these were the most important questions.

The class was then introduced to the Master Map for *Who*—Story Analysis (Unit 17, page 137). Students first worked on the character analysis in small groups. Later they shared the group responses and worked as a class to review and finalize a map with representative responses. They synthesized their impression of Jean, the main character, and then worked on differentiating her appearance from her behavior and personality. The class referred to Jean as "an all-American girl." Students from different ethnic and cultural backgrounds volunteered to describe what typical Chinese, Japanese, or Pakistani girls might be like. This resulted in a lively class discussion filled with evidence of critical thinking by the students.

A colleague of the teacher thought of an extended activity for using the *Who*—Story Analysis maps. She suggested a carousel jigsaw activity. For this activity, the words *looks, acts, feels,* and *says* were written on separate posters on the four walls of the classroom. Students were divided into four groups. In two- or three-minute periods, each group was told to discuss and write about a character, using the category listed on its poster. The groups rotated to each poster station. At the conclusion, the four groups gathered to discuss the contents of each poster and arrive at a consensus on the analysis of the character.

The field-test teacher reported that her class began to expect this type of work. She felt that she got concrete evidence of the students' thinking processes during the instructional activities. Furthermore, the students became able to evaluate the products that resulted from conceptual mapping for critical thinking. They could develop appropriate and valid questions for tests and use these to prepare for exams.

Appendix B

A Language Intervention Example

Background

This clinical example describes the authors' intervention process and outcomes with Jane—a girl with communication disorders who received individual language intervention with conceptual mapping and cognitive mediation. The background information indicated that Jane had normal visual and auditory functioning. Her prenatal, natal, and early developmental history followed normal expectations, and major milestones were reached within normal time limits. Jane had a history of respiratory illnesses during her early years. She was also diagnosed as exhibiting borderline attention-deficit, adjustment, and school-related anxiety disorders during Grade 3 and was placed on Ritalin. The reports from her classroom teachers supported the medical diagnosis and treatment.

Jane was referred the summer following Grade 3 for clinical services by a private-school teacher at age 10 years, 1 month. She had repeated kindergarten, causing her to be one year older than her classmates. The referring teacher met with the parents to discuss Jane's problems in following the curriculum in Grade 3. The problems the teacher mentioned were associated with listening, paying attention, following directions, and reading comprehension. Jane appeared to be an appropriate candidate for language intervention, and comprehensive psycho-educational and language assessments were initiated immediately after the referral. The results of the assessments are reported below. After the initial psycho-educational and language assessments, Jane was enrolled for language intervention beginning in August 1997. She received individual therapy for 2½ hours per week during the 1997–98 school year.

Baselines for Intervention

Before intervention, Jane was evaluated with a broad-based, psycho-educational battery of tests to determine levels of intellectual ability, academic achievement, and language and communication abilities. The Reading subtests of Part 2: Tests of Achievement of the Woodcock-Johnson Psycho-Educational Battery (Woodcock and Johnson, 1977) were administered, and the result was a percentile rank of 36 (confidence interval from 31 to 46 at 90%). The conclusion was that while Jane's general reading ability was within the average normal range, she read words and nonsense syllables and comprehended paragraphs at levels below average for her age.

Appendix B

On the Wechsler Intelligence Scale for Children–III (WISC–III) (Wechsler, 1992), Jane obtained a Full IQ of 99 (Verbal IQ of 110 and Performance IQ of 87). The difference of 23 points between Verbal IQ and Performance IQ was judged to be significant and indicated much stronger verbal than nonverbal abilities.

On the Matrix Analogies Test–Expanded Form (MAT–EF) (Naglieri, 1985), Jane obtained a Total score of 89 (confidence interval from 83 to 95 at 90%), indicating that Jane' nonverbal reasoning and problem-solving abilities fell within the low normal range.

The Clinical Evaluation of Language Fundamentals–3 (CELF–3) (Semel, Wiig, E.H., and Secord, 1989) was also administered. Jane's CELF–3 Total Language score was 78, the Receptive Composite score was 69, and the Expressive Composite score was 90. The difference between the Receptive and Expressive Composites was significant (21 points), indicating greater facility with aspects of expressive language than with aspects of receptive language. The score of 3 for the subtest, Listening to Paragraphs, indicated severe difficulties in listening to and interpreting short, social-context-based paragraphs.

Level 2 of the Test of Word Knowledge (TOWK) (Wiig, E.H. and Secord, 1992) was used to examine Jane's understanding of the meaning components of language. Jane's Total (89), Receptive Composite (86), and Expressive Composite (93) scores indicated performances within the average normal range. The standard score of 3 for the supplementary subtest, Conjunctions and Transition Words, indicated severe difficulties in integrating semantics and syntax and achieving logical cohesion in short paragraphs.

The Clinical Evaluation of Language Fundamentals–3: Observational Rating Scales (CELF–3 ORS) (Semel, Wiig, E.H., and Secord, 1996), completed by Jane's classroom teacher, identified several areas of difficulty. In the area of Listening, the ratings for how often problems occurred paying attention and remembering classroom instructions were Always. In Speaking, the ratings were Always for difficulties in asking for help when needed, expanding an answer or giving details, and using correct grammar. In Reading, the ratings were Always for questions about difficulties in understanding what was read, identifying the main idea of what was read, remembering details from what was read, and following written directions (e.g., on worksheets). In Writing, the ratings were Always for difficulties in writing what she was thinking and expanding an answer in writing or providing details. These observations supported the areas of difficulties identified by formal test results.

Intervention Scope and Sequence

The lessons and units used in language intervention centered around social stories from *Room 14: A Social Language Program* (Wilson, 1993) and assigned texts from the curriculum. The content and materials were selected to meet Jane's needs as indicated by tests, observations, and teacher and parent reports. The scope of intervention covered four central domains: (1) pragmatics, (2) semantic processing, (3) listening and reading comprehension, and (4) narrative production.

Intervention began by emphasizing the concepts that are basic to listening. This included analysis of observable listening behaviors (e.g., body language) as well as of behaviors associated with processing (e.g., focusing attention, interpreting content, and forming associations). After the initial requirements for listening were met, the intervention focus shifted to the semantic processing and reading comprehension domains. At this point, assigned texts from the language arts curriculum provided the content for intervention. Prior knowledge; making meaning for keywords and concepts; and analysis of characters, settings, time lines, episodes, and themes were emphasized first. The emphasis then shifted to synthesizing, evaluating, applying the given information, and constructing new knowledge. The narrative and pragmatic components were introduced last. The emphasis was on writing a sequel to a story or using social skills to write a story about how a given character solved a specific problem in units from *Room 14* (Wilson, 1993).

A Model for Intervention with Conceptual Mapping

The intervention goal was to support the construction of new knowledge about language and communication effectively and quickly. Therefore a macromodel for intervention using conceptual mapping and cognitive mediation was developed. This model has its basis in top-down learning, where underlying principles, schema, or strategies can be detailed and made usable by developing an understanding of underlying concepts (e.g., trust), scripts (e.g., introducing yourself and others), or routines (e.g., catching a bus). At the same time, the model is based on bottom-up learning, where instances or events are observed using contextual illustrations (Wilson, 1993) or modeling and integrated to form concrete representations (e.g., scripts). This is useful for interpreting and dealing with familiar and novel situations in social and academic problem-solving contexts.

The intervention process contains several stages with examples and activities and uses conceptual mapping and cognitive mediation as tools. With Jane, the first stage focused on eliciting prior knowledge about social or story themes, highlighting key vocabulary, and making basic predictions.

Appendix B

The second stage used thinking aloud, guided questioning, and scaffolding procedures to create an awareness and understanding of, among others, concepts, associations, relationships, and cause-effect chains. The activities focused on concrete information and knowledge (e.g., characterization and analysis of context and relations).

The third stage focused on using conceptual mapping and cognitive mediation, developing questions and answers, and using related activities for practice and transfer to new contexts. Conceptual maps were used to analyze content, structure, process, and sequence; compare and contrast critical aspects (e.g., changes in relationships before and after a turning point); and synthesize the new knowledge to plan for future applications. The questions and answers and extended activities focused on comparing and contrasting, eliciting descriptions, identifying primary and secondary information, and summarizing.

The fourth stage focused on applying the old and new knowledge to new contexts (e.g., Jane's home life), representations (e.g., tables or charts), media (e.g., email messages), or goals (e.g., developing her own test). This stage was designed to develop metaknowledge (i.e., knowledge about what knowledge has been gained), metastrategies (i.e., novel and innovative ways of using the new knowledge), and metacognition (i.e., knowledge of which reasoning approaches will be most effective for solving a given problem). All activities used at this stage were related to a unit theme and brought the new knowledge to a higher level of complexity, abstraction, or both.

Within each stage, there was movement toward building Jane's knowledge to a high point and then bridging to the next stage of intervention with examples, modeling, and related activities. This allowed for continued growth and further generalization of targeted domains.

Postintervention Assessments and Observations

After one year of language intervention, Jane—now 11 years, 0 month old—was re-evaluated. The language tests that were used to assess baselines were also used to assess progress. On the Reading subtests of Part 2: Tests of Achievement of the Woodcock-Johnson Psycho-Educational Battery (Woodcock and Johnson, 1977), Jane's reading level was now within the average normal range (a percentile rank of 44 with a confidence interval of 36 to 52 at 90%). The CELF–3 (Semel, Wiig, E.H., and Secord, 1989) Total Language, Receptive Composite, and Expressive Composite scores (all 102) placed her performance in the average normal range. On Level 2 of TOWK (Wiig, E.H., and Secord, 1992), Jane's Total (97), Receptive Composite (100), and Expressive Composite (93) scores also indicated performances within the average normal range. Jane's new classroom teacher rated her behaviors in the areas of Listening, Speaking, Reading, and Writing with the CELF–3 ORS (Semel, Wiig, E.H., and Secord, 1996). In the areas of Listening, Speaking, and Reading, the majority of the ratings were either Never or Sometimes, indicating that earlier difficulties were no longer in evidence in the classroom. In Writing, all ratings were Never. These observations support the progress identified by the formal test results.

Ongoing Behavioral Observations

The observations of Jane's behaviors and reactions were ongoing during intervention with conceptual mapping and cognitive mediation. The clinical observations are summarized within the *Garden of Knowledge* metaphor (see pages 27–29). Even during the early intervention sessions, few, if any, of Jane's behaviors and responses using negative behaviors from the Garden of Knowledge (e.g., "You seem to be closing the gate. What is happening?") were observed. Instead Jane's responses were in the positive category. Jane gave behavioral responses that belonged to the category "What's in your garden?" She was cautious and yet expressed hopeful interest in the concept maps and the conceptual mapping process. Throughout intervention, her behavioral responses concurred with the category "Open the gate." These responses indicated a willingness to be taught and allow new knowledge into the "garden."

As Jane gained more experience with conceptual mapping, her responses expressed that there were "Too many gaps or spaces in the rows." This reflected a recognition of the need to add to or complete a specific area or domain and provide more supporting details. She also gave responses that matched the category "Let's get rid of that weed," meaning that something did not fit the conceptual map focus and needed to be deleted. As she became more competent, executive behaviors (e.g., self-monitoring, self-evaluation, revision, and repair) became more apparent. Jane could always come up with ideas, but as intervention progressed she often indicated "Let that rabbit go." This response showed that she monitored and evaluated herself spontaneously and realized that an idea might take her totally off course.

During the later stages of intervention, more positive behavioral responses emerged. Jane would make comments that fell in the category "Lovely garden!" These comments indicated an emerging and growing appreciation for the organization of knowledge that came with conceptual mapping. Later her behavioral responses were in the category "Wow! What a garden!" or "I'm so proud of our garden!" These behaviors demonstrated excitement about the process, empowerment, and ownership. Finally Jane asked "What kind of garden next year?" This indicated that Jane realized that the conceptual map formats could be used for different concepts, themes, or contexts and therefore gave further evidence of metaknowledge.

Jane's confidence grew during the conceptual mapping and cognitive mediation process. In the beginning, she relied on the authors to supply a great deal of scaffolding or model the process. Gradually she recognized what was needed within each task before the need was mentioned. That was when Jane realized that she owned the information and knowledge. With that realization, Jane made the discovery that not only were her ideas valued but her ideas were necessary. As a result, the traditional educator-student relationship changed to one in which the educator and student became partners in a learning and discovery process. This relationship enabled Jane to accept more and more responsibility for her own learning. She assumed the responsibility and took charge with excitement. This growth in critical thinking was shown by her creations. Once, after Jane had constructed and completed her own conceptual map on the computer, she exclaimed, "I am so proud of our work!" Another time she brought in a test on levers, an assignment in physical science, that she had written and typed herself on her home computer. Jane also showed a hand drawn conceptual map she had made to organize her study notes for a future science test.

Evidence of Critical Thinking

Observations before, during, and after intervention with conceptual mapping that showed changes in the quality and level of Jane's critical thinking were also gathered. The observations were grouped using labels: attitude, attention, inner authority, and concreteness.

Before intervention, Jane's attitude demonstrated a lack of confidence; she was discouraged and obsessed with getting good grades. After intervention, Jane expressed confidence; she was encouraged, felt the joy of learning, expressed excitement about her discoveries, and took pride in "our work."

In the area of attention, she was easily distracted by visual or auditory stimuli. Following intervention, Jane was focused, not easily distracted, and embedded in her work.

Before intervention, there was little evidence of inner authority. Jane depended on others for external evaluation, acknowledgment, and rewards. After intervention, Jane worked on completing activities for the sake of getting finished.

In the concreteness category, Jane interpreted everything at the surface level, did not make inferences or extrapolate knowledge, and provided literal interpretations of figurative uses. After intervention, she showed remarkable changes. She was able to transfer the new knowledge to a variety of situations at home and school. She wrote organized stories and related themes and discoveries to her own social experiences.

Summary of Observed Benefits

Based on the ongoing observation of Jane's attitudes, comments, and reactions to conceptual mapping for language intervention, the authors perceived many benefits. First the visual aspects of conceptual mapping helped focus Jane's attention. Conceptual mapping provided a way for her to focus on details associated with a concept, theme, or process in a natural way instead of as a meaningless drill. This may be because only details that were necessary

Map It Out

for categorizing, comparing and contrasting, identifying relationships and changes, or developing procedural steps in a process were elicited.

Second the conceptual maps aided Jane's memory and made for quick reviews in preparation for classes and tests. The conceptual mapping process resulted in a shift from dependence on cognitive mediation to independence with minimal facilitation. The process seemed to foster greater independence and responsibility for her own learning.

Third the conceptual mapping and cognitive mediation process increased Jane's vocabulary, improved concept formation, and developed her critical thinking abilities. The organization and sequence of the intervention models provided Jane with structure, flexibility, and direction.

Appendix C

Behavioral Observations of Critical Thinking in Context

Subject Area: _____   Task(s): _____

Name: _____   Date: _____

	Always	Often	Sometimes	Rarely
1. Analysis (The student...)				
• Recognizes major components, elements, or dimensions				
• Identifies major parts of components				
• Categorizes the parts of components				
• Sees patterns within major elements				
• Identifies relevant facts and details for the various components				
2. Synthesis (The student...)				
• Forms basic, concrete connections or associations				
• Forms high-level, abstract connections or associations				
• Understands the whole picture on a concrete or literal level				
• Understands the whole picture on an abstract or figurative level				
• Constructs new meanings and understandings				
• Broadens the scope and application of prior knowledge				
3. Prediction (The student...)				
• Predicts or hypothesize the outcomes				
• Identifies other inferences that can be drawn from the content				

© 2001 by E.H. Wiig and C.C. Wilson
Duplication permitted for educational use only.

Map It Out

	Always	Often	Sometimes	Rarely
• Identifies several possibilities for extending or following up on the content				
• Imagines and describe scenarios that respond to "What if…?" questions				
• Identifies which hypotheses can be formulated in response to the content				
4. Evaluation (The student…)				
• Forms opinions on a concrete or literal level				
• Substantiates his or her opinions or points of view concretely				
• Makes appropriate links to new situations				
• Forms and substantiate high-level opinions or perspectives				
• Identifies what information is missing				
• Modifies, edits, or elaborates by using critical thinking approaches				
5. Application (The student…)				
• Uses new knowledge in simple and concrete ways				
• Uses new knowledge in simple yet connected ways				
• Uses knowledge in complex or abstract applications				
• Uses knowledge in unique and creative ways				
• Applies critical thinking strategies to new subjects				

_____ + _____ = _____ ÷ 27 × 100 = _____% of top ratings
   Always   Often

100%–80% = Level 4   49%–30% = Level 2
79%–50% = Level 3   29%–0% = Level 1

Appendix D

Critical Thinking Guide

Subject Area: _____   Task(s): _____

Name: _____   Date: _____

1. Analysis

- What do I know? _____

- What is important? _____

- What is not important? _____

- What are the parts? _____

- What else do I need to know? _____

- What previous knowledge can I use? _____

2. Synthesis

- What patterns do I see? _____

- What do these patterns mean? _____

- What relationships do I see? _____

- How can the patterns and relationships be organized? _____

3. Prediction

- What will the outcomes be? _____

- What other inferences can I make? _____

© 2001 by E.H. Wiig and C.C. Wilson
Duplication permitted for educational use only.

Map It Out

- What are all the possibilities? _____
- What if…? _____
- What hypotheses can I formulate? _____

4. Evaluation

- Have I considered all the elements? _____
- Do my conclusions make sense? _____
- Could there be any other conclusions? _____
- Have I identified all my options for action? _____

5. Application (How can I use this for…)

- Problem solving _____
- Decision-making _____
- Planning _____
- Evaluating or judging _____
- Creating or designing _____
- Editing or revising _____
- Improving my performance, the product, or my understanding _____
- Other _____

Bibliography

Evans, H., and Dansereau, D.F. (1991). Knowledge maps as tools for thinking and communication. In R.F. Mulcahy, R.H. Short, and J. Andrews (Eds.), *Enhancing learning and thinking* (pp. 97–102). Westport, CT: Greenwood.

Margulies, N. (1991). *Mapping inner space: Learning and teaching mind mapping.* Tucson, AZ: Zephyr Press.

Wiig, E.H. (1992). *Language intervention for school-age children: Models and procedures that work.* Chicago: Applied Symbolix.

Wiig, E.H., and Freedman, E. (1993). *The word book: Building concepts for thinking and learning.* Austin, TX: Pro-Ed.

Wiig, E.H., and Wilson, C.C. (1997). *Ladders to interpretation: Assessing and developing text comprehension.* Chicago: Applied Symbolix.

Wilson, C.C., Lanza, J., Evans, J., and Wiig, E.H. (1997). *Concept power.* Chicago: Applied Symbolix.

References

Bloom, B. (Ed.). (1956). *Taxonomy of educational objectives: The classification of educational goals. Handbook I—Cognitive domain.* White Plains, NY: Longman.

Bruner, J.S. (1973). *Beyond the information given: Studies in the psychology of knowing.* New York: W.W. Norton.

Bruner, J.S. (1983). *In search of mind: Essays in autobiography.* New York: Harper and Row.

Buzan, T. (1991). *Use both sides of your brain* (3rd ed.). New York: Dutton.

Caine, R.N., and Caine, G. (1991). *Making connections: Teaching and the human brain.* Alexandria, VA: Association for Supervision and Curriculum Development.

Caine, R.N., and Caine, G. (1997). *Education on the edge of possibility.* Alexandria, VA: Association for Supervision and Curriculum Development.

Costa, A.L. (Ed.). (1991). *Developing minds: A resource book for teaching thinking* (2nd ed.). Alexandria, VA: Association for Supervision and Curriculum Development.

Dansereau, D.F., and Cross, D.R. (1990). Knowledge Mapping: Cognitive Software for Thinking, Learning, and Communicating [Computer software]. Fort Worth, TX: Texas Christian University, Department of Psychology.

De Bono, E. (1992). *Serious creativity: Using the power of lateral thinking to create new ideas.* New York: Harper Business.

Elkind, D., and Flavell, J. (Eds.). (1969). *Studies in cognitive development: Essays in honor of Jean Piaget.* New York: Oxford University Press.

Feuerstein, R. (1980). *Instrumental enrichment: An intervention program for cognitive modifiability.* Baltimore: University Park Press.

Finke, R.A., Ward, T.B., and Smith, S.M. (1992). *Creative cognition: Theory, research, and applications.* Cambridge, MA: MIT Press.

Gardner, H. (1991). *The unschooled mind: How children think and how schools should teach.* New York: Basic Books.

Gilhooly, K.J. (1988). *Thinking: Directed, undirected and creative* (2nd ed.). New York: Academic Press.

Glasgow, J., Narayanan, N.H., and Chandrasekaran, B. (Eds.). (1995). *Diagrammatic reasoning: Cognitive and computational perspectives.* Cambridge, MA: MIT Press.

Halpern, D.F. (1989). *Thought and knowledge: An introduction to critical thinking* (2nd ed.). Hillsdale, NJ: Erlbaum.

Hyerle, D. (1996). *Visual tools for constructing knowledge.* Alexandria, VA: Association for Supervision and Curriculum Development.

Map It Out

Inspiration Pro 5.0 [Computer software]. (1997). Portland, OR: Inspiration Software.

Lakoff, G., and Johnson, M. (1980). *Metaphors we live by.* Chicago: University of Chicago Press.

Microsoft PowerPoint [Computer software]. (1998). Redmond, WA: Microsoft Corporation.

Naglieri, J.A. (1985). Matrix Analogies Test–Expanded Form (MAT–EF). San Antonio, TX: The Psychological Corporation.

Semel, E.M., Wiig, E.H., and Secord, W.A. (1989). Clinical Evaluation of Language Fundamentals–3 (CELF–3). San Antonio, TX: The Psychological Corporation.

Semel, E.M., Wiig, E.H., and Secord, W.A. (1996). Clinical Evaluation of Language Fundamentals–3: Observational Rating Scales (CELF–3 ORS). San Antonio, TX: The Psychological Corporation.

Senge, P.M. (1990). *The fifth discipline: The art and practice of the learning organization.* New York: Doubleday.

Vygotsky, L.S. (1986). *Thought and language* (A. Kozulin, Ed.) (Rev. ed.). Cambridge, MA: MIT Press.

Wechsler, D. (1992). Wechsler Intelligence Scale for Children–III (WISC–III). San Antonio, TX: The Psychological Corporation.

Wiig, E.H. (1989). *Steps to language competence: Developing metalinguistic strategies.* San Antonio, TX: The Psychological Corporation.

Wiig, E.H., and Kusuma-Powell, O. (2001). *Visual tools for critical thinking in classrooms: Conceptual mapping and cognitive mediation.* Arlington, TX: Schema Press.

Wiig, E.H., and Secord, W.A. (1992). Test of Word Knowledge (TOWK). San Antonio, TX: The Psychological Corporation.

Wiig, E.H., and Wiig, K.M. (1996, October). *Mental models, conceptual maps, and organizers for language and communication.* Paper presented at the regional meeting of the Association of International Schools in Africa (AISA), Dar es Salaam, Tanzania.

Wiig, K.M. (1994a). *Knowledge management foundations: Thinking about thinking—How people and organizations represent, create, and use knowledge.* Arlington, TX: Schema Press.

Wiig, K.M. (1994b). *Knowledge management: The central focus for intelligent-acting organizations.* Arlington, TX: Schema Press.

Wiig, K.M. (1995). *Knowledge management methods: Practical approaches to managing knowledge.* Arlington, TX: Schema Press.

Wilson, C.C. (1993). *Room 14: A social language program.* Moline, IL: LinguiSystems.

Woodcock, R.W., and Johnson, M.B. (1977). Woodcock-Johnson Psycho-Educational Battery. Itasca, IL: Riverside.

Wykoff, J. (1991). *Mindmapping: Your personal guide to exploring creativity and problem-solving.* New York: Berkley.